ISSUES IN REPRODUCTIVE TECHNOLOGY I: AN ANTHOLOGY

Garland Reference Library of the Social Sciences
(Vol. 729)

ISSUES IN • • • • REPRODUCTIVE TECHNOLOGY I

AN ANTHOLOGY

Helen Bequaert Holmes, editor

GARLAND PUBLISHING, INC.
New York & London, 1992

Library of Congress Cataloguing-in-Publication Data

Issues in reproductive technology I: an anthology / Helen Bequaert Holmes, editor.
p. cm. — (Garland reference library of social science; vol. 729)
Includes index.
ISBN 0-8153-0035-2
1. Human reproductive technology—Social aspects. 2. Human reproductive technology—Psychological aspects. 3. Human reproductive technology—Moral and ethical aspects. I. Holmes, Helen B. II. Series: Garland reference library of social science; vol. 729.
RG133.5.I77 1992
362.1'981'78—dc20 92–9929
CIP

Printed on acid-free, 250-year-life paper
Manufactured in the United States of America

Contents

Part II. New Facets to the Abortion Debate

Part III. Cryopreservation of Human Embryos

Part IV. Psychosocial Dimensions to the Search for Fertility Through IVF

Preface

The healing arts are heavily dependent on technology for diagnosis and for most "cures" of the sick—technology such as cleverly extracted antibiotics or tunnel-like machines for visualizing slices of the human body. And the natural, normal process of human reproduction has slowly but surely become medicalized and thus technologized. Yet *Homo sapiens* reproduced long before the species created even sling shots or wheels.

Because it is a natural phenomenon, reproduction will take place without technology. Technology is sometimes put to use to prevent or control that natural process; or, on the other hand, to help people who find they cannot reproduce. Since reproduction is an expected part of being human, those who cannot may feel that they are not truly human. Centuries ago such persons might have turned to priests or shamans with their misery—now they turn to medicine, and medicine then turns to technology.

That I call reproduction "natural" and raise questions about the role therein of medicine and technology certainly does not mean that I endorse naturalism, subscribe to any naturalistic fallacy, or believe in the wisdom of evolution. I make no claim that what is natural is morally right or physically perfect. Mother Nature can be cruel and heartless; evolution, relying as it does on chance, cannot be wise. Yet both are formidable foes when we attempt to "fool" them, and we need to take care not to bungle our attempts at improving the natural condition. Although medicine often technically outwits nature in morally acceptable ways, medical technology in *reproduction* needs especially careful assessment. To this end, the authors in this volume have applied their sensitive analyses.

All facets of the healing arts have their social, psychological, ethical, legal, and political dimensions. Yet when medicine adopts a nonmedical process, many more issues in those areas are raised. People from specific disciplines (such as political science or sociology) who are concerned about these issues often find no outlet for analyses that of necessity are cross-disciplinary. The present serial was conceived, therefore, to give such authors an opportunity to write outside the binds of disciplinary constraints, to share their views with other concerned scholars and with the general public.

I have defined "reproductive technology" very broadly, to comprise methods that prevent conception, that stop reproduction after conception, that cause conception when it does not occur naturally, that monitor or attempt to "improve" the conceptus, that are used during labor and delivery, and that handle problems with compromised newborns. For each volume I plan to select four or five specific areas to be discussed in depth by an eclectic group of scholars and health activists: This inaugural volume covers contraception, abortion, cryopreservation of embryos, psychosocial studies of in vitro fertilization, and contract motherhood. Although most of the authors come from the United States, stimulating international perspectives appear in contributions from Australia, Canada, Denmark, England, and the Netherlands.

Each piece in this collection turns out to demonstrate that the effect of technology development and use in reproduction is far from neutral. Human reaction may run from exaggerated avoidance to fanatical adoption, via a myriad intermediate stances.

The introductory essay in each section highlights some issues and hints at the richness to be found in the other essays in that section. In this preface, however, I shall point out two themes that seem to run under the surface throughout the entire book.

First, several authors have used the term "feminist"—so is this a feminist anthology? Yes, it is in the sense that many authors here write their essays as if based on the premise that society continues to oppress women as a class: for example, by exploitation, restricted role expectations, marginalization, and maleness as a norm. Reproduction and the oppression of women are closely connected. This interconnection can include expecting women (at best) or forcing them (at worst) to use their bodies to produce more humans. When technology is brought into play, does it enhance a woman's ability to liberate herself from these expectations or demands? This query may well prove to have been the central theme of the book. In my view, most of the technologies throughout the spectrum outlined above generally have not liberated women from role expectations but instead have enhanced society's control over when women reproduce and the quality of the product. Yet women can be enthusiastic advocates and lobbyists for those very technologies, as is brought out clearly in all the essays in the section on psychosocial dimensions of in vitro fertilization.

A second theme is "rights." After the Civil Rights and the Women's Movements in the United States, everyone has adopted a rhetoric of rights; frequently one hears the phrase "reproductive rights." Unfortunately, when everyone claims rights for one or another entity, a nonproductive competition between rights arises. Although this theme lies beneath the surface in many essays, Thomas Shevory in his contribution explicitly and lucidly discusses the indeterminacy of rights analysis.

This book would not exist without the hard work and cooperation of many people. My editor at Garland Publishing, Marie Ellen Larcada, had the vision that sparked the whole project; through her continuing support she encouraged me as I tried to follow that vision. Also at Garland, Chuck Bartelt valiantly and cheerfully struggled with some 20 different interpretations of the guidelines for preparing diskettes, and Shirley Cobert put the final polishing touches on the prose.

Of course, no anthology could exist without its authors. Ours are singularly hard-working: they revised and rerevised stoically. At least five authors conscientiously delayed or cut short professional trips in order to rework a sentence I had questioned.

Authors who also assisted by reading some manuscripts include Betsy Hartmann, Ruth Lucier, and Hilde Nelson. In addition, Casey Miller, Kate Smith, Thomas Shannon, and Francis Holmes commented on portions of essays. I thank my editorial assistants, Susan Shaw, Haleh Pazwash, Robyn Gingold, and Jessica Bloom for their efforts in planning, organizing, and proofreading—and for library detective work. The reference and interlibrary loan librarians at the University of Massachusetts Library merit praise for their undaunted assaults on incomplete citations.

Yet the person really responsible for the book's very existence is my husband Francis. He was vital to its success, both through his active assistance (reviewing manuscripts, carrying texts to photocopy, financial support—and, of course, shopping, cooking, and dishwashing) and by his patience (never a gripe over a room heaped high with manuscripts or those delayed vacation trips). Thank you, Francis.

Helen Bequaert Holmes

CONTRIBUTING AUTHORS

MINA ALIKANI is Senior Embryologist at the Center for Reproductive Medicine and Infertility, Cornell University Medical Center, New York City. In 1983 she began her training in in vitro fertilization in California. At the center she has both clinical and research responsibilities. Her main areas of research are fertilization failure, assisted fertilization by micromanipulation techniques, and cryopreservation of embryos. She published a review of clinical results after cryopreservation, in a 1990 issue of *Current Opinion in Obstetrics and Gynecology.*

ELIZABETH BARTHOLET is a Professor of Law at Harvard Law School, where she has taught since 1977. Previously she was involved in civil rights and public interest litigation, first as a staff attorney with the NAACP Legal Defense Fund and later as Director of the Legal Action Center, a public interest law firm in New York City. She now teaches, writes, and serves as a consultant, on legal and policy issues related to adoption, reproductive technology, and surrogacy.

MARGE BERER has been a writer, editor, and activist on reproductive health and rights in Britain and internationally for the past twelve years. She is editing an international resource book on women and HIV/AIDS and co-editing an anthology of feminist perspectives on international population and family planning policies. She has been newsletter editor for the Women's Global Network for Reproductive Rights in London and in Amsterdam and was a co-founder of the Women's Reproductive Rights Information Centre in London.

ANDREA L. BONNICKSEN is Professor of Political Science at Northern Illinois University. She is the author of *In vitro fertilization: Building policy from laboratories to legislatures* (Columbia University Press) and *Civil rights and liberties: Principles of interpretation* (Mayfield). She is the co-editor of *Emerging issues in biomedical policy: Annual volumes* (Columbia University Press) and the Book Review Editor for Public Policy for the journal *Politics and the Life Sciences.*

SARAH S. BOONE is a Ph.D. candidate in anthropology at the University of Virginia. She has an M.A. in social and political philosophy from Rutgers University and has special interest in the relationships between identity constructs, representation, and oppression. In the fall of 1989 she worked with a small American company in Rome, doing preliminary research on Italy's "new racism," which targets African immigrants.

CHERYL D. CHILDS is a 1991 graduate of Bennett College with a dual major in English and history. A member of the Bennett Scholars Honors Program, she was a lead participant in Bennett's 1989 Humanities Symposia—Ethics, Family Values, and Innovative Technologies—and was chosen to represent the college in the Bennett/Randolph-Macon College Program for a year of study in England. She plans to pursue a career in public interest law.

HEATHER DIETRICH trained in biology and later became a researcher and teacher in science and technology policy in England and Australia. Currently on leave from the University of Technology in Sydney, she is an adviser in the Environment Policy Section of the Federal Department of Industry, Technology and Commerce. An active feminist, she focuses on policy issues in reproductive technology and genetic engineering. She represented New South Wales and social science perspectives (and informally, women's interests) on Australia's National Bioethics Consultative Committee.

KATHLEEN FORD holds a Ph.D. in sociology from Brown University and is an Associate Research Scientist with the School of Public Health of the University of Michigan. She is the principal investigator for a study of AIDS risk behaviors and condom use among African-American and Hispanic adolescents and young adults in Detroit and for a study of AIDS risk behaviors and condom use among commercial sex workers and their clients in Indonesia.

DANA GALLAGHER has an M.P.H. degree and expects to complete training as a Physician Assistant in 1992. She has fitted cervical caps since 1979 and assisted the Vermont Women's Health Center in setting up its investigational study of cervical caps. She was a member of the now defunct National Cervical Cap Advisory Committee (a national organization of preapproval cap providers) and the Medical Advisory Board of Cervical Cap Ltd.

ANITA HARDON is the research coordinator of the Women and Pharmaceuticals Project of WEMOS, a Dutch public interest group that monitors medical developments. From 1985 to 1988 in the Philippines she conducted research for her dissertation on pharmaceutical use and distribution for the community-based health programs; she developed an action-oriented and participatory research methodology. Also affiliated with the medical anthropology unit of the University of Amsterdam, she conducts and coordinates applied studies in the fields of drugs, reproductive health, and AIDS.

BETSY HARTMANN is Director of the Population and Development Program at Hampshire College. She is the author of *Reproductive rights and wrongs: The global politics of population control and contraceptive choice* (Harper & Row) and co-author of works on Bangladesh including (with James Boyce) *A quiet violence: View from a Bangladesh village* (Food First; Zed Books) and (with Hilary Standing) *The poverty of population control: Family planning and health policy in Bangladesh* (Bangladesh International Action Group). She is active in the international women's health movement.

HELEN BEQUAERT HOLMES is an independent scholar, and editor with a Ph.D. in genetics. She co-edited *Birth control and controlling birth: Women-centered perspectives, The custom-made child? Women-centered perspectives* as well as *Feminist perspectives on medical ethics*, a book derived from two special issues of the journal *Hypatia*. She has done research on feminist technology assessment and ethical analysis in reproductive medicine in the United States, in the Netherlands, and, with a Fulbright grant, in New Zealand.

HOWARD W. JONES, JR., is currently Professor of Obstetrics and Gynecology at the Eastern Virginia Medical School and Chairman of the Board of the Jones Institute of the school's Department of Gynecology. He is Professor Emeritus of Gynecology and Obstetrics at Johns Hopkins University. With his wife, he founded the Jones Institute for Reproductive Medicine in Norfolk and initiated the first in vitro program in the United States, from which over 900 children have been born. His interest in ethical aspects of assisted reproduction is evident by his views on cryopreservation.

LENE KOCH has an M.A. in Anglo-Saxon studies and history and a Ph.D. in the history of medicine. A senior research fellow at the University of Copenhagen, Institute of Social Medicine, she has published books and papers in women's studies and reproductive technologies. Her most recent book, *Ønskebørn. Kvinder og reagensglasbefrugning* (The wish for a child. Women and in vitro fertilization) (Rosinante) describes her interviews with IVF patients. She is writing a book on the history of genetics.

ELAINE A. LISSNER is a resident of Santa Cruz, California, an independent scholar and a women's health activist with a special interest in researching and publicizing male contraception. A synopsis of her chapter in this volume appeared in the January 1992 issue of *Ms.* magazine.

RUTH M. LUCIER is Director of Interdisciplinary Studies, Professor of Philosophy and Religion, and Coordinator of the Institute for Ethics in the

Professions at Bennett College. Her interests include knowledge theory and cross-cultural ethics. She is President of the American Society for Value Inquiry, serves on the Executive Committee of the International Development Ethics Association, and chaired the 1991 International Society of Value Inquiry sessions in Nairobi. She is working on a book on ethical values in African traditional thought.

HILDE LINDEMANN NELSON is the associate editor of the *Hastings Center Report*. She is a member of the Hastings Center projects on feminism and on bioethics and the family and has published essays in feminist ethics and the ethics of assisted reproduction. She is at working on a book with James Lindemann Nelson on medicine and the ethics of the family.

ELIZABETH O'DAIR is a researcher in a study of AIDS risk behaviors and condom use among African-American and Hispanic adolescents and young adults in Detroit. She is completing a Master of Public Health degree in health behavior and health education at the University of Michigan. As a member of the Peace Corps, she was involved in health education activities in Latin America.

KELLY OLIVER is Assistant Professor of Philosophy at the University of Texas at Austin. She has published articles on Nietzsche, poststructuralist theory, and various aspects of feminist theory. She co-edited a special issue of *Hypatia: A Journal of Feminist Philosophy* on feminism and language and is the author of *Unraveling the double-bind: Julia Kristeva's theory of the subject on trial* (Indiana University Press, 1992).

CHRISTINE OVERALL is Associate Professor of Philosophy at Queen's University, Kingston, Ontario. She is the author of *Ethics and human reproduction: A feminist analysis* (Allen & Unwin), the editor of *The future of human reproduction* (Toronto Women's Press), and the co-editor of *Feminist perspectives: Philosophical essays on method and morals* (University of Toronto Press) and *Perspectives on AIDS: Ethical and social issues* (Oxford University Press).

SHAWNDA M. PARKS in the fall of 1991 was a junior in the Bennett College Interdisciplinary Studies Program. She has worked as a researcher for the Bennett Women's Studies Program, has been actively involved in community service projects aimed at strengthening public libraries, and has tutored students in logic for critical thinking courses. She is preparing for work in journalism and mass communications.

LAURA M. PURDY is an Associate Professor at Wells College; she has also held the Irwin Chair at Hamilton College and has taught at Cornell University. Most of her research has been in applied ethics, particularly in reproductive ethics, in which field she has published such articles as "Genetic disease: Can having children be immoral?" and "Are pregnant women fetal containers?" Her book, *In their best interest? The case against equal rights for children* was published by Cornell University Press in 1992.

SUSAN RUBINSTEIN is a researcher in a study of AIDS risk behaviors and condom use among African-American and Hispanic adolescents and young adults in Detroit. She holds an M.P.H. degree in population planning and international health and in health behavior and health education from the University of Michigan. She has worked as a health educator in a women's clinic in California.

ANGELINE FAYE SCHRATER is an independent scholar with the Project on Women and Social Change at Smith College. After serving with the Peace Corps (Guatemala 1966-1968) she earned a Ph.D. in immunology (University of Pennsylvania) and then did basic research on tolerance and responses to parasites. She resigned from Smith's biology faculty to pursue interests in women's roles in science, the impact of reproductive technologies on women's health, and the important but murky interface between development and deployment of those technologies.

SUSAN SHAW is a women's health activist and independent scholar. She graduated from Hampshire College, with a concentration in medical anthropology and women's studies. She is assistant editor of the PWA Newsline for the People With AIDS Coalition in New York City and is struggling to get more recognition for the needs of women with AIDS, especially women of color.

THOMAS C. SHEVORY has a Ph.D. in political science from the University of Iowa. He is an assistant professor of politics at Ithaca College, specializing in public law, public policy, and legal history. His publications include, "Rethinking public and private life via the surrogacy contract," *Politics and the Life Sciences*, February 1990, and *John Marshall's Law and politics: A critical analysis* (Greenwood Press, forthcoming).

TJEERD TYMSTRA is a medical sociologist at the University of Groningen, The Netherlands. He studies the psychosocial impact of new medical technologies, especially controversial ones. His research interests include reproductive technologies, organ donation and transplantation, and clinical screening procedures. In 1991 he conducted a survey of health professionals at the request of the Dutch national commission set up to study what limits ought to be drawn in applying new medical techniques in their country.

MARY ANNE WARREN teaches in the Philosophy Department at San Francisco State University. She earned her doctorate at the University of California at Berkeley. She has published many articles in applied ethics and feminist philosophy and two books: *The nature of woman: An encyclopedia and guide to the literature* (Edgepress) and *Gendercide: The implications of sex selection* (Littlefield Adams).

DOROTHY C. WERTZ is a medical sociologist with an interdisciplinary background in social ethics, social anthropology, and the study of religion and society. She is Senior Scientist at the Shriver Center for Mental Retardation and Research Professor in the Health Services Section at the Boston University School of Public Health. Her publications include *Lying-in: A history of childbirth in America* (Yale University Press); and articles on interpersonal communication and interpretation of risk in genetic counseling.

LINDA S. WILLIAMS works in Ottawa as a consultant for the Royal Commission on New Reproductive Technologies and teaches in the Sociology Department of Carleton University. Her previous work has included studies of commuter marriage and rape victim reporting to the police. In 1990 she completed a background paper for the Canadian Human Rights Commission on the human implications of the new reproductive technologies in Canada.

ROSALIE A. YEMBA in 1991 was a junior at Bennett College. A native of Kinshasa, Zaire (Central Africa), with a major in biology and a minor in chemistry. She plans to study medicine and specialize in pediatrics. At Bennett she is secretary of the International Students Association, and a researcher in the Women's Studies Program, and is an active community service volunteer.

PART I

ISSUES RAISED BY NEW CONTRACEPTIVES

Chapter 1

CONTRACEPTIVE CHOICE: A MULTITUDE OF MEANINGS

Betsy Hartmann

Commentators on contraceptive technology frequently decry the fact that women in the United States have fewer contraceptive choices than women in Europe and even in developing countries. A combination of strict regulatory procedures, high liability payments and insurance costs, and opposition from conservatives and feminists alike are obstacles to the speedy development and marketing of new contraceptives (Hilts 1990). Implicit in this analysis is the belief that more technologies automatically equal more choices.

Contraceptive choice, however, is not such a simple matter, for it involves complex power relationships at almost every social level. Choice is defined and constrained by the following factors:

Women's need for children. For many poor women especially, bearing a large number of children is vital to economic and psychological survival. In this context women may actively choose *not* to use contraception.

Issues of control in the sexual relationship. Even if a woman wants to control births, her male partner or other family members may object, either forcing her to use no method at all or a method that can be used surreptitiously such as the injectable Depo Provera.

The availability of methods. For women who are able to use contraception, choice may be limited by cost, access to a family planning provider, and the range of available methods. In many population control programs, for example, only one or two of the more effective contraceptive methods, e.g., sterilization and the IUD, are promoted, since the overriding goal is to lower birth rates, not to meet the individual woman's reproductive health needs (Hartmann 1987). In many places the crucial backup of safe, legal abortion is not an option.

Uninformed consent. Lack of sex education, heavy-handed or coercive treatment of women in population control programs, and inadequate information about contraceptive risks and benefits are a few of the elements that diminish informed contraceptive choice. The 1989 United States Supreme Court ruling that federally funded family planning clinics cannot even counsel women on abortion shows how access to information can involve power relationships at the very highest level of government (*Webster v. Reproductive Health Services*).

Research priorities. Since the inception of the birth control revolution in the 1950s, contraceptive research and development have focused overwhelmingly on female methods, so that women have had to shoulder the burden of risk. In addition, systemic and surgical birth control methods have received much higher priority than safer though less profitable and effective barrier technologies, such as the condom and diaphragm (Hartmann 1987, Chap. 9).

These biases are no accident. Not only do they reflect deeply ingrained sexism—the management of *women's* fertility is seen as the goal—but also the population control imperative that underlies a substantial portion of contraceptive research. In the design of technology, effectiveness in preventing pregnancy has taken precedence over other important concerns, such as absence of side effects, cultural suitability, individual control, and prevention of sexually transmitted diseases (STDs).

Today the United States is still the major actor in the field, contributing an estimated 75 percent of worldwide funding for reproductive research and contraceptive development (Mastroianni, Jr., et al. 1990, 83). However, in the last two decades the locus of U.S. contraceptive research has shifted from large pharmaceutical companies to public agencies, universities, and private nonprofit organizations, notably the Population Council and Family Health International, both of which pursue a population control agenda (Mastroianni, Jr., et al. 1990, Chap. 5). Internationally, the World Health Organization (WHO) now plays a leading role.

A major question currently facing the international women's health movement is to what extent this shift affords women greater opportunity to influence contraceptive research. For example, feminist groups are debating whether they should agree to participate in postmarketing surveillance of new contraceptives such as Norplant. Many activists fear the groups will either be coopted or sidetracked from other important work (personal observation).

Risk/Benefit Calculations and Regulatory Procedures

Contraceptive safety is a relative term, and whoever determines which methods are acceptable has enormous authority. According to the recent U.S. National Research Council contraceptive study:

> All active drugs cause adverse effects in some users. If safety were understood as the total absence of adverse effects, then no drug could be called "safe." Safety of a drug is conceived as a favorable ratio of benefits to risks for the population of users of the drug as a whole (Mastroianni, Jr., et al. 1990, 102).

Given this definition, the issue then becomes how risks and benefits are calculated.

Population control agencies typically measure the risk of women dying from a contraceptive side effect against the risk of women dying in pregnancy or childbirth. In poor countries with high maternal mortality rates, this in effect makes all contraceptives look "safe" and provides the agencies with a defense against charges that they promote contraceptives without adequate medical screening and follow-up. In many social marketing programs in developing countries, for example, the pill is advertised widely and made available without prescription or screening in retail outlets (Hartmann 1987, Chaps. 9 & 10; Hartmann & Standing 1989, Chap. 4).

For a variety of reasons, the use of high rates of maternal mortality to justify contraceptive risk is wrong. It penalizes poor women for their poverty since high maternal mortality rates generally result from inadequate nutrition and health care; it minimizes other harmful but not necessarily life-threatening contraceptive side effects, such as IUD-related anemia, infection, and infertility; and it places the burden of risk entirely on women, neglecting male contraceptive methods, such as the condom and vasectomy (Hartmann 1987, Chap. 9). In addition, as Judith Bruce notes:

> The health risks of women seeking to become pregnant and bear children *cannot be exchanged* for the health risks of women seeking to avoid conception and childbearing. These two groups of women should be viewed as carrying *distinct* risks derived from their reproductive intentions (Bruce 1987, 364).

The maternal mortality method of calculating contraceptive risk in part explains why women in developing countries are sometimes seen to have more contraceptive "choices" than women in the United States, where the Food and Drug Administration (FDA) takes a more cautious approach to contraceptive safety. Interestingly, there is considerable pressure on the FDA to relax its standards. The National Research Council study, for example, recommends that the FDA increase the weight it assigns to contraceptive effectiveness and convenience. "Given the potentially serious health consequences of an unwanted pregnancy resulting from contraceptive failure, methods with fewer side effects are not necessarily safer if they have higher failure rates" (Mastroianni, Jr., et al. 1990, 2). Perhaps this type of reasoning underlies the FDA decision to classify the cervical cap as a Class III (significant risk) device. (See Gallagher, this volume.)

Clearly, for women to exercise meaningful contraceptive choice, they need to have a significant voice in the formulation of risk/benefit standards.

Technology Is Seldom Neutral

The six essays in this section explore these critical aspects of contraceptive choice in more depth. Anita Hardon's piece on the hormonal implant Norplant raises many of the controversial issues surrounding this method. Designed by the Population Council to have "significant personal and demographic impact" (Greenslade & Brown 1983, 10), Norplant is now used in 44 developed and developing countries, including the United States. It is part of a new generation of provider-dependent, long-acting contraceptive technologies that, while minimizing user failure, also minimize women's control.

Hardon criticizes the methodology of the acceptability studies used to promote Norplant and exposes how its "minor" side effects can be a major problem for some women. She also draws attention to the way Norplant lends itself to coercive use, since women cannot take it out themselves.

Her analysis is supported by a 1990 Population Council study of Indonesia, where over a half million women have had Norplant inserted by the country's population control program. The study documents that the program has failed to give women adequate information about the drug, refused many women removal on demand, and failed to train enough practitioners in removal technique. Many women were not even told that they should have Norplant taken out after five years when its efficacy declines; failure to remove it at this point increases the risk of life-threatening ectopic pregnancy (Ward et al. 1990).

Angeline Faye Schrater examines what may prove, after hormonal implants, to be the next major wave of contraceptive technology: antifertility vaccines that act on the immune system. The most advanced thus far is vaccination of women against the placental hormone human chorionic gonadotropin (hCG). Two different hCG vaccines have been tested in clinical trials. The first, and more problematic one, was developed by Indian scientist G.P. Talwar and colleagues with assistance from the Population Council; the second, by Vernon Stevens and colleagues under the auspices of the WHO.

Although Schrater is careful to present both the pros and cons of the two vaccines, one is left with a disturbing sense of the potential for abuse and harmful side effects resulting from their mass use. Will they prove reversible when used by a woman over a period of years? If a woman is vaccinated while pregnant, could it have an adverse effect on the fetus? How can one be sure vaccines will not induce autoimmune disease in some women in the long term? Will women be vaccinated without informed consent?

Contraceptive vaccines could also put considerable stress on already inefficient, underfunded health systems, such as those found in many parts of Africa and southern Asia. Schrater notes that, as the efficacy of the vaccine wanes, women will need to have blood drawn to determine when they are no longer protected from pregnancy. Aside from the time and money blood tests involve, there is also the risk of HIV transmission from unsterile instruments. Blood tests and injections may already be responsible for significant transmission of HIV in Africa (Minkin 1991).

Indeed, in this age of AIDS and cutbacks in health care spending, infertility vaccines as well as contraceptives such as Norplant that require surgical insertion and removal seem to be particularly *inappropriate* technologies for mass use in developing countries. If health systems are not even delivering adequate primary care, how can they be expected to comply with the informed consent procedures and sophisticated safety standards required for ethical use of these drugs?

Elaine Lissner's article on frontiers in nonhormonal male contraception indicates some of the alternative directions research could take. She describes a number of promising vas-based and heat-based methods now undergoing meager study and concludes that more resources should be devoted to their development. More male contraceptive options will not only increase men's choices, but women's as well, and will also allow men to share the burden of risk. Indeed, it is a sad commentary on the state of contraceptive research that there are currently only three male methods widely available: irreversible vasectomy, the condom, and withdrawal.

Making more male technologies available is not sufficient, however; major changes in values and behavior are necessary to ensure their use. Such is the case with the condom, which, given the current epidemic of HIV and other

STDs, is a particularly appropriate technology. In their article on condom effectiveness and acceptability, Susan Rubinstein, Kathleen Ford, and Elizabeth O'Dair document the considerable social barriers to condom use among different communities and age groups. Sustaining condom use can also be a problem, as demonstrated by the relapse to riskier sex practices among some sections of the gay community. The authors write positively of the new female condom currently under clinical trial.

In respect to women's influence over the direction of contraceptive research, Dana Gallagher's article on the Prentif Cavity Rim cervical cap describes how the U.S. feminist health community pressured and worked with the FDA for the study and ultimate approval of the device. Although the relationship was difficult at times, the cap's approval shows that such cooperation is possible and desirable.

Finally, Susan Shaw's paper on sexuality, contraception and pregnancy among black teenage women takes on many of the myths that currently surround the issue, both in the white and black communities. In particular, she criticizes the view originated by New York Senator Daniel Patrick Moynihan that adolescent pregnancy is a symptom of a crisis in the black, matriarchal family. This matriarchy is in turn blamed for perpetuating poverty and high rates of unemployment among black males.

There are intriguing parallels between Moynihan's view, still very much in force today, and the logic of population control, which blames poverty on high birth rates, and not the other way around. Indeed, as Hardon discusses in her article, various state legislatures in the United States have proposed that incentives be given to welfare mothers to use Norplant. A now infamous editorial in the *Philadelphia Inquirer*—entitled "Poverty and Norplant: Can contraception reduce the underclass?"—stated: "It's very tough to undo the damage of being born into a dysfunctional family. So why not make an effort to reduce the number of children . . ." (Kimelman, 1990).

This focus on contraception as the technical fix or cure for social disease is likely to increase as inequality worsens in the years ahead. "If only there were fewer of them" has long been a rallying cry of the rich and privileged, who do not hesitate to use racism and nationalism to galvanize political support. Although men and women certainly need more contraceptive choices, one must be vigilant about who is doing the choosing, as the articles in this section so amply demonstrate.

References

Bruce, Judith. 1987. Users' perspectives on contraceptive technology and delivery systems: Highlighting some feminist issues. *Technology in Society* 9:359–383.

Greenslade, Forrest C., and George F. Brown. 1983. Contraception in the population/development equation. Background paper to the presentation by George Zeidenstein, Population Council, New York.

Hartmann, Betsy. 1987. *Reproductive rights and wrongs: The global politics of population control and contraceptive choice.* New York: Harper & Row.

Hartmann, Betsy, and Hilary Standing. 1989. *The poverty of population control: Family planning and health policy in Bangladesh.* London: Bangladesh International Action Group.

Hilts, Philip J. 1990. Birth-control backlash: Years of litigation and agitation have left America in the dark ages of contraception. *New York Times Magazine* 16 Dec.:41, 55, 70, 72, 74.

Kimelman, Don. 1990. Poverty and Norplant: Can contraception reduce the underclass? *Philadelphia Inquirer* 12 Dec.:A18

Mastroianni, Luigi, Jr., Peter J. Donaldson, and Thomas T. Kane, eds. 1990. *Developing new contraceptives: Obstacles and opportunities.* Washington, D.C.: National Academy Press.

Minkin, Stephen. 1991. Iatronic AIDS: Unsafe medical practices and the HIV epidemic. *Social Science and Medicine* 30(7):786–787.

Ward, Sheila J., Ieda Poernomo Sigit Sidi, Ruth Simmons, et al. 1990. Service delivery systems and quality of care in the implementation of Norplant in Indonesia. Report prepared for the Population Council, New York.

Webster v. Reproductive Health Services. 1989. 109 S.Ct. at 3044.

Chapter 2

NORPLANT: CONFLICTING VIEWS ON ITS SAFETY AND ACCEPTABILITY

Anita Hardon

Introduction

Norplant is a long-acting contraceptive technology that has led to heated public debates among women's health advocates and reproductive researchers. Norplant, a hormonal implant, consists of six silastic rods, each containing 36 milligrams of the progestin levonorgestrel, which can be effective for a period of five years. It was developed by the Population Council and has been produced by Leiras Pharmaceuticals, Finland, since 1983. By mid-1990, Norplant clinical and preintroductory trials had been conducted in 44 developed and developing countries. The new contraceptive technology had been registered and approved for marketing in 15 countries. The U.S. Food and Drug Administration (FDA) approved its use on December 10, 1990. Since its introduction over half a million women have used Norplant worldwide (Population Council 1990b).

This chapter reviews the development of Norplant, highlighting the controversies that have arisen concerning its safety and its introduction in developing countries. Special attention is paid to the so-called acceptability studies

---

This essay is partially based on the article "Norplant: A critical review" in the *Women and Pharmaceuticals Bulletin* (Amsterdam), November 1990:14–18.

that have been done to assess how women accept the use of Norplant. The design, results, and conclusions of these studies are considered against the background of the concerns raised by women's health advocates.

Development of Norplant

The Population Council (PC), a U.S.-based international nonprofit organization established in 1952, conducts social and health science research relevant to developing countries, including biomedical research on contraceptive technology. In 1967, it initiated the research that led to the creation of Norplant. At that time pharmaceutical companies were less inclined than formerly to develop new contraceptive methods because of the long-term toxicity trials required by the U.S. FDA.

The contraceptive effect of Norplant was initially based on the principle that a microdose of progestins suppresses fertility but does not suppress ovulation. The PC researchers expected fewer side effects than with the contraceptive pill due to the continuous release of low doses of progestin. Between 1970 and 1975, many clinical trials were carried out to determine the most effective combinations of capsules and hormones. The Norplant system was developed in 1974. While testing implants containing megestrol acetate in Chile, Brazil, and India, the researchers were confronted with ovarian hypertrophy and an increased number of ectopic pregnancies (pregnancy outside the uterus) among the contraceptive failures. The numbers were higher than would be expected in a comparable group not using contraceptives. These sequelae were caused by the low-dose progestin (Liukko et al. 1977; Segal 1983), which inhibits the transportation of the egg through the fallopian tubes. By 1975 the PC decided to increase the dose, thus reducing the chance of pregnancy as well as diminishing the risk of ectopic pregnancy. The dose of progestins was increased to a level that is still much lower than that of oral contraceptives.

The initial multinational clinical trials of levonorgestrel implants were conducted in 1975 in Brazil, Chile, Denmark, the Dominican Republic, Finland, and Jamaica, monitored by the International Committee for Contraceptive Research (ICCR), a network of collaborating centers founded by the PC.

In July 1975, the ICCR began a study to compare the safety and efficacy of levonorgestrel, norgestrienone, and megestrol acetate implants. Megestrol acetate was later withdrawn from the studies because it was associated with an increased risk of breast nodules in beagle dogs. Norgestrienone was found to have slightly higher pregnancy rates after one year's use than levonorgestrel, while bleeding disturbances occurred more frequently among levonorgestrel users (Segal 1983). The PC chose levonorgestrel as the progestin for their implants for the following reasons:

It was the longest-working reliable progestin.

It had already been approved by the FDA and had been used in oral contraceptives since the sixties.

It had, as implant, the highest continuation rates, that is, relatively few women had their implant removed within the first three years of use.

Mechanisms of Action and Side Effects

The two main mechanisms of action of Norplant are suppression of ovulation and thickening of the cervical mucus to make it impermeable. This method suppresses ovulation in a little more than 50 percent of the menstrual cycles. Although its working mechanisms are not completely understood, the implants are very reliable.

The accurate pregnancy (failure) rates are as follows: 0.2 per 100 women for the first year, 0.5 for the second year, and 1.2, 1.6, and 0.4 per 100 women for the subsequent three years. The overall (cumulative) pregnancy rate for the entire five years was 3.9 per 100 users. There is a correlation between effectiveness and a woman's weight. After the second year heavier women, particularly those who weigh more than 70 kilograms, have a proportionally higher probability of becoming pregnant than lighter women. For women over 70 kilograms, the cumulative gross pregnancy rate per 100 continuing users through five years was 8.5 (WHO 1990).

Once the implants are removed, the contraceptive effect ceases quickly and the woman can become pregnant as rapidly as women who have used an IUD or have not used any method. Rates of pregnancy for women who have Norplant removed for planned pregnancy are similar to those for women using no contraception, according to the PC (Population Council 1990b).

In a manual for clinicians the Population Council (1990b) lists the contraindications for Norplant use. These include women who suffer from cardiovascular disorders, women with undiagnosed abnormal vaginal bleeding, women with benign or malignant liver tumors, and women with known or suspected breast cancer. In addition, WHO guidelines (WHO 1990) warn that women with certain conditions such as diabetes, anemia, and high blood pressure should receive regular medical checkups.

Both the WHO guidelines and the PC manual note that women who are pregnant should not use Norplant and that Norplant should not be considered a method of first choice in lactating women. The WHO guidelines advise that

Norplant not be used earlier than six weeks after birth. Both manuals also point out that clinicians should consider whether the woman smokes or takes any other medications.

The most frequently reported side effects according to both manuals are changes in menstrual bleeding patterns. Irregularities vary widely and may include:

Prrolonged menstrual bleeding during the first months of use (more days than a woman would normally experience)

Untimely bleeding or spotting between periods

No bleeding at all for several months or even for a year or more in a few cases

A combination of these patterns (WHO 1990)

In addition, both manuals mention other complaints that are likely to be "method-related":

headaches (the most frequent complaint after menstrual irregularities)

nervousness

vomiting

dizziness

inflammation of the skin

acne

change of appetite

weight gain

breast tenderness

excessive facial hair growth or hair loss

infection, pain, or itching at the implant site, and

functional ovarian cysts

The manuals mention a number of other complaints reported by some users or physicians that may or may not be associated with the method: breast discharge, inflammation of the cervix, mood change, depression, general malaise, weight loss, itching, and hypertension.

Reactions of Women's Health Advocates

An important issue raised by women's health advocates is the tendency of complex contraceptive technologies to make women more dependent on medical professionals for their administration and removal. A potential for abuse of Norplant exists in family planning programs that do not acknowledge a woman's right to a free choice of existing methods and that do not acknowledge a woman's right to removal of the method whenever she desires. Women's health advocates also stress that the long-term effects of the method are not yet known. Removal problems have occurred when the rods had not been inserted properly and in situations in which health personnel had not been sufficiently trained in removal.

A further concern is fetal exposure to progestins in the case of method failure or when the method is inserted in pregnant women. Furthermore, the safety of Norplant use by lactating women has not yet been determined. In Bangladesh and Brazil women's health advocates opposed the introduction of Norplant on the above grounds. In Brazil the Ministry of Health decided to discontinue further enrollment in the ongoing trials (Reis 1990).

Evaluation by WHO

In 1985, the World Health Organization (WHO) presented its evaluation report on Norplant. The report concluded that the Norplant system is an "effective and reversible long-term method of fertility regulation . . . particularly advantageous to women who wish an extended period of contraceptive protection" and is considered "suitable for use in family planning programs along with other methods of fertility regulation." At the same time WHO pointed to the need for:

A training program for medical personnel

More research on long-term side effects

Research into the use of implants during lactation

Postmarketing surveillance studies and continuation of acceptability studies (WHO 1985)

In accordance with WHO's recommendation, the Population Council established three international centers for training physicians in Norplant insertion and removal techniques in the Dominican Republic, Indonesia, and Egypt. Leiras also trained a number of clinicians in Finland. All the principal investigators for the preintroduction trials were trained at these centers; after returning to their countries, they trained others. In addition, PC, in collaboration with Family Health International (FHI), the Association for Voluntary Surgical Contraception (AVSC), and the Program for Appropriate Technology in Health (PATH), prepared a five-day Norplant curriculum, which was to serve as a prototype for in-country training of physicians, nurses, and counselors. The curriculum has been tested in several countries.

Rare and long-term side effects cannot be detected before a method is widely used because such research requires a large group of users. Thus, WHO, in collaboration with the PC and FHI, in 1987 initiated postmarketing surveillance of Norplant in seven countries to learn about rare events associated with implant use. For five years 7500 to 8000 Norplant users and the same number of controls will be followed in the first long-term internationally coordinated and controlled postmarketing surveillance of a contraceptive's safety in developing countries. Data from all the participating centers are collected and analyzed at WHO's headquarters in Geneva. The study investigates what happens to women even if they switch to another method or become pregnant and focuses not only on commonly recorded events, but also on rare events, such as tubal pregnancies. Most of the women in the control group use IUDs. The study began in June 1987 with pilot projects in Chile, Sri Lanka, and Thailand, and the full surveillance project was launched in autumn 1988 at multiple centers in Bangladesh, Chile, China, Egypt, Indonesia, Sri Lanka, and Thailand.

After several studies on lactation, the PC now recommends:

> Steroids are not considered the contraceptives of first choice for breastfeeding women. Studies have shown no significant effects on the growth or health of infants whose mothers used levonorgestrel implants beginning six weeks after childbirth (Population Council 1990b, 33).

As for the acceptability studies that WHO recommended, the PC initiated research on the determinants of user satisfaction with the method and the service delivery system through which it is offered. The PC reports that user and program studies are underway in Bangladesh, Brazil, Colombia, Dominican Republic, Egypt, Ghana, Haiti, Indonesia, Kenya, Mexico, Nepal, Nigeria, Philippines, Senegal, Singapore, Thailand, the United States, and Zambia.

Norplant Acceptability Studies

Norplant has been subjected to more acceptability studies than any other fertility regulating method currently on the market. Tables 2–1 and 2–2 present an overview of the aims, methods, results, and conclusions of Norplant acceptability studies that have been published in the journals *Studies in Family Planning* and *International Family Planning Perspectives* in the past decade

TABLE 2–1

Norplant Acceptability Studies: Aims and Methods

Country	Aims	Respondents No.
Indonesia Lubis et al. 1983	assess performance of Norplant provide data on acceptability	813
Thailand Satayapan et al. 1983	determine how Norplant is perceived measure continuation rate	887
Egypt Shaaban et al. 1983	evaluate acceptability of Norplant compare with IUD	250
Ecuador Marangoni et al. 1983	determine acceptability of Norplant	283
Sri Lanka Basnayake et al. 1988	evaluate safety, efficacy, and acceptability of Norplant	400
USA Darney et al. 1988	identify personal perceptions of Norplant define determinants of and levels of user-satisfaction	205
Four country I Kane et al. 1990	determine level of interest in trying Norplant determine impact of social and demographic factors	2586
Four country II Zimmerman et al. 1990	look at Norplant from perspective of users and nonusers understanding concerns and motivations of users	279

(Basnayake et al. 1988; Darney et al. 1988; Kane et al. 1990; Lubis et al. 1983; Marangoni et al. 1983; Satayapan et al. 1983; Shabaan et al. 1983; Zimmerman et al. 1990). More studies have been done by or with support from the Population Council, but these have not yet been published in the above journals, and are therefore not considered in this review.

Table 2–1 shows that the formulation of the aims varies somewhat but always includes how users view Norplant. Sometimes additional aims, such as studying safety and efficacy or studying factors that influence acceptability, are given. The number of respondents varies between 2586 (in a four-country study, Zimmerman et al. 1990) and 205 (in San Francisco, USA, Darney et al. 1988).

Most studies have focused on the acceptability of Norplant to users and to women who discontinued use. One four-country study (Kane et al. 1990) has also assessed acceptability to potential users, i.e., people coming to a family planning service in search of a suitable fertility regulating method; and another comparative study (Zimmerman et al. 1990) has looked into acceptability to husbands and family planning program personnel.

Usually, the studies are done in university-based health clinics or mother and child clinics in urban centers, where the service delivery system is likely to be better than in small village clinics. It is important to realize that the clinic environment may affect the responses of women to the interview questions. They probably identify the interviewers with the health services and, because of this, may not be inclined to talk about problems that they encountered with the service delivery system itself. An alternative environment for discussion about advantages and disadvantages of the methods would be the community and the homes of users and nonusers. In such situations, one could also talk about the method with others involved, such as husbands or mothers of the users, thereby getting more insight into sociocultural aspects that affect contraceptive use.

None of the reviewed studies make explicit what criteria and indicators are used to assess if a method is acceptable or not. Implicit criteria appear to be (1) the degree to which women continue to use the method and (2) the degree to which women decide to stop using the method because of side effects (see Table 2–2). The studies in Indonesia (Lubis et al. 1983), Thailand (Satayapan et al. 1983), and Sri Lanka (Basnayake et al. 1988) mention which inclusion and exclusion criteria were used in the selection of the research sample. The others do not give details other than that the respondents were Norplant users or potential users. One of the four-country studies (Zimmerman et al. 1990) cautions that, in addition to the formal criteria, other selection processes may occur. The authors report that clinic staff may pick women who are likely to

Respondents Type	Research site	Criteria for in/exclusion
users	2 urban clinics	PC criteria
users	3 urban clinics	PC criteria
users	1 urban clinic	not given
users	2 urban clinics	not given
users	2 urban clinics	married 18–40 years no contraindications not pregnant
users	1 urban clinic	not given
potential users	10 clinics	start/change contraceptive use
users nonusers husbands service providers in focus group discussions (FGD)	urban clinics	countries with more than five years experience with Norplant no specifics on selection of participants in FGDs

TABLE 2–2

Norplant Acceptability Studies: Main Results and Conclusions

Country	1-year continuation rate	Main reasons for discontinuing	Main side effects
Indonesia Lubis et al. 1983	95.3	menstrual problem skin problem husband objection	irregular menstruation amenorrhea skin irritation
Thailand Satayapan et al. 1983	88.4	menstrual problem skin infection other medical	menstrual change weight change severe headache
Etypt Shaaban et al. 1983	89.6	bleeding/pain personal pregnancy	menstrual change headache depression
Ecuador Marangoni et al. 1983	87.4	menstrual problem skin infection acne and headache	not given
Sri Lanka Basnayake et al. 1988	98.7	pregnancy menstrual problem	menstrual change headache and dizziness back, stomach pain
USA Darney et al. 1988	2-year rate 77	side effects fears inefficacy (end of 5 years) medical reasons	menstrual change weight change headache
Four country I Kane et al. 1990	no data	*reasons not to try Norplant:* prefer other method fear of side effects husband disapproves	
Four country II Zimmerman et al. 1990	no data	*perceived disadvantages:* irregular, prolonged bleeding weight loss headaches dizziness	*reported advantages:* nothing to remember effective long-term duration

[a]At 3-month follow-up. At 12-month follow-up this was 30%.

[b]This was at 3-month follow-up. At 12 months 75% complained of menstrual change.

% of users	Other important results	Conclusion
52 21 11	frequency of side effects increases with education	Norplant may be acceptable to women
57 6 2	11% of discontinuation is due to infections at implant site	Results are strong indication of acceptability
67[a] 6 1	continuation rate—Norplant is better than IUD	Norplant is an acceptable method that deserves wider use.
	first few removals proved to be difficult	There is substantial demand for a contraceptive like Norplant
71.8[b] 19 16	40% users mention long-acting as advantage of Norplant	The study suggests that Norplant is a safe, effective, acceptable method
82 32 24	other side effects include decreased libido, chest pains, numbness of arms	This study found Norplant an acceptable method of contraception
	reported advantages of Norplant: effectiveness newness promise safety	The study reveals a relatively high level of interest in using Norplant
	rumors in all countries: causes sterility and cancer capsules migrate affects breast milk reports that removal on demand does not always occur to satisfaction of user	Findings permit program planners to identify resistance points

keep the method in. The preintroductory trial in Ecuador also reports that clinic staff play a role in client selection:

> Staff were worried mainly about the women's reactions to the pronounced bleeding disturbance associated with the implants. . . . The staff was initially overselective in choosing users, but as the trial progressed they became more confident and the rate of acceptance increased (Marangoni et al. 1983, 79).

In sum, the process of selecting research samples for Norplant acceptability studies is problematic, first because clinics in urban centers are selected and then because local investigators use certain inclusion and exclusion criteria in selecting which potential users will participate. Thus the population in all studies is far from representative of the general population that will use the method when it is on the market and distributed through health care channels. Despite this methodological shortcoming, the researchers tend to draw conclusions such as the following about the general acceptability of the methods in the countries concerned (see also Table 2–2).

> The data presented in this article are encouraging and indicate that Norplant implants may be acceptable to Indonesian women (Lubis et al. 1983, 183).

> We interpret these continuation rates, and the perceptions and experiences of the users of the method to date, as a strong indication of the acceptability of the implant methods (Thailand—Satayapan et al. 1983, 176).

> Norplant implants are an effective acceptable method of contraception with minimal side effects, and definitely deserve wider use in Egypt (Shaaban et al. 1983, 167)

> Our experience shows that there is a substantial demand for a contraceptive with the characteristics of the Norplant system . . . (Ecuador—Marangoni et al. 1983, 179).

> The study of 205 women who received Norplant contraceptives at an urban family planning clinic in the USA found Norplant to be a highly acceptable method of contraception for women of different ethnic and economic groups, despite the occurrence of side effects (Darney et al. 1988, 158)

In addition to the research population not being representative, the lack of explicit indicators and criteria for determining acceptability to potential users makes it difficult to judge the validity of the general conclusion that Norplant is acceptable for a wider population.

The studies indicate relatively high continuation rates. Menstrual change, skin irritations, and headaches are reportedly the main side effects and the main reasons for discontinuing the method. In interpreting the results, the researchers tend to define disorders such as headaches, dizziness, and weight gain as minor side effects, of which the relationship with Norplant has not been proven. According to the Sri-Lankan acceptability study, for example:

> Of the 189 women who were followed up at 12 months, one reported that she had been hospitalized for prolonged headache and dizziness, no medical problems could be found (Basnayake et al. 1988, 43).

Women's fears of long-term effects, effects on the fetus, and the like are classified as rumors that form obstacles to the expansion of Norplant use. One study notes:

> Rumors reported by participants in all countries were (1) Norplant causes cancer and sterility, (2) the capsules migrate to other parts of the body, and (3) the breast milk of Norplant users negatively affects Norplant offspring (Zimmerman et al. 1990, 97).

Understanding the User Perspective

Apart from the above-mentioned methodological shortcomings of the studies, perhaps the most important limitation of the studies is their failure to discover people's own ideas of reproductive physiology, their own perception of the mode of action of the methods, and their own cost-benefit analysis in choosing a birth control method. Beliefs about reproductive physiology clearly affect people's perceptions of the methods. The Nichters in an essay on modern fertility regulating methods, for example, have shown how people explain the effects of oral contraceptives in Sri Lanka:

> A pervasive notion among informants was that the pill worked because of its heating effect in the body. . . . Some informants noted that taking these pills every day raised the heat level of the body to such an extent that male and female *dhatu*, a substance associated with vitality and strength, was burned up. . . . Another health concern noted by Sinhalese women was that the excess heat in a woman's body caused by taking the pill rendered the womb dry. Over time a dry womb becomes incapable of accepting male seed (Nichter & Nichter 1989, 60–61).

The Nichters stress that the issues of "rumors" and "side effects" have to be recast, calling for a more profound analysis of why these concerns exist.

With respect to Norplant, it is remarkable that so little has been written about the consequences of menstrual disturbances for the day-to-day life of the users. Anthropological research suggests that such consequences can be far-reaching. Menstruation is an important event in any woman's life. The meaning that is attributed to this event or its loss varies, affecting, among other things, cooking procedure, sexual interaction, and religious practices (Buckley & Gottlieb 1988; DelVecchio Good 1980; WHO 1981). Douglas (1988) has described how menstrual blood is often perceived to be a dangerous element for men. Among the Enga of New Guinea, for example:

> [C]ontact with it, or with a menstruating woman will, in the absence of appropriate counter-magic, sicken a man and cause persistent vomiting, "kill" his blood so that it turns black, corrupt his vital juices so that his skin darkens and hangs in folds as his flesh wastes, permanently dull his wits, and eventually lead to a slow decline and death (Douglas 1988, 147).

Delay or absence of menstruation in many societies is considered unhealthy for woman (Newman 1985). In Colombia, Browner (1985), found that the stopping of expected blood flow is perceived as an illness. In Malaysia, too, Ngin (1985) reported a prevailing perception among the Chinese Malays that irregular menstruation is unclean and bad for woman's health and that remedies should be taken to ensure the expected onset. Laderman (1983) describes that to increase the flow of scanty menstruation, women in East Malaysia are encouraged to eat sweet things. Menstruating women in her research areas may not pray during menses, and men are not supposed to have sexual intercourse with their wives at this time.

The reproductive researchers have a technical answer to the irregular menstruation resulting from Norplant use: they recommend that potential acceptors be "counseled" about the possibility of suffering from menstrual disorders, especially in the first few months after Norplant implantation, and that they be told that this adverse effect is not serious in medical terms for hemoglobin levels do not decrease. Some family planning programs give estrogens to women who suffer from serious bleeding; however, WHO (1990) advises against this.

How the Technology Affects the User-Provider Relationship

Another limitation of the reviewed acceptability studies is that they do not show how the new technology affects the relationship between the provider and user of the method. As noted in the above, Norplant is a technology that makes women dependent on health workers for removal, and thus for reversal of its effects. In the preintroductory trials there were reports of providers denying removal to women. In 1990, the four-country accessibility study, for example, stated:

> In all four countries there were reports that removal on demand did not occur to the satisfaction of the user. Women participating in the clinical

> study who asked for removal because of irregular bleeding experienced the greatest difficulty, as clinicians often suggested waiting to see whether the menstrual flow would normalize. Both service providers and discontinuers reported that when faced with a clinician that would not remove the implants, women in the Dominican Republic, Egypt, and Indonesia learned to give reasons that they knew the clinician would accept, such as the spouse's requesting another baby. In Thailand, because of the cost of the method, women are routinely informed when choosing Norplant that the implants are appropriate for long-term spacing and will not be removed for minor side effects (Zimmerman et al. 1990, 99).

Such findings can be understood within the framework of diverging interests of providers and users. The family planning workers and clinicians may have an interest in achieving high continuation rates. In Thailand the cost of Norplant is used as a reason. In the other countries the interest of providers in continued Norplant use may be related to the preoccupation of family planning programs with achieving high acceptor rates and low fertility rates or with the feeling of clinicians that "high continuation rates" are a successful outcome of the trial.

Information Provision and Contraceptive Choice

None of the reports on acceptability studies describes the information that was provided to women about Norplant prior to acceptance of the method, though such information is likely to affect woman's perceptions of effects and side effects of the method. The Ecuadorian study does refer to this information, but it gives no insight into its content: "the professionally designed educational materials directed to both the users and the clinic personnel were especially effective informational tools" (Marangoni et al. 1983, 179).

Because of the missing information on the content of the "effective" informational tools, it is not clear to what extent women were provided with an opportunity to become aware of the variety of birth control methods that exist and of the relative advantages and disadvantages of each, nor is it clear if the trials have followed an appropriate "informed consent" procedure.

Health groups and women in Brazil and Bangladesh have seriously criticized these acceptability studies (Reis 1990; UBINIG 1988). To them the preintroductory trials do not genuinely test the acceptability of the method in the countries concerned but appear to be forms of early marketing of the method, designed to overcome "resistance points." A study in Bangladesh among a few Norplant users, pointed to a newspaper call for participants in a trial, that described Norplant as early as 1981 as follows:

> A new birth control method, NORPLANT. A wonderful innovation of modern science.
>
> This method is for women
> This can be implanted under the skin of arm
> This will ensure sterility for five years
> When removed, can have children again
>
> Get more information from: Bangladesh Fertility Research Programme. 3/7 Asad Avenue (1st floor), Mohammadpur, Dhaka (UBINIG 1988).

The Potential for Misuse

Women's health advocates the world over are, in fact, most concerned about the last two points raised, i.e., the effect of the technology on the user-provider relationship and the manner in which the method affects women having a genuine free and informed choice. As mentioned, these concerns are related to the provider-dependent and complex nature of the technology: women cannot take the implants out themselves.

That these concerns are not unrealistic became clear in a number of different widely publicized "Norplant cases" in the United States, which emerged shortly after the approval of the method by the U.S. Food and Drug Administration in December 1990.

The first, and perhaps most serious, case is the proposal of a Kansas state legislator to pay $500 to any mother on welfare who uses Norplant. Under the bill, believed to be the first of its kind considered by a state, Kansas would also pay for implanting the device and for annual checkups. The rationale of the bill, according to its sponsor Kerry Patrick R. Leawood, is to save taxpayers the $205,000 of basic public assistance that each child costs from birth to adulthood. Leawood stresses that "something has to be done to reduce the number of unwanted pregnancies, and this type of voluntary program, where the public is given a strong financial incentive to use a safe reversible contraceptive device that has a useful life of five years represents the best way to prevent them" (Lewin 1991).

Whereas the Kansas bill has little chance of passing, it certainly demonstrates the potential for misuse of the method. Clearly, providing certain population groups—welfare mothers—with incentives to use certain contraceptive methods interferes with the right to privacy under the First Amendment of the U.S. Constitution as interpreted by the Supreme Court in the 1950s to include contraception. For the welfare mothers who do not want to use the method, the legislation could be considered "cruel and unusual punishment."

Another case that induced controversy was the order of Judge Howard Broadman of Tulare County, California, to implant Norplant as part of a plea bargain in the case of a woman who had pled guilty of child abuse. The woman was ordered to have the capsules inserted on her release from jail. The implants would have to be kept in for the entire probation period. In sentencing the woman, the judge made Norplant sound no more complex than a condom. "It's a new thing," he reportedly said. And "easily removable" (Cantwell 1991).

Upon hearing about this incident, one of the original developers of Norplant, Dr. Sheldon Segal, protested, citing the infringement of the defendant's reproductive rights (Norplant easy . . . 1991). When other critics argued that the defendant might have medical conditions that would make Norplant harmful, the judge left it up to doctors to decide whether the device would be safe (MacKenzie 1991).

In this case, again, a woman is given an incentive to use Norplant—a shorter jail sentence. This incentive interferes with her reproductive rights. The fact that doctors are given the right to decide whether the method is suitable for the woman reinforces the fears of women's health advocates about the provider-dependent nature of the method. The woman's own ideas on what a suitable contraceptive would be are not considered.

It is ominous that in a country with relatively accessible health and family planning services these issues arise so shortly after the method's approval. They pose serious questions as to the manner in which the methods are used in countries where more people are poor and underprivileged and where family planning programs have the explicit aim of reducing population growth—not for the "benefit" of the individual but for the development of the state. Though not yet systematically documented, the introduction of Norplant in such countries is likely to have a negative effect upon women's and men's rights to a free and informed choice of birth control method.

Conclusion

Women's health advocates are concerned about the widespread distribution of Norplant in family planning programs in developing countries, while issues concerning ethical administration, safety of the method, and service delivery have not yet been resolved. This review of Norplant makes clear that appropriate use of such a new contraceptive technology depends on the context in which the method is used. If the method is, for example, administered in a relatively coercive family planning program, then a woman's right to choose freely from a range of contraceptives and a woman's right to stop the method are likely to be violated. Norplant, in my view, is a sophisticated technology that requires a high standard of health care if it is to be administered safely. It is questionable whether such standards can be achieved in many developing countries. Women in developing countries living in remote areas, moreover, are more likely to suffer from anemia and to have or have had liver diseases. These conditions, which require extra medical attention, make rational use of implants especially difficult.

Before distributing the method on a wider scale, long-term health-related, economic, and social consequences of the method ought to be examined, and prerequisites and conditions for safe use ought to be determined.

The postmarketing surveillance of the WHO will produce substantial information on the health-related consequences of Norplant marketing. The economic and social consequences, however, do not appear to be studied as rigorously. One wonders, for example, how the extensive training that is needed for safe Norplant delivery and use will be financed. Can this effort be sustained when the initial international funding stops? Does the financial burden on family planning programs in developing countries not lead to a deterioration of other services? Even in a rich country like the United States, these issues have been raised. A review of Norplant in the *Contraceptive Technology Update* comments, "Perhaps the most significant is the problem of cost." The review points out that the price of Norplant will prevent many low-income women from using it. Not only are they likely to have to pay about $300 for the device, they also have to pay for the insertion and, if required, the removal (Arrival of . . . 1991).

Continuous monitoring of the implementation of the Population Council and WHO guidelines seems to be needed because safe use can be assured only when such guidelines are implemented. Yet the economic consequences of such monitoring and supervision mechanisms also need to be assessed. Concerning the social consequences, more attention should be paid to the ethical issue of a woman's right to removal of the implants in relatively aggressive family planning programs, and a woman's right to objective and balanced information on all contraceptive options. The sociocultural consequences of bleeding disturbances also require more systematic attention.

In determining the conditions and prerequisites for Norplant's safe use, women's health advocates and women users in a variety of sociocultural settings should play an important role and should be involved from an early stage.

Acknowledgments

I thank Sandra Waldman of the Population Council for sending detailed information and a commentary on an earlier draft and Judy Norsigan of the Boston Women's Health Book Collective for providing accounts of Norplant usage situation in the United States in 1991. I wish to thank as well many other women who have voiced their experiences with and ideas and opinions on Norplant during workshops on new reproductive technology at women and health gatherings. They have inspired me to write this essay.

References

Arrival of Norplant may be bittersweet for clinics. 1991. *Contraceptive Technology Update* 12(1):1–5.

Basnayake, S., S. Thalpa, and S.A. Balogh. 1988. Evaluation of safety, efficacy and acceptability of Norplant implants in Sri Lanka. *Studies in Family Planning* 19(1):39–47.

Browner, C.H. 1985. Traditional techniques for diagnosis, treatment and control of pregnancy in Cali, Colombia. In *Women's medicine: A cross-cultural study of indigenous fertility regulation,* ed. L.F. Newman. New Brunswick, NJ: Rutgers University Press.

Buckley, T., and A. Gottlieb, eds. 1988. *Blood magic: The anthropology of menstruation.* Berkeley: University of California Press.

Cantwell, M. 1991. Coercion and contraception. *New York Times* 27 January:E16.

Darney, P.D., E. Atkinson, S. Tanner, et al. 1988. Acceptance and perceptions of Norplant among users in San Francisco, USA. *Studies in Family Planning* 21(3):153–160.

DelVecchio Good, M.-J. 1980. Of blood and babies: The relationship of popular Islamic physiology to fertility. *Social Science and Medicine* 14B(3):147–156.

Douglas, M. 1988. *Purity and danger: An analysis of concepts of pollution and taboo.* London: Ark Paperbacks (original text 1966).

Hansen, E.B., and L. Launsø. 1987. Development, use and evaluation of drugs: The dominating technology. *Social Science and Medicine* 25:65–73.

Kane, T.T., G. Farr, and B. Janowitz. 1990. Initial acceptability of contraceptive implants in four developing countries. *International Family Planning Perspectives* 16(2):49–54.

Laderman, C. 1983. *Childbirth and nutrition in rural Malaysia.* Berkeley: University of California Press.

Lewin, T. 1991. A plan to pay welfare mothers for birth control. *New York Times* 9 February:8,9.

Liukko, P., R. Erkkola, and L. Laakso. 1977. Ectopic pregnancy during use of low-dose progestagens for oral contraception. *Contraception* 16:575–580.

Lubis, F., J. Prihartono, T. Agoestina, et al. 1983. One-year experience with Norplant implants in Indonesia. *Studies in Family Planning* 14(6/7):181–184.

MacKenzie, J.P. 1991. Whose choice is it, anyway? *New York Times* 28 January:A18,A22.

Marangoni, P., S. Cartagena, J. Alvarado, et al. 1983. Norplant implants and the TCu 200 IUD: A comparative study in Ecuador. *Studies in Family Planning* 14(6/7):177–180.

Newman, L.F., ed. 1985. *Women's medicine: A cross-cultural study of indigenous fertility regulation.* New Brunswick, N.J.: Rutgers University Press.

Ngin, C. 1985. Indigenous fertility regulating methods among two Chinese communities in Malaysia. In *Women's medicine: A cross-cultural study of indigenous fertility regulation*, ed. L.F. Newman. New Brunswick, N.J.: Rutgers University Press.

Nichter, M., and M. Nichter. 1989. Modern methods of fertility regulation: When and for whom are they appropriate? In *Anthropology and international health. South Asian case studies*, ed. M. Nichter. Dordrecht, Neth.: Kluwer.

Norplant easy to use, easier to abuse. 1991. *CDRR News* January/February:1.

Population Council. 1990a. Approvals rise to 15 countries. *Norplant Worldwide* 14 May. New York: The Council.

Population Council. 1990b. Norplant contraceptive subdermal implant. *Manual for clinicians*. New York: The Council.

Reis, A.G. 1990. Norplant in Brazil. (Unpublished report submitted to WEMOS.)

Satayapan, S., K. Kanchanasinith, and S. Varakamin. 1983. Perceptions and acceptability of Norplant implants in Thailand. *Studies in Family Planning* 14(6/7):170–176.

Segal, S.J. 1983. The development of Norplant implants. *Studies in Family Planning* 14 (6/7):159–163.

Shaaban, S.M.M., M. Salah, A. Zarzour, et al. 1983. A prospective study of Norplant implants and the TCu 380Ag IUD in Assiut, Egypt. *Studies in Family Planning* 14(6/7):163–169.

UBINIG. 1988. The Norplant trial: An investigative study on the methodology and ethical issues. *Hygiea* 3(1 & 2):19–34.

World Health Organization (WHO). 1985. Facts about an implantable contraceptive. *WHO Bulletin* 33(3):485–494.

World Health Organization (WHO). 1990. *Norplant contraceptive subdermal implants. Managerial and Technical Guidelines.* Geneva: WHO.

World Health Organization Task Force on Psychosocial Research in Family Planning. 1981. A cross-cultural study of menstruation: Implications for contraceptive development and use. *Studies in Family Planning* 12(1):3–16.

Zimmerman, M., J. Haffey, E. Crane, et al. 1990. Assessing the acceptability of Norplant implants in four countries: Findings from focus group discussions. *Studies in Family Planning* 21(2):93–103.

Chapter 3

CONTRACEPTIVE VACCINES: PROMISES AND PROBLEMS

Angeline Faye Schrater

Introduction

The search for effective and acceptable contraceptives is a millennia-old quest. Zatuchni (1989) writes that in ancient times a potion for men contained burned mule testicles, willow bark, and cottonseed. Chemicals and devices used by women have included ointment of lead, potions of willow leaves and barrenwort in wine, suppositories containing crocodile dung, and goat bladder condoms. Little change in contraceptives occurred until the middle of the twentieth century. Now, however, available at the global level are a plethora of birth control methods that include oral and injectable hormones, spermicides, barrier devices, surgical techniques, and IUDs, all in great variety. These modern contraceptives are used by nearly 500 million women (excluding those not in marital unions), and the trend toward increased use is expected to continue (United Nations 1989, 36).

Although modern methods are vastly improved over ancient ones, they are, nonetheless, often inadequate, unsafe, or unacceptable (Bell 1984; Hartmann 1987; Lee et al. 1989; Vessey 1986). No method is ideal or even suitable for every woman, nor for any particular woman at all points during her years of reproductive potential. Thus the search for effective, acceptable, and safe contraceptives continues, in part to provide greater choice for women and in part to increase the effectiveness of family planning programs.

Vaccines are among the newest of the technologies to be added to the contraceptive cornucopia. Until now, most birth control methods have been variations on two themes, barrier and hormone. Antifertility vaccines are unique from all other contraceptives in that vaccines utilize innate physiological processes, immune responses, to regulate fertility. Researchers began developing vaccines nearly two decades ago after realizing that some cases of infertility in women and in men were due to an immune response to sperm, a response that prevented fertilization (Menge 1980; Mathur et al. 1987). If an "accident of nature" could cause infertility, then it might be possible to develop vaccines to induce infertility by immunological pathways. Thus was born the concept of immunocontraception.

Immunity and Traditional Vaccines

For those unfamiliar with the immune system this section provides a background for understanding the promises and problems associated with contraceptive vaccines.

The immune system is a functionally integrated collection of vessels, organs, cells, and molecules that help protect an individual from disease and illness caused by a "foreign" substance or microorganism. For example, it recognizes microorganisms such as viruses and bacteria to be foreign antigens, then generates specific, protective responses. To the immune system foreign is nonself, i.e., anything chemically unique from one's own cells and molecules. An antigen is any substance that induces an immune response; it is the ultimate, specific target as well.

Immunity can be classified into two broad categories, antibody-mediated and cell-mediated. In the first, specialized cells, B cells (in concert with other cells and molecules), recognize antigen, then synthesize and secrete protein molecules called antibodies (immunoglobulins). Antibodies induced by a particular antigen recognize and bind to that antigen. If the affinity (tightness of binding) of antibody is sufficiently high, binding initiates a chain of events culminating in removal of antigen from the system.

The second type of immunity is mediated by various subpopulations of other specialized cells known collectively as T cells. For example, cytotoxic T cells can recognize antigen on a cell and cause death of that cell, again resulting in antigen removal. In some individuals and under ill-defined conditions of antigen presentation, delayed-type hypersensitivity T cells produce hormonelike factors upon antigen contact and cause allergic responses that can range from itching to skin eruptions to shock. Both antibody- and cell-mediated immunity can be elicited by the same antigen.

Protective levels of immunity are not reached until two to three weeks after initial contact with antigen. In the case of severe illness and/or infection with extremely pathogenic organisms, death can occur before immunity is effective. Generally, however, immune responses help one recover from the consequences of exposure to foreign antigens, then prevent reinfection. The three cardinal features of an immune response are specificity, self/nonself discrimination, and memory. These features determine vaccine design as well as govern assumptions about efficacy and safety.

Specificity

Immune responses and the subsequent molecular reactions are exquisitely specific. Antibody and immune-reactive cells match up with their inducing antigens like pieces of a jigsaw puzzle. Antibody and immune-reactive cells induced by one antigen can react with a different antigen only if the latter displays recognition sites identical or similar to those on the eliciting antigen. Immune recognition of the same or similar sites on two different molecules is called cross-reactivity.

Self/Nonself Discrimination

Cells capable of reacting to self are either continuously deleted during one's lifetime or are functionally suppressed by immunoregulatory cells (Burnet 1959; Goodnow et al. 1990; Ramsdell & Fowlkes 1990). Without this self-tolerance, autoimmune disease ensues, i.e., the destruction by the immune system of one's own cells and molecules. Occasionally, self-tolerance does break down; some forms of anemia, diabetes, and rheumatoid arthritis are autoimmune-induced. Autoimmune diseases seldom are fatal but often are debilitating. In general, women suffer a higher incidence of autoimmune disease than do men (Sinha et al. 1990).

Intentional bypass of the immunological injunction against self reactivity can be achieved by presenting self antigens physically linked to nonself antigens; the immune system acts upon the entire complex as if it were nonself. This ability to induce autoimmune responses provides the immunological basis for contraceptive vaccines.

Memory

Immunological memory prevents reinfection or illness upon subsequent exposure to the original inducer of a response. Initial contact causes proliferation of specific immune-reactive cells, thereby increasing the numbers of cells recognizing that antigen. Qualitative changes also occur. Under complex conditions of stimulation and antigen deposition, some cells (of both B and T lineage) become long-lived, with functional life spans ranging from years to decades (Beverley 1990; Klinman & Linton 1990). Memory B cells synthesize antibodies with a higher average affinity for antigen than that of antibodies synthesized by primary cells. The expanded, qualitatively different, yet highly specific cell populations provide immunological memory. When the individual re-encounters the original antigen (or a cross-reactive one), the immune system responds with more speed and vigor than it could upon initial exposure. The most important point to remember is this: because of memory, immunity is seldom reversible though it may wane to low activity.

Traditional Vaccines

Quite possibly the best-known vaccine is the one against smallpox. Inoculation to prevent smallpox was prevalent in China by the tenth century A.D., and by the seventeenth century the practice had reached Persia (Temple 1986). Tradition credits Lady Mary Montague (1689–1762), wife of the British ambassador to Constantinople, with introducing the technique to England in 1717. The World Health Organization (WHO) declared war on smallpox in 1973, mounted an intensive vaccination campaign, and declared in 1980 that smallpox was eradicated.

The development and use of vaccines to prevent many common infectious diseases stands as a prime accomplishment of twentieth-century biomedical research. Traditional vaccines are directed against nonself, against the immunologically relevant but noninfectious/nontoxic antigens of disease-causing microorganisms. They prime the immune system for future encounters with infectious agents and prevent life-threatening or debilitating disease. Traditional vaccines owe their effectiveness to immunological memory.

Antifertility Vaccines

An Overview

Vaccines to regulate fertility differ from traditional ones in several important aspects. Contraceptive vaccines prevent pregnancy rather than disease. They induce immune responses against internal self antigens, one's normal molecular constituents, rather than against external nonself antigens. (The exceptions to self in this context would be anti-sperm vaccines designated for women.) Because their immunological targets are self, they carry the potential for inducing disease, i.e., autoimmunity, rather than preventing it. Lastly, vaccines to regulate fertility are intended to induce a functionally reversible response rather than the irreversible memory generally induced by traditional vaccines.

Several different vaccines designed to control or regulate fertility are being developed (reviewed in Ada et al. 1985; Griffin 1986; Naz & Menge 1990; Stevens 1986b, 1990a; Talwar & Raghupathy 1989). Some induce immune responses that affect gametes, i.e., sperm and ova (or eggs). Depending on the target antigen they could immobilize sperm, destroy sperm, or prevent union of sperm and egg at the egg's surface. Anti-gamete vaccines would control fertility by preventing fertilization.

Other vaccine candidates are the hormones that participate in reproductive processes. Two pituitary gonadotropins, follicle-stimulating hormone (FSH) and human lutenizing hormone (hLH), control development of gametes in women; FSH controls gamete development in men. Secretion of both hormones is regulated by gonadotropin-releasing hormone (GnRH), a small peptide synthesized in the brain by the hypothalamus. All three hormones transit via the bloodstream and so are vulnerable to interception by antibody molecules. Immunity to these hormones could prevent development of sperm and eggs. The most promising candidate, the hormone human chorionic gonadotropin (hCG), is first synthesized by the fertilized egg and ultimately by the placenta. hCG stimulates production of progesterone, a hormone necessary for implantation, and for establishment and maintenance of the early stages of pregnancy. The hCG vaccines could control fertility by antibody-mediated and/or by cell-mediated mechanisms (Stevens et al. 1981). In the former, antibodies would bind to hCG and neutralize its pregnancy-sustaining effect, resulting in resumption of an apparently normal menstrual cycle. If cell-mediated immunity were operative, cytotoxic T cells could destroy the cells that produce hCG. A combination of mechanisms is likely.

Sperm Vaccines

Sperm antigens are potential vaccine candidates because spermatozoa can accidentally induce antibody responses in both men and women and because deliberate immunization of male and female animals with sperm antigens reduces fertility (Naz 1988; Naz & Menge 1990; Talwar & Raghupathy 1989). Some sperm antigens, however, cross-react with brain and kidney tissues and with lymphocytes and red blood cells (Naz 1988). Clearly, only those antigens unique to sperm can be used to develop an anti-sperm contraceptive vaccine. A brief description of four sperm-specific candidate antigens follows.

The isozyme lactate dehydrogenase (LDH-C_4) is one of the best characterized sperm-specific antigens. In a 1986 study, female mice, rabbits and baboons immunized with this antigen had fewer pregnancies than did control animals (Goldberg & Shelton 1986); in a later study of female mice, fertility was unaffected (Mahi-Brown et al. 1990). Male mice immunized with LDH-C_4 produced sperm with an impaired ability to penetrate mature eggs in vivo; unfortunately, the animals also developed orchitis, an inflammation and cellular infiltration of the testes (Mahi-Brown et al. 1990).

A second antigen, the human sperm protein SP-10, has been designated a primary vaccine candidate by a WHO Task Force on Contraceptive Vaccines (Anderson et al. 1987). SP-10 is unique to the sperm head, and a monoclonal antibody against it inhibits human sperm penetration of hamster ova, a common test for sperm function. Baboons and macaques have a similar sperm antigen and may provide appropriate models for testing a vaccine (Herr et al. 1990).

A third candidate is the fertilization antigen FA-1 (Naz 1987; Naz et al. 1984; Naz & Menge 1990). FA-1 induces infertility in female rabbits, and antisera to FA-1 inhibit in vitro fertilization of mouse and hamster eggs. Because sera from some infertile men and women react with FA-1, it has been implicated as an agent of involuntary infertility (Naz & Menge 1990).

The fourth possibility is PH-20, a surface protein on guinea pig sperm needed for sperm adhesion to mature ova. All male and female guinea pigs immunized with PH-20 became infertile but regained fertility when antibody titers waned, 6–15 months after immunization (Primakoff et al. 1988). Primakoff (1991) reported similar results in a later study, but also noted that all immunized males developed cell-mediated autoimmune orchitis.

Egg Vaccines

Most research has focused on antigens associated with the zona pellucida, the outer coating of the mature ovum (Caudle & Shivers 1989; Dunbar 1983, 1989; Sacco 1987; Sacco et al. 1989). Zona antigens induce infertility in various mammals; when tested in vitro, anti-zona antibodies inhibit sperm attachment to the zona pellucida. Immunization with egg antigens can also cause autoimmune damage to egg follicles, although pathology may depend on the agent used to enhance immunity (Dunbar et al. 1989). Results from mice immunized with a synthetic zona peptide antigen suggest that the use of a purified antigen and a highly immunogenic, nonself carrier are important factors in eliciting a reversible contraceptive response while avoiding ovarian damage (Millar et al. 1989).

Hormone Vaccines

By far the greatest effort toward development of contraceptive vaccines has been directed toward the placental hormone hCG (reviewed in Stevens 1986b, 1990a; Talwar & Raghupathy 1989). Because an antifertility vaccine against hCG will most likely be the first approved for family planning (Stevens 1990a), that research will be discussed in detail in the following sections.

Human Chorionic Gonadotropin Vaccines

An Overview

Chorionic gonadotropin is the one antigen that fulfills criteria for an ideal contraceptive vaccine. (1) It is present but transiently during reproductive processes. (2) Its biological function is understood, so questions of efficacy and safety are more easily answered. (3) Its antigenic determinants are defined, thereby enabling design of a vaccine whose response is restricted to the target antigen. (4) Its chemical characteristics are known, thus manufacture would be easy. (Points modified from Ada 1985.)

The native hormone hCG consists of two subunits, alpha and beta. Alpha is structurally similar to alpha subunits of the pituitary hormones. Beta likewise is similar to pituitary hormone beta subunits, especially to that of hLH. Were the intact hormone used as immunogen, it could induce cross- reactivity with all three pituitary hormones. When the entire beta subunit is used, it induces antibodies cross-reactive with hLH. Since a consequence of antibodies binding to antigen is removal of that antigen from the system, cross-reactivity could alter pituitary hormone levels and disturb menstrual cycles and/or gamete formation. One end of beta hCG, however, has a 35 amino acid sequence (peptide region) that is not shared by hLH. The peptide provides beta hCG with antigenic determinants distinct from those of hLH, thereby eliminating cross-reactivity to pituitary hormones.

Two hCG vaccines exist, differing mostly in the molecules used as primary immunogen. One, the hCG beta subunit vaccine, utilizes the entire beta subunit. The second, the synthetic hCG peptide vaccine, uses a synthetic peptide of the 35 amino acid sequence unique to beta hCG. Both vaccines have been tested in several animal species for safety and efficacy. Both have undergone Phase I (safety) clinical trials in women in India and Australia.

Preclinical Animal Studies

Animal species as diverse as rabbits, rats, goats, and nonhuman primates have been immunized with the prototype vaccines and with their individual components (reviewed in Rao et al. 1988; Stevens 1986a–c; Talwar et al.

1988; Talwar & Raghupathy 1989). With one exception, no adverse effects were observed, even in animals given antigen more frequently and in higher doses than would be intended in human clinical trials. As experiments in nonhuman primates have the most relevance, only those studies are summarized.

In rhesus monkeys immunization with ovine LH-hCG beta subunit complex induced reversible infertility (Rao et al. 1988; Talwar et al. 1986). Antibody affinity was more important than titer; the higher the affinity, the more efficient the neutralization of the intact hormone. Female baboons immunized with synthetic hCG peptide vaccine developed protective immunity that also was affinity- and titer-dependent (Stevens 1986c; Stevens et al. 1981).

Tissues from immunized animals showed no autoimmune-induced pathology, although sera from some immunized animals did react with tissues from non-immunized animals (Burek et al. 1986). The reactivity may not reflect autoimmunity; healthy individuals often have low levels of autoantibodies (Burek et al. 1986; Sinha et al. 1990; Thau et al. 1987).

The only documented instance of adverse effects occurred with female marmoset monkeys given the beta subunit vaccine (reviewed in Thanavala et al. 1979). The marmosets developed contraceptive antibody titers lasting for up to a year in some animals. If, however, the affinity of antibodies decreased (rather than increased) as the titer declined, some animals became pregnant then suffered miscarriages. (In no studies have immunized baboons and rhesus monkeys had miscarriages after titers declined and pregnancy was established (Stevens 1986c, 1990b; Talwar et al. 1986).) The marmosets were immunized with human chorionic gonadotropin, however, and cross-reactivity to marmoset CG (or other hormones) may have been responsible.

Given that chorionic gonadotropin acts early in pregnancy, it is unlikely that antibodies to hCG would disrupt a late-stage pregnancy. Indeed, pregnant marmosets given anti-hCG antibodies late (after week 12 of a 20-week gestation period) were unaffected (Hearn et al. 1975). Obviously, the possibility of recurring miscarriage after immunization would make hCG vaccines unacceptable. Although researchers do not expect the situation to arise during clinical trials, all fertile volunteers would be advised of the possibility and be closely monitored (Stevens 1990b).

The hCG Vaccines and Human Clinical Trials

hCG Beta Subunit Vaccine: Phase I Trials in India

Under the auspices of the International Committee for Contraceptive Research, the Population Council, and the Indian National Institute of Immunology, G.P. Talwar and colleagues designed and tested three formulations, A, B, and M, of an hCG beta subunit vaccine (Singh et al. 1989; Talwar et al. 1988, 1990; Talwar & Raghupathy 1989). In all three, hCG is physically joined either to tetanus toxoid or to cholera toxin chain B, bacterial antigens that are excellent carriers for self antigens. Tetanus toxoid is the preferred carrier, but some individuals are allergic to it and some respond poorly. The simplest formulation is B, whose sole immunogen relevant to contraception is beta hCG. Formulation A contains alpha oLH, which binds with beta hCG, forming a complex similar to native hCG and therefore considered a superior antigen. Formulation M is a mixture of beta oLH and beta hCG, each linked to the same carrier. Clinical trials were approved by the Drug Controller of India and the Institutional Ethics Committee and were conducted in five institutions across India (Singh et al. 1989; Talwar et al. 1990).

One hundred and one women gave written consent and participated in the safety trials. Volunteers were 25–35 years old and had previously undergone tubal ligation. After baseline clinical chemistry and hematology values were established, the women received three injections at monthly intervals and a fourth injection 6 to 8 months after the first. Each formulation was tested at two doses, with 14–15 women per group; the 13 women in the control group received only the vaccine vehicle (an oil emulsion). Blood was drawn monthly for antibody analysis and clinical exams were given at 4- to 6-week intervals. The major trial period encompassed 52 weeks.

By 6 to 8 weeks after primary immunization all women had developed high-affinity anti-hCG antibody with titers above the threshold level calculated as necessary to interrupt pregnancy. Generally, the higher vaccine dose induced longer-lasting responses. For formulation M (beta-oLH-beta-hCG) the above-threshold titers only lasted 17 to 20 weeks. Formulation A induced protective titers with a mean duration of 35 to 37 weeks, whereas both doses of B elicited protective titers lasting 34 weeks. A year after initial immunization titers were below threshold in 62 of the 88 women from the experimental groups, "suggesting the reversibility of the antibody response" (Singh et al. 1989, 741). Within the next 2 to 12 months titers in the other 26 women had dropped below this level.

All women who received vaccines developed antibodies that cross-reacted with LH but did not significantly alter menstrual regularity (Kharat et al. 1990). This cross-reactivity with LH is considered desirable, providing an additional factor to control fertility (Talwar et al. 1986).

Most women reported no side effects after the first injection. However, 25 women (28 percent) from the experimental groups reported "minor complaints such as erythema, pain at site of injection, fever, oedema, generalized rash, transient joint pain, nausea, muscle pain and giddiness" (Talwar et al. 1990, 305). Three women (23 percent) in the control group reported weakness, fever, and pain at the injection site. Of the 101 women in the study, 49 reported at least one side effect after injections; 18 did so more than once. Prior to the last immunization, 11 women became allergic to tetanus toxoid. Their final injection was therefore given either without the carrier or with antigens linked to cholera toxin.

The authors conclude that none of the hCG beta subunit formulations elicit adverse effects and that A and B induce reversible, protective responses, "thus further work can be undertaken to study the efficacy of these vaccines in humans for preventing pregnancy" (Talwar et al. 1990, 302).

Synthetic hCG Peptide Vaccine: Phase I Trial in Australia

Vernon C. Stevens designed the peptide vaccine (reviewed in Stevens 1986c; Stevens et al. 1981) and with his colleagues developed it under the auspices of the WHO (Griffin 1986; Jones 1986; Jones et al. 1988; Stevens 1986a, 1990a). Because the peptide carries the antigenic "signature" unique to beta hCG, it avoids the risk of autoimmune-induced hormonal imbalance and menstrual cycle disturbance that is possible with the beta subunit vaccine. The peptide is linked to diphtheria toxoid, a bacterial antigen that induces fewer allergic reactions than does tetanus toxoid (Stevens 1986a). The vaccine was approved for use in Phase I clinical trials by the Australian Department of Health and the United States Food and Drug Administration. The WHO and the Clinical Investigation and Drug and Therapeutics Committees of the Flinders Medical Centre in Adelaide gave ethical approval (Jones 1986).

Thirty women gave written, informed consent to participate in the study (Jones 1986; Jones et al. 1988). They were 26–43 years old and had earlier elected surgical sterilization for personal reasons; prior to entering the trial they were given thorough medical exams. The vaccine was tested at five dosages, with the lowest dose at 1/20 of the highest (full) dose. Four women in each dosage group received vaccine; two per group received only the emulsion vehicle and were controls. The second injection was given 6 weeks after the first. The study lasted 9 months, a 3 month preinjection interval and a 6 month period following the first injection. Clinical assessment and laboratory tests were done at various intervals, and the women were hospitalized for 48 hours observation after each injection.

By the sixth week after initial immunization all women had developed the level of anti-hCG antibody Jones and his colleagues had calculated as necessary to interrupt pregnancy (Jones et al. 1988). Those who received the highest antigen dose had adequate titers by the fifth week. Contraceptive titers persisted for 12 to 24 weeks in women given the two highest doses; in two women immunized with the highest dose, titers persisted for 9 to 10 months. No women developed antibodies cross-reactive with LH or FSH.

None of the women experienced serious side effects. Several had mild and transient muscle pain; two reported itching and redness at the injection site. Only one woman (4 percent of the vaccine group) became allergic to diphtheria toxoid; she was replaced with another volunteer. Of the 30 women, 25 had unaltered menstrual patterns; 1 woman from the control group had early menopause. Three vaccine recipients had intermenstrual spotting; one had an abnormally heavy flow.

The authors state that the synthetic hCG peptide vaccine "gives promise of being an acceptable means of birth control in that the target antigen is present transiently . . ., the immune response appears specific . . ., and the effect is potentially reversible" (Jones et al. 1988, 1298). They conclude that immunosafety studies in baboons (Burek et al. 1986; Stevens et al. 1981) and this clinical trial provide sufficient evidence of safety to proceed to efficacy studies, i.e., Phase II clinical trials.

Discussion

Gamete Vaccines

Because some infertile men and women have anti-sperm antibodies, researchers have assumed that sperm-specific proteins would be excellent antigens for contraceptive vaccines. Given the results of two studies published in 1989, however, the presumed efficacy of sperm vaccines might be pondered with the proverbial grain of salt. In one study both men and women, fertile or infertile, had similar frequencies of anti-sperm antibodies (J.K. Critser et al. 1989), and the authors questioned whether the antibodies were clinically significant. Moreover, after a prospective study of 235 couples with long-standing infertility (median five years), Eggert-Kruse and coworkers (1989) concluded that the presence of anti-sperm antibodies in infertile men or women did not affect fertility prognosis.

In theory, sperm vaccines could be given to men as well as to women. Unfortunately, the high probability of inducing autoimmune orchitis with attendant testicular damage makes it unlikely these vaccines can be used as male contraceptives. As for women, they would not develop autoimmunity, but some might develop permanent immunity from antigen "boosting" as a consequence of intercourse. Relevant to this concern are reports that some women undergoing intraperitoneal insemination as therapy for infertility developed anti-sperm antibodies (E.S. Critser et al. 1990; Livi et al. 1990). Lastly, to design sperm vaccines for use in women would incur yet another instance of what Mary Brown Parlee describes as "women being the primary targets of the technologies and [experiencing] at first hand the broad range of the effects of their use" (Parlee 1986, 34).

Zona pellucida vaccines also have an uncertain future. No one agrees on the incidence or significance of anti-zona antibodies in women who are involuntarily infertile (Caudle & Shivers 1989; Dunbar 1989). Indeed, some infertile women who tested positive for anti-zona antibodies became pregnant after being treated for other fertility problems such as endometriosis (Caudle & Shivers 1989). Another major obstacle to zona pellucida vaccines lies in the potential for eradicating all of a woman's eggs, despite careful selection of agents to enhance immunity and use of purified antigens.

Chorionic Gonadotropin Vaccines

Most likely hCG vaccines will undergo further clinical trials in women in the near future and merit considerable discussion. The section on promises is short, in part because they are considered at great length in the primary literature and in part because Jones (1986) has succinctly and ably summarized them. To evaluate the promises, it is important to understand the problems, which are biological as well as social/cultural in nature. This detailed discussion of problems and some possible solutions is intended to enlighten and to provide some balance to the many scientific discourses on contraceptive vaccines.

The Promises

Researchers generally agree that hCG vaccines hold the promises of being safer than oral contraceptives and IUDs, and of providing relatively long-lasting but reversible protection with a minimum of effort by both providers and users. Vaccines are considered especially attractive for use in developing nations, which lack a solid and extensive medical infrastructure and which are under severe social and economic pressures generated in part by rapidly increasing populations. Warren Jones, who headed the WHO clinical trial, cites the following advantages of contraceptive vaccines:

> (1) The use of a non-pharmacologically active agent. (2) Ease and convenience of administration making it suitable for distribution by paramedical personnel. (3) Long-lasting (12 months) but potentially reversible effect. (4) Acceptability of the "vaccine" principle—of particular importance in developing countries. (5) Reduced patient failure, since protection is not dependent on constant positive action by the recipient.

(6) Large-scale synthesis and manufacture of a vaccine at low cost (Jones 1986, 184).

The Problems

Writing from the user's perspective, Anita Hardon of the WEMOS/HAI Women and Pharmaceuticals Group defined several problems with hCG vaccines (Hardon 1989). These include (a) the difficulty of "switching off" the immune response; (b) the unknown consequences if a woman is pregnant when given the vaccine, or becomes pregnant after immunization; (c) the need for a blood test to determine whether a woman still has a protective titer; (d) the need for additional protection during the immunological lag period; (e) the possibility of inducing cross-reactivity to other hormones; (f) the short period of effectiveness; and (g) the shortage of adequate health care settings in most Third World countries. To these I would add (h) the probability of allergic responses to the carrier proteins and (i) the potential for coercive abuse by population control programs. I have integrated Hardon's concerns with mine and those of some scientists. They are expressed in a series of comments and caveats directed toward the advantages enumerated by Jones (1986). Some will be dealt with individually, others together because they are related.

Point (1). Contraceptive vaccines *are* pharmacologically inactive compared to oral contraceptives and implants. Although the antigen used in the vaccines is a portion of hCG, it is not biologically active in the same way as the native, intact hormone. Rather, it induces an immune response that alters the levels of native hCG. Perhaps more important to safety are the differences in the two types of vaccines tested in the Phase I clinical trials. Only the synthetic hCG peptide vaccine used in Australia induces responses that do not cross-react with pituitary hormones. The hCG beta subunit vaccine tested in India was designed to induce responses to hLH as well as to hCG. Immunization with this vaccine results in interference not only with the hormone necessary to maintain pregnancy but also with lutenizing hormone, necessary for a normal menstrual cycle. Many of our hormones work within interactive loops, and immunologically induced modulation of hormone levels could ultimately disrupt several organ systems.

A related concern is auto-induced tissue damage. Although results from long-term studies (4.5–7.7 years) in monkeys (Thau et al. 1987) and from the trials in India (Talwar et al. 1990) indicate that cross-reactivity to LH is not harmful, some researchers have stressed the need to carefully monitor women for evidence of autoimmunity (Stevens 1986b). Health care systems in most countries are stretched thin. Aside from clinical trials it is unlikely that immunized women and men would be as closely monitored as were the experimental animals, and serious side effects could go undetected and unchecked. Because women have a greater predilection to develop autoimmune disease than do men (Sinha et al. 1990), the synthetic peptide vaccine is the safer one.

An additional safety problem arises from the three bacterial antigens used as carriers. Although protection against tetanus, cholera, and diphtheria is considered a positive side benefit, women can become allergic to any of the carriers. If the individual is safely to be given the vaccine, vaccination and booster injections must be preceded *each time* by tests for allergic reaction to the carrier molecule. Tests for hypersensitivity, or allergies, generally require a 48–hour waiting period, thus adding another complication to vaccine use. That complication is necessary: although most allergic responses simply cause discomfort, in rare instances they can be fatal.

Points (2), (4), and (5). These involve personal control. Because vaccines must be administered by medical personnel, women can be denied a major element of control over whether and when to regulate their own fertility. "Reduced patient failure" achieved by removing a woman's responsibility for birth control may be advantageous to doctors and population control councils, but its advantage to women is not an automatic corollary. Thus far, once a woman is vaccinated, she cannot, with any effect, change her mind about contraception until the response has run its course. There is hope that further research will eliminate this problem. Preliminary studies in rabbits indicate that injection of hCG peptides (not the vaccine) will neutralize antibodies without boosting the response, and this method may be useful in the future to reverse the contraceptive effect (Stevens 1990b).

The "acceptability of the 'vaccine' principle" in developing nations could be considered a danger to women rather than an advantage. The widespread use of vaccines to prevent infectious disease opens the door for abuse and direct or indirect coercion by the state. Contraceptive vaccines could be given without consent, informed or otherwise. In Bangladesh women have been forced to use contraceptives (Akhter 1988; Hartmann 1987). Recent reports from Indonesia document sterilization abuse of men (Hull 1991) and coercive use of Norplant with subsequent refusal to remove the implant (Ward et al. 1990). Hartmann and Fried (1991) point out that coercion is not only a problem in the Third World: a California judge proposed Norplant use for three years as a condition of probation for a woman convicted of child abuse. Policies of coercion exist in the world, and are unlikely to disappear.

Point (3). There are actually three issues here, the first being duration of protective immunity. The effect is not yet long-lasting and the 12–month duration of contraceptive antibody levels pertains to a "best case scenario."

Since immunological responses vary among individuals, the protective titer and its duration cannot be known with certainty for any woman. In neither clinical trial did mean protective levels persist for more than 37 weeks; a safe, conservative estimate of effectiveness lies closer to 20 weeks. Results from rabbit experiments, however, indicate the duration may be increased by giving vaccine in a slow-release, biodegradable delivery system (Stevens et al. 1990). The slow release of antigen helps induce high-affinity antibodies, which may be more important than high titer for immunocontraception.

The second issue involves the need to recognize the time span of protective immunity. The response requires five to six weeks to reach a protective level, so women must rely on an alternate method of contraception until that level is reached. A more serious problem lies in the absence of overt physiological signals to let women know when their immunity "runs out". As the response wanes, they must have blood drawn and tests run to determine whether their antibody levels are sufficiently low to risk unwanted pregnancy or to attempt a desired one. Kits currently being developed to determine antibody levels with just a drop of blood from a finger-prick sample could alleviate this problem (Griffin 1990; Stevens 1990b). But without adequate distribution, rural and poor women may need to return to the clinics for blood tests. If so, how will they get to the clinics? How long must they wait for results? Who will pay for the tests? An added concern is that regardless of method of drawing blood, the dangers of AIDS transmission are always high if stringent safety rules concerning reuse of lancets and needles are not followed.

The final comment directed to point (3) is the unresolved question of reversibility. The evidence for reversibility comes from an earlier efficacy trial with six women (Talwar et al. 1976) and from extensive animal studies in which nonhuman primates immunized with contraceptive vaccines became pregnant after antibody titers waned to low levels (Stevens 1986c; Stevens et al. 1981; Talwar et al. 1979). With regard to the clinical trials in women, Talwar and his colleagues state that the *response* to beta hCG vaccine is reversible, citing as evidence the decline of antibody levels to that below the calculated protective titer (Talwar et al. 1990). Stevens and his colleagues are both accurate and conservative, stating only that the *effect* is "potentially reversible" (Jones et al. 1988, 1298).

The issue is not one of semantics, for immune *response* and contraceptive *effect* are distinct though related aspects of contraceptive vaccines. Without periodic antigenic stimulus, every immune response will decline. At best, with contraceptive vaccines only the effect, not the response, is reversible. Yet, resolving this question is crucial, for, as Stevens insists: "From an ethical view, it is imperative that a fertile woman receiving this treatment for birth control be informed that she is using either a reversible or an irreversible antifertility method" (1986b, 373).

Concerning reversibility, it is unlikely that hCG synthesized during pregnancy would act as a "booster." Immunological specificity involves not only exquisitely specific antigen-antibody interactions but also the requirement by memory cells that they be boosted with the *original* antigen complex in order to respond. The evidence that hCG synthesized during the early stages of pregnancy does not stimulate the immune-reactive cells that responded to the hCG antigens in the vaccines (Ramakrishnan et al. 1976; Stevens 1990b; Talwar et al. 1976) is central to the concept of reversibility .

The above comments and caveats are directed specifically toward the advantages cited by Jones. The following comment pertains to questions that *must* be answered before the vaccines can be used beyond the closely monitored clinical trials. As Stevens carefully pointed out (1986b), one ethical issue is whether the vaccine will cause deleterious effects in children born of mothers who were immunized before they knew they were pregnant, or who had low-level immunity, or who lost protective immunity prior to a booster shot. If immunization under those conditions affects an embryo or fetus, and if they are manifest on a time scale similar to those caused by diethylstilbestrol (DES) (Brown 1984), then only when those children reach puberty will the consequences be known.

The problems cited above require serious consideration and thoughtful resolution. Paul David Griffin, scientist with the WHO program responsible for development and testing of the peptide vaccine, wrote a thoughtful reply to Hardon's 1989 article. He attested to the developers' enthusiasm and optimism for the vaccine's future "if the ongoing animal studies and clinical trials prove satisfactory" (Griffin 1990, 6). He gave strong assurances that the WHO would halt testing and further development of the peptide vaccine should serious side effects occur during expanded safety and efficacy trials, and cited ongoing research aimed at answering the expressed concerns. Griffin also expressed support for the continued participation of women's organizations and consumer groups in WHO-sponsored meetings to assess vaccine safety and efficacy.

Conclusion

Immunocontraception, i.e., the deployment of one's own immune system to regulate fertility, may well provide a safe and effective means of fertility regulation and expand the range of choices for contraception. In their present stage vaccines against sperm and eggs are too dangerous for use in humans, and may never be reliably effective. Vaccines against chorionic gonadotropin hold great promises—those of safety, ease of use, noninvasiveness, and reversibility; they also carry considerable risks—those of allergy, autoimmunity, irreversibility, and teratology, especially for women who lack access to basic health care. Nonetheless, the biological problems can most likely be resolved to nearly everyone's satisfaction. More research with nonhuman primate models will help solve some of the problems; use of vaccines only in areas with a solid infrastructure to provide medical care will prevent others.

Women of all nations need access to a variety of safe and effective contraceptives. Yet the realities of their choices are determined mostly by the political, cultural, and economic environments that surround them. Therefore, I direct the strongest caveat about antifertility vaccines toward the enormous potential for political coercion and abuse. Inherent in most methods of birth control are elements and undercurrents of racism and sexism, power and prestige, risk and safety, and informed consent. Those who wield power and influence must challenge assumptions, fight abuse, and promote knowledge. Women as well as men, whether as direct or indirect consumers of reproductive technology, or as educators and policy makers, need to understand its physiological and technological aspects. Without that, effective challenge is difficult, informed consent is meaningless.

Acknowledgments

I wish to thank Betsy Hartmann, Vernon Stevens, Robert Woodland, and Richard White for critical reading, constructive criticism, and encouragement.

References

Ada, Gordon R., Anthony Basten, and Warren R. Jones. 1985. Prospects for developing vaccines to control fertility. *Nature* 317:288–289.

Akhter, Farida. 1988. The state of contraceptive technology in Bangladesh. *Reproductive and Genetic Engineering* 1:153–158.

Anderson, D.J., P.M. Johnson, N.J. Alexander, et al. 1987. Monoclonal antibodies to human trophoblast and sperm antigens: Report of two WHO-sponsored workshops, June 30, 1986, Toronto, Canada. *Journal of Reproductive Immunology* 10:231–257.

Bell, Susan. 1984. Birth control. In *The new our bodies, ourselves*, ed. Boston Women's Health Book Collective, 220–262. New York: Simon & Schuster.

Beverley, Peter. 1990. Human T-cell memory. *Current Topics in Microbiology and Immunology* 159:111–122.

Brown, Kris. 1984. Some common and uncommon health and medical problems: DES. In *The new our bodies, ourselves,* ed. Boston Women's Health Book Collective, 496–500. New York: Simon & Schuster.

Burek, C. Lynne, Julian Smith, and Noel R. Rose. 1986. Immunosafety studies with the WHO hCG vaccines. In *Reproductive immunology 1986*, ed. D.A. Clark and B.A. Croy, 170–177. Amsterdam: Elsevier Science (Biomedical Division).

Burnet, F. Macfarlane. 1959. *The clonal selection theory of acquired immunity.* London: Cambridge University Press.

Caudle, Michael R., and C. Alex Shivers. 1989. Current status of anti-zona pellucida antibodies. *American Journal of Reproductive Immunology* 21:57–60.

Critser, E.S., P.M. Villines, M. Gentry, et al. 1990. Sperm antibodies after intraperitoneal insemination of sperm: A preliminary report. *American Journal of Reproductive Immunology* 21:143–146.

Critser, J.K., P.M. Villines, C.B. Coulam, and E.S. Critser. 1989. Evaluation of circulating anti-sperm antibodies in fertile and patient populations. *American Journal of Reproductive Immunology* 21:137–142.

Dunbar, Bonnie S. 1983. Antibodies to zona pellucida antigens and their role in infertility. In *Immunology of reproduction*, ed. T.G. Wegmann and T.J. Gill, 507–534. New York: Oxford University Press.

Dunbar, Bonnie S. 1989. Ovarian antigens and infertility. *American Journal of Reproductive Immunology* 21:28–31.

Dunbar, Bonnie S., C. Lo, John Powell, and Vernon C. Stevens. 1989. Use of a synthetic peptide adjuvant for the immunization of baboons with denatured and deglycosylated pig zona pellucida glycoproteins. *Fertility and Sterility* 52:311–318.

Eggert-Kruse, W., M. Christmann, I. Gerhard, et al. 1989. Circulating anti- sperm antibodies and fertility prognosis: A prospective study. *Human Reproduction* 4:513–520.

Goldberg, Erwin, and J.A. Shelton. 1986. Immunosuppression of fertility by LDH-C_4. In *Immunological approaches to contraception and promotion of fertility*, ed. G.P. Talwar, 219–230. New York: Plenum Press.

Goodnow, Christopher, Stephen Adelstein, and Anthony Basten. 1990. The need for central and peripheral tolerance in the B cell repertoire. *Science* 248:1373–1379.

Griffin, Paul David. 1986. The WHO Special Programme of Research, Development and Research Training in Human Reproduction and its Task Force on Vaccines for Fertility Regulation. In *Reproductive immunology 1986*, ed. D.A. Clark and B.A. Croy, 154–161. Amsterdam: Elsevier Science (Biomedical Division).

Griffin, Paul David. 1990. Letter to the Editor. *Women's Global Network for Reproductive Rights Newsletter* 32:6–7.

Hardon, Anita. 1989. An analysis of research on new contraceptive HCG vaccines. *Women's Global Network for Reproductive Rights Newsletter* 29:15–16.

Hartmann, Betsy. 1987. *Reproductive rights and wrongs. The global politics of population control and contraceptive choice.* New York: Harper & Row.

Hartmann, Betsy, and Marlene Gerber Fried. 1991. Norplant: Notes of caution on new contraceptive. Letter to the Editor. *Boston Globe* 14 Jan.:10.

Hearn, John P., R.V. Short, and S.F. Lunn. 1975. The effects of immunising marmoset monkeys against the beta subunit of HCG. In *Physiological consequences of immunity against hormones*, ed. R.G. Edwards and M.F. Johnson, 229–247. Cambridge: Cambridge University Press.

Herr, John C., Richard M. Wright, Edward John, et al. 1990. Identification of human acrosomal antigen SP-10 in primates and pigs. *Biology of Reproduction* 42:377–382.

Hull, Terrence H. 1991. Reports of coercion in the Indonesian vasectomy program: A report to AIDAR. Department of Political and Social Change, Australian National University, Canberra. February 21, 1991.

Jones, Warren R. 1986. Phase I clinical trial of an anti-hCG contraceptive vaccine. In *Reproductive immunology 1986*, ed. D.A. Clark and B.A. Croy, 184–187. Amsterdam: Elsevier Science (Biomedical Division).

Jones, Warren R., S.J. Judd, R.M.Y. Ing, et al. 1988. Phase I clinical trial of a World Health Organisation birth control vaccine. *Lancet* 1:1295–1298.

Kharat, I., N.S. Nair, K. Dhall, et al. 1990. Analysis of menstrual records of women immunized with anti-hCG vaccines inducing antibodies partially cross-reactive with hLH. *Contraception* 41:293–299.

Klinman, Norman R., and P.J. Linton. 1990. The generation of B-cell memory: A working hypothesis. *Current Topics in Microbiology and Immunology* 159:19–35.

Lee, Nancy C., Herbert B. Peterson, and Susan Y. Chu. 1989. Health effects of contraception. In *Contraceptive use and controlled fertility. Health issues for women and children*, ed. Allan M. Parnell, 48–95. Washington, D.C.: National Academy Press.

Livi, Claudia, Elisabetta Coccia, Laura Versari, et al. 1990. Does intraperitoneal insemination in the absence of prior sensitization carry with it a risk of subsequent immunity to sperm? *Fertility and Sterility* 53:137–142.

Mahi-Brown, Cherrie A., Catherine Vandevoort, Ryan P. McGuinness, et al. 1990. Immunization of male but not female mice with the sperm-specific isozyme of lactate dehydrogenase (LDH-C_4) impairs fertilization in vivo. *American Journal of Reproductive Immunology* 24:1–8.

Mathur, Subbi, Mark R. Neff, H. Oliver Williamson, et al. 1987. Sperm antibodies and human leukocyte antigens in couples with early spontaneous abortions. *International Journal of Fertility* 32:59–65.

Menge, Alan C. 1980. Clinical immunologic infertility, diagnostic measures, incidence of antisperm antibodies, fertility and mechanisms. In *Immunological aspects of infertility and fertility regulation*, ed. D. Dhindsa and G.B. Schumacher, 205–224. Amsterdam: Elsevier/North-Holland.

Millar, Sarah E., Steven M. Chamow, Anne W. Baur, et al. 1989. Vaccination with a synthetic zona pellucida peptide produces long-term contraception in female mice. *Science* 246:935–938.

Naz, Rajesh. 1987. The fertilization antigen (FA-1) causes reduction of fertility in actively immunized female rabbits. *Journal of Reproductive Immunology* 11:117–133.

Naz, Rajesh. 1988. The fertilization antigen: Applications in immunocontraception and infertility in humans. *American Journal of Reproductive Immunology and Microbiology* 16:21–27.

Naz, Rajesh, Nancy J. Alexander, Mohamed Isahakia, and Marilyn S. Hamilton. 1984. Monoclonal antibody to a human germ cell membrane glycoprotein that inhibits fertilization. *Science* 225:342–344.

Naz, Rajesh, and Alan Menge. 1990. Development of antisperm contraceptive vaccine for humans: Why and how? *Human Reproduction* 5:511–518.

Parlee, Mary Brown. 1986. Women and reproductive technologies. *Frontiers* 9:32–35.

Primakoff, Paul. 1991. Sperm surface proteins as antigens for a birth control vaccine that blocks sperm function. Paper presented at the Annual Meeting of the American Association for the Advancement of Science, Washington, D.C. 14–19 February.

Primakoff, Paul, William Lathrop, Laura Woolman, et al. 1988. Fully effective contraception in male and female guinea pigs immunized with the sperm protein PH-20. *Nature* 335:543–546.

Ramakrishnan, S., S.K. Dubey, C. Das, et al. 1976. Influence of HCG and tetanus toxoid injections on the antibody titers in a subject immunized with Pr-Beta- HCG-TT. *Contraception* 13:245–251.

Ramsdell, Fred, and B.J. Fowlkes. 1990. Clonal deletion versus clonal anergy: The role of the thymus in inducing self tolerance. *Science* 248:1342–1348.

Rao, L.V., Om Singh, and Gursaran P. Talwar. 1988. Immunological cross-reactivity of antibodies with species chorionic gonadotropin is a critical requirement for efficacy testing of human gonadotropin vaccines in sub-human primates. *Journal of Reproductive Immunology* 13:53–63.

Sacco, Anthony G. 1987. Zona pellucida: Current status as a candidate antigen for contraceptive vaccine development. *American Journal of Reproductive Immunology and Microbiology* 15:122–130.

Sacco, Anthony G., Edward C. Yurewicz, and Marappa G. Subramanian. 1989. Effect of varying dosages and adjuvants on antibody response in squirrel monkeys (*Saimiri sciureus*) immunized with the porcine zona pellucida M_r = 55,000 glycoprotein (ZP3). *American Journal of Reproductive Immunology* 21:1–8.

Singh, Om, L. Venkateswara Rao, Amitabh Gaur et al. 1989. Antibody response and characteristics of antibodies in women immunized with three contraceptive vaccines inducing antibodies against human chorionic gonadotropin. *Fertility and Sterility* 52:739–744.

Sinha Animesh, A., M. Theresa Lopez, and Hugh O. McDevitt. 1990. Autoimmune diseases: The failure of self-tolerance. *Science* 248:1380–1388.

Stevens, Vernon C. 1986a. An infertility vaccine. In *Progress towards better vaccines*, ed. Rosemary Bell and G. Torrigiani, 133–155. Oxford: Oxford University Press.

Stevens, Vernon C. 1986b. Current status of antifertility vaccines using gonadotropin immunogens. *Immunology Today* 7:369–374.

Stevens, Vernon C. 1986c. Development of a vaccine against human chorionic gonadotropin using a synthetic peptide as the immunogen. In *Reproductive immunology 1986*, ed. D.A. Clark and B.A. Croy, 162–169. Amsterdam: Elsevier Science (Biomedical Division).

Stevens, Vernon C. 1990a. Birth control vaccines and immunological approaches to the therapy of noninfectious diseases. *Infectious Disease Clinics of North America* 4:343–354.

Stevens, Vernon C. 1990b. Personal communication with the author.

Stevens, Vernon C., John E. Powell, Arthur C. Lee, and David Griffin. 1981. Antifertility effects of immunization of female baboons with c-terminal peptides of the beta- subunit of human chorionic gonadotropin. *Fertility and Sterility* 36:98–105.

Stevens, Vernon C., John E. Powell, Michael Rickey, et al. 1990. Studies of various delivery systems for a human chorionic gonadotropin vaccine. In *Gamete interaction: Prospects for immunocontraception*, ed. Nancy J. Alexander et al., 549–563. New York: Wiley-Liss.

Talwar, Gursaran P., C. Das, A. Tandon, et al. 1979. Immunization against hCG: Efficacy and teratological studies in baboons. In *Non-human primate models for study of human reproduction*, ed. T.C. Anand Kumar, 190–201. Basel: Karger Verlag.

Talwar, Gursaran P., V. Hingorani, Sneh Kumar, et al. 1990. Phase I clinical trials with three formulations of anti-human chorionic gonadotropin vaccine. *Contraception* 41:301–316.

Talwar, Gursaran P., and Raj Raghupathy. 1989. Anti-fertility vaccines. *Vaccine* 7:97–101.

Talwar, Gursaran P., N.C. Sharma, S.K. Dubey, et al. 1976. Isoimmunization against human chorionic gonadotropin with conjugates of processed beta subunit of the hormone and tetanus toxoid. *Proceedings of the National Academy of Sciences, USA* 73: 218–222.

Talwar, Gursaran P., Om Singh, A.K. Bamezai, et al. 1986. Potential of new technologies for development of fertility regulating vaccines. In *Reproductive immunology 1986*, ed. D.A. Clark and B.A. Croy, 178–183. Amsterdam: Elsevier Science (Biomedical Division).

Talwar, Gursaran P., Om Singh, and L. Venkateswara Rao. 1988. An improved immunogen for anti-human chorionic gonadotropin vaccine eliciting antibodies reactive with a conformation native to the hormone without cross-reaction with human follicle stimulating hormone and human thyroid stimulating hormone. *Journal of Reproductive Immunology* 14:203–212.

Temple, Robert. 1986. *The genius of China*. New York: Simon & Schuster.

Thanavala, Yasmin, John P. Hearn, Frank C. Hay, and Martin Hulme. 1979. Characterisation of the immunological response in marmoset monkeys immunized against hCG beta subunit and its relationship with their subsequent fertility. *Journal of Reproductive Immunology* 1:263–273.

Thau, Rosemarie B., C.B. Wilson, K. Sundaram, et al. 1987. Long-term immunization against the beta subunit of ovine lutenizing hormone (oLHβ) has no adverse effects on pituitary function in rhesus monkeys. *American Journal of Reproductive Immunology and Microbiology* 15:92–98.

United Nations. 1989. *Levels and trends of contraceptive use as assessed in 1988*. No. E.89.XIII.4. New York: United Nations.

Vessey, M.P. 1986. Benefits and risks of contraception. In *Reproduction in mammals. Book 5. Manipulating reproduction*, ed. C.R. Austin and R.V. Short, 121–147. Cambridge: Cambridge University Press.

Ward, Sheila J., Ieda Poernomo Sigit Sidi, Ruth Simmons, and George B. Simmons. 1990. Service delivery systems and quality of care in the implementation of Norplant in Indonesia. Report prepared for the Population Council, New York. February.

Zatuchni, Gerald. 1989. Advances in contraception. *Advances in Contraception* 5:193–196.

Chapter 4

FRONTIERS IN NONHORMONAL MALE CONTRACEPTIVE RESEARCH

Elaine A. Lissner

Introduction

We speak of a "contraceptive supermarket" for women—the concept that since no one method is right for everybody, a variety of methods should be available (Djerassi 1981). We argue that the pill's unsuitablity for older women does not mean it should be kept from younger women, that the diaphragm is right for some women despite its messiness and restriction of spontaneity, and that the sponge's relatively low effectiveness rate does not mean it should be taken off the shelf.

But when we think about contraceptive availability this way and what contraceptive supermarket is available to men, the answer is that only three purely male methods exist—withdrawal, the condom, and vasectomy. This contrasts with the list for women—the diaphragm, the sponge, IUDs, the pill, cervical caps, "morning after" pills, Norplant, natural methods, ovulation detectors, the female condom, foams, jellies, suppositories, sterilization, and more (Hatcher et al. 1988, Chap. 9). And when we consider that of the three male methods, withdrawal has low effectiveness, the condom faces psychological resistance, and vasectomy is not reliably reversible (Engelmann et al. 1990), the selection for men seems paltry indeed.

One common argument against providing a male contraceptive supermarket is that there is no expressed demand among the men of our society (Corea 1985, Chap. 9). However, similar statements could have been made 30 years ago about women and the pill. As seen with the introduction of the pill, the availability of a convenient method can create unprecedented demand. Besides, many men are *already* using male contraception in the form of vasectomy, both in the United States and elsewhere. Currently, male sterilization makes up 10 to 12 percent of the world's contraceptive use (and up to 16 percent in countries such as the United States and United Kingdom) (Hatcher et al. 1989; Pop. Crisis Comm. 1987). Clearly, demand can be high for even the far from ideal methods of today.

An additional reason to create a better male contraceptive supermarket is that doing so actually augments the choices available to women. Women in relationships with men have more contraceptive options when their partners can also take responsibility. With easy and safe male methods, their partners would have that option. This increased ability to control reproduction and space children can substantially improve women's and children's health, survival rates, and economic status (World Bank 1984, 87). Such ability may also help reduce the pressure to push unsuitable and unsafe contraceptives in the name of population stabilization.

If a male contraceptive supermarket is clearly a good thing, the difficult question is how to create one. Most researchers and funding sources believe that the only new male contraceptive on the horizon is the "male pill," which would take years to formulate and years to approve (Djerassi 1981, Chap. 5). Male hormonal contraceptives, moreover, have many of the same complex effects as female hormonal preparations. Therefore, since the prospects seem somewhat dim, little effort is being put into male contraception (Wilmore 1988).

However, there *are* other possibilities. They are not well known, and most people who know of them assume that they are not well researched. After more than 70 years of isolated pieces of research and related discoveries, the evidence, however, has begun to build.

This chapter will introduce these methods, describe some of their history, and present the current state of research. Many methods are surprisingly viable with only small difficulties remaining. In view of the enormous technological progress made by our society in the last few decades, these comparatively modest challenges should provoke interest and effort in the scientific community. These methods will be divided into two types: vas-based methods (no-scalpel vasectomy, chemical injection, injectable plugs, the Shug, and SMA) and heat methods (simple wet heat, artificial cryptorchidism, and ultrasound).

Vas-based Methods

Vas-based methods rely on cutting, blocking, or otherwise limiting fertility in the vas deferens, the passage through which sperm travel from the epididymis (where they mature) to the penis.

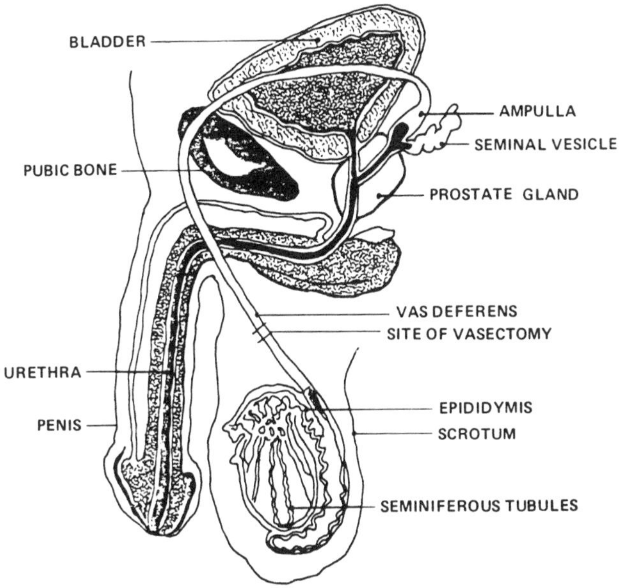

Figure 4–1
Male reproductive system, showing the site of vasectomy.

Vasectomy, currently the main vas-based method in use, is an important worldwide method of male contraception, as described earlier. Many researchers understand that improved vasectomy would have a huge market. Exactly *how* large is not known, although studies about tubal sterilization in women show that the availability of safe and sure reversal would double the percentage of women who consider sterilization and that a non-surgical procedure would add another 5 to 15 percent (Shain 1980). Clearly, the equivalent changes in men would have an enormous impact on worldwide contraceptive patterns.

Despite what seems to be a clear need for research on vas-based methods, very little work has been done since 1977 (Free 1978; Thomas 1988), a situation due partly to lack of funding, partly to technical difficulties, and partly to improved techniques of vasectomy reversal (Droegemueller 1978).

Vasovasostomy (vasectomy reversal), however, still results in pregnancy in only about 50 percent of the cases (Engelmann et al. 1990) and is a surgical procedure that requires skilled microsurgeons and thousands of dollars—clearly not a technique available to most men. Therefore, the need for simpler vas-based methods remains great.

Researchers have long dreamed of creating new vas-based methods. In the 1970s, a variety of elaborate metal valves were created, most of which either punctured the vas (due to their inflexibility) or insufficiently prevented sperm passage (Free 1978). Most of these methods (some of which had only minor problems) died for lack of funding or proponents. The past decade, however, has brought a new crop of advances. Although these advances may seem less flashy than the magnetic valves and biogalvanic cells of old, they show many times the promise for practical and immediate application.

An ideal male contraceptive method would have five characteristics in addition to the usual criteria of safety, efficacy, and convenience. It would be (1) easily reversible, (2) nonsurgical (Davis 1980; Zaneveld et al. 1978;); (3) reversible many times, as in the valve concept (Lynne & Politano 1978); (4) reversible nonsurgically (Misro et al. 1979); and lastly, (5) nonocclusive. Vas occlusion (such as in vasectomy) has been associated with antibodies to sperm and the formation of sperm granulomas (inflammatory reactions to sperm leakage from the reproductive tract into surrounding tissue). Granulomas and antibodies may make reversal more difficult (Herr et al. 1989; Urry et al. 1990).

Although only one of the following vas-based methods meets all of the criteria for an ideal male contraceptive, note that traditional vasectomy meets none of the five criteria. Therefore, each of these methods would be an improvement over vasectomy.

Advances in Reaching the Vas Deferens

Two new methods of accessing the vas deferens have been developed: no-scalpel vasectomy and percutaneous injection.

No-Scalpel Vasectomy

"The no-scalpel vasectomy technique is the way all vasectomies should be done. If a vasectomy can be accomplished with this minimal surgery, then any surgeon doing more surgery should justify why more is necessary." According to Dr. Douglas Huber, the former medical director of the Association for Voluntary Surgical Contraception, "These were the conclusions of one surgeon on the AVSC team of experts visiting [China] . . ." (Huber 1989, 217). No-scalpel vasectomy, originally developed in China, is gaining worldwide recognition. It is described by Huber:

> The Chinese have been using a refined method of vasectomy that eliminates the scalpel, results in fewer hematomas, and leaves a much smaller wound than conventional techniques used in other countries. The [no-scalpel vasectomy] has been performed for 4–8 million men in Sichuan Province since its introduction in 1974. After application of local anesthesia, a specially designed vas fixing forceps encircles and firmly secures the vas without penetrating the skin. A curved hemostat with sharpened points is used to puncture the skin and vas sheath and stretch a small opening in the scrotum. The vas is lifted out and occluded as in other vasectomy techniques. This same midline puncture site is used to deliver the other vas in an almost bloodless procedure. The first [no-scalpel vasectomy] training outside China took place in November 1986 in Bangkok. Through May 1987, approximately 1,500 [no-scalpel vasectomies] were performed in Thailand, Sri Lanka, Nepal, and the U.S. Each surgeon reported a significant reduction in bleeding from the wound. The client response is favorable, the elimination of the scalpel and the smaller wound apparently being important to men in these countries just as in China (Huber 1987, 176).

Although it is a new technique and requires training, no-scalpel vasectomy is ultimately faster and safer than traditional vasectomy (Nirapathpongporn et al. 1990). Because it is also "semisurgical," rather than "surgical," it results in fewer complications and is more to men's liking. These are important advantages for such a widely used method of contraception.

The no-scalpel technique can be either a way to access the vas deferens in order to sever it (vasectomy) or a way to access the vas deferens in order to limit fertility by other means, such as chemical injection, insertion of plugs, or injection of a temporary fertility-limiting agent. Discussed here as an aid to vasectomy, it should *immediately replace* the standard vasectomy procedure. Its use to access the vas for other fertility-limiting procedures is discussed later in this chapter.

Percutaneous Injection

While the no-scalpel technique is a semisurgical method of accessing the vas, percutaneous (through the skin) injection is completely nonsurgical. It is thus less threatening and less risky than even the no-scalpel method (Goldsmith et al. 1985b). This advantage, however, comes with a drawback: percutaneous injection is a delicate procedure, requires training and precision, and must be done exactly right.

In percutaneous injection, the vas deferens is first secured and kept from moving around under the scrotal skin by the placement of a gentle clamp, which encircles the section of vas and skin. Once the vas is secured, a puncture needle is inserted into the vas and then replaced by an injection needle.

Two tests are performed to make sure that the needle is correctly placed, and then the fertility-limiting substance is injected (Shunquiang & Jinbo 1986).

Although the procedure is delicate and the needle must be placed accurately, percutaneous injection becomes reasonably fast (about 10 minutes) with practice (Goldsmith et al. 1985b). The training is worthwhile, since percutaneous injection has the potential to be much more widely accepted than vasectomy in cultures with a taboo about or a fear of skin incisions. For example, over 512,000 percutaneous injections have been performed in China (Goldsmith et al. 1985a, b), the majority with sclerosing chemicals as the injectable. In the next section these chemicals (along with some alternatives) are discussed.

Advances in Fertility Limitation Inside the Vas

There are four new approaches to limiting fertility once inside the vas.

Chemical Injection

A number of substances can cause permanent sterilization by injection. Since 1964, researchers have tested at least 26 different combinations of chemicals (Davis 1980; Goldsmith et al. 1985a). The only two requirements for the chemical are that it be nontoxic and be a sclerosing agent (an agent that will produce enough scarring of the vas wall to block the vas).

The Chinese have performed chemical sterilization with a combination of carbolic acid and n-butyl alpha cyanoacrylate in over 500,000 men with satisfactory results (azoospermia in 96 percent of cases) (Goldsmith et al. 1985b) with, however, no data on safety. Two sets of American researchers have done similar experiments in men with different chemicals and reported satisfactory safety results, but they obtained azoospermia in only 7 of 8 and 17 of 21 cases, respectively (Goldsmith et al. 1985a, b). As the Chinese and Americans begin to collaborate, these discrepancies will presumably be resolved. So, although the research on permanent injection methods needs to be systematized and the most effective chemical needs to be determined, it appears that permanent chemical sterilization will be a fairly effective nonsurgical substitute for vasectomy.

Injectable Plugs

Injectable plugs are designed for one-time reversibility. They are ideal for men who believe they want permanent sterilization but would like the possibility of reversal in case of death of a child or some other unforeseen circumstance.

In China over 512,000 men have received injectable plugs. Such plugs involve the same procedure as chemical injection, except that instead of a sclerosing chemical, polyurethane or silicone is injected and hardens to form a plug.

Tests have shown a 98 percent effectiveness rate, and all the men who have had their plugs removed for at least a year have fathered children (Shunquiang & Jinbo 1986; Zhao 1990). Encouraged by these results, the World Health Organization started trials in 10 men in 1990 (Nullis 1991). Continued success will reportedly lead to a trial in 3500 men around the world (and availability in some parts of the world within two years).

Injectable plugs seem reliably *reversible* but, like chemical injection, slightly less *effective* than vasectomy (98 percent instead of 99 percent). This tradeoff will appeal to some men but not others. Injectable plugs should be made available around the world so individuals (and not policy makers) can decide what best meets their needs.

The Shug

The Shug (short for silicone plug) is a noninjectable plug alternative. Its only advantage over injectable plugs is its double design, which gives it the potential to be more leak-free. A double silicone plug connected by nylon suture in the middle, the Shug is inserted into the vas deferens using the no-scalpel method. Like injectable plugs, it results in reversible sterilization. Test monkeys have shown nearly full return of fertility after seven months of Shug use (Zaneveld et al. 1988). Arguably, however, this is not enough time for an immune reaction to sperm to develop. Since immune reactions tend to lower slightly the chances of reversibility, long-term testing is the next crucial step for Shug development.

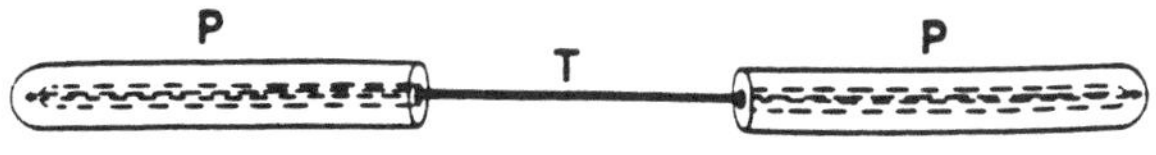

Figure 4–2
Schematic representation of the Shug. The plugs (*P*) are hollow except at the ends where the nylon thread (*T*) is bonded. Reprinted with permission from Zaneveld et al. 1988.

The Shug's double design means that any sperm that leak past the first plug are likely to stay in the space between the plugs rather than leak past the second plug. This important principle could be applied to injectable plugs; double injectable plugs would probably be more reliable than single ones.

The Shug has recently undergone clinical trials. After researchers found about a 97 percent decrease in motile sperm count in the men studied (Zaneveld 1990), they subsequently decided that a properly sized Shug would be two to

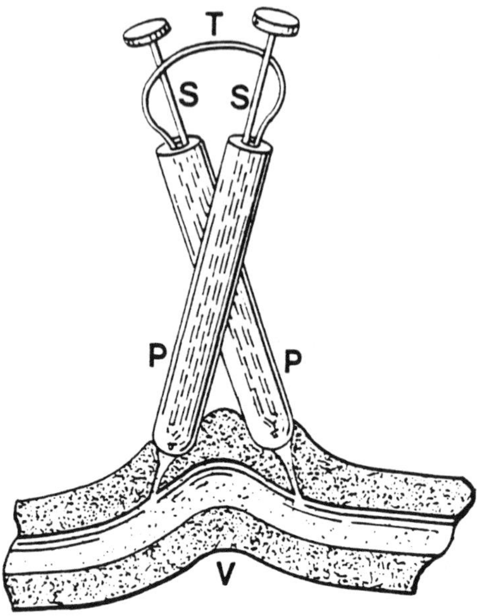

Figure 4–3
Implantation of the Shug. P, plug; T, connecting thread; S, metal stylus; V, vas deferens. Reprinted with permission from Zaneveld et al. 1988.

four times larger than the ones they used and are repeating the trials with larger devices. This change should make the Shug as effective in humans as it was in monkeys.

If test results remain positive, the Shug potentially could replace many standard vasectomies. In such a use, it could remain in place for a man's whole adult lifetime. Although the prospect of testing for safety for such long-term use may seem daunting, this problem, which incidentally applies to most contraceptive methods, can be circumvented. Initially, as was done with the pill, use of the method can be time-limited (Djerassi 1988). For example, a man can be told that the Shug has been tested for only 8 years and that it is approved for 3-year use. After 3 years, he will be told that he may safely use it for another 3 years. This approach can continue until the original volunteers find that, for example, the silicone begins to degrade after 40 years. The public could then be safely informed that this is a 35-year method. Men could have their old plugs removed, thus avoiding health danger.

Although the Shug's only advantage over no-scalpel vasectomy is increased reversibility, this is a big advantage which would be an attractive feature to many men. The Shug should be researched and perfected as soon as possible.

SMA

A temporary means of contraception to be used with either the percutaneous or no-scalpel technique, SMA uses the new polymer stryrene maleic anhydride. When injected into the vas deferens, this polymer lowers the pH of the vas deferens enough to kill sperm passing through. To achieve the initial effect, just enough SMA is injected to coat the vas, not block it. The polymer immediately attaches itself to the walls of the vas in a thin film and then kills the sperm passing by it instead of blocking all sperm passage. Because it kills passing sperm and does not block the vas, this method is not occlusive and keeps the vas in an essentially undamaged and natural state.

Fertility can be restored at any time. Since the polymer remains primarily whole, it can be flushed out at any time by an injection of dimethyl sulfoxide (DMSO), a bioacceptable solvent in the small quantities necessary (Rubin 1983). Thus fertility can be limited by one simple injection or restored by another (Misro et al. 1979). Alternatively, since the polymer itself dissolves very slowly in the process, fertility can be returned by just allowing the SMA to dissolve. Depending on the dosage administered, the time can be set anywhere from three months to five years (Guha et al. 1990). This method is thus ideal for child spacing.

SMA can be injected either percutaneously or by exposing the vas with the no-scalpel method. Thus the procedure can be semisurgical or completely nonsurgical, depending on the training of the physician.

This method has been completely safe and effective in more than 10 years of rat and monkey trials. From studies that tested SMA's length of action in monkeys, its reversibility in rats, its teratogenic potential in rabbits, and its toxicity in rats and monkeys, results show excellent effectiveness and reversibility and no toxicity or teratogenicity (potential to cause birth defects) (Guha et al. 1985, 1990; Misro et al. 1979; Sethi et al. 1989, 1990a,b,c).

The literature reports nothing negative or discouraging about this method. As described above, it meets the five criteria. If it continues to prove safe and pass long-term tests, it appears to be THE most promising vas method to date.

Heat Methods

The deleterious effect of heat on male fertility has been known since the time of Hippocrates (Adams 1939, 312). Much as aspirin was "discovered" in the 1800s from a bark that Native Americans had long been accustomed to chewing to relieve pain, heat methods are now being "discovered" as the newest method of male contraception.

These methods derive their effectiveness from the simple fact that the testes must be several degrees cooler than normal body temperature in order to maintain proper spermatogenesis (Fukui 1923; Rock & Robinson 1965). One biological advantage for this has been hypothesized. Since men with high fevers are infertile until they are well again (Kandeel & Swerdloff 1988), newborns will then be more likely to have healthy fathers, thus increasing infant survival rate.

The body conveniently provides cooling by enclosing the testes in the scrotum. The scrotum performs a twofold function by keeping the testes outside the body wall and by creating a heat exchange, much like the one in a modern refrigerator, between incoming and outgoing blood vessels (Kandeel & Swerdloff 1988). When this twofold function is impeded by the wearing of jockey shorts (as many advice columnists have warned their readers), by high environmental temperatures, or by one of the three methods presented here, fertility will be impaired.

All of the following contraceptive methods (with the exception of permanent ultrasound) are easily reversible, nonsurgical, reversible nonsurgically, reversible multiple times, and nonocclusive. Therefore, discussion will focus mainly on safety, efficacy and convenience, with an occasional note on psychological and economic factors.

Simple Wet Heat

Simple wet heat in the form of hot water, which is inexpensive and available to everyone, was the first contraceptive heat method discovered by the scientific community. In 1921, Dr. M. Voegli, after 10 years of experimentation with nine male volunteers, reported on this method. Although time-consuming, the method was perfectly effective and resulted in normal offspring after cessation (Corea 1985, Chap. 9).

Voegli's program for temporary sterilization is as follows: "A man sits in a [shallow or testes-only] bath of 116 degrees Fahrenheit for forty-five minutes daily for three weeks. Six months of sterility results, after which normal fertility returns. For longer sterility, the treatment is repeated" (Corea 1985, 179). Voegli, a Swiss doctor practicing in India, taught the method to Indian men during famines between 1930 and 1950. During that 20-year period the doctor reported no substantial adverse side effects (Segal 1962, 347).

The simple wet heat method in use today is not substantially different from what Voegli reported in 1921, although combinations of lower temperatures and more frequent treatment have also been studied. More research needs to be done in this area. For example, treatment at a lower temperature with a booster treatment every three weeks may be effective (Kandeel & Swerdloff

1988). Further research could identify the most efficient and comfortable combination.

Some might consider Voegli's method inconvenient. However, it lasts six months, is separate from the sex act, appears to be safe and effective, and is readily available to everybody. Challenges to its implementation are that (1) not enough research funds have been directed toward this "folk" method to accumulate the huge body of evidence of safety that is required of a "new" method and, more importantly, (2) since money can be made only from creative applications of the method (not from patenting the method itself), no large pharmaceutical firms will sponsor it (Segal 1988). Both of these problems could be solved by backing and research efforts by government and nonprofit agencies.

In 1949, Voegli began a 20-year campaign to publicize the heat method so that, if the results of further studies were favorable, the method could be widely used (Corea 1985, Chap. 9; Robinson et al. 1968). Her attempts to publicize it were generally unsuccessful, although in 1954 the Japanese government requested the information and conducted several successful experiments (Corea 1985, Chap. 9).

Artificial Cryptorchidism

In the United States, among the few who picked up Voegli's work were John Rock and Derek Robinson of Harvard University. Their work on the effect of insulated underwear (Robinson & Rock 1967) and hot water (Rock & Robinson 1965) on spermatogenesis forms the basis of a related new method of contraception: artificial cryptorchidism.

The idea of artificial cryptorchidism is simple. Researchers combined two pieces of information: (1) raising the temperature of the testes to body temperature (by using insulated underwear or hot water) results in subfertility (as found by Robinson, Rock, and others) and (2) men with cryptorchid (undescended) or retractile testes are often infertile (Nistal & Paniagua 1984). By putting these two facts together, the pioneers in this area concluded that the testes can be raised to body temperature with less trouble than with insulated underwear by simply maintaining the testes within the inguinal canal (the tube into which retractile testes withdraw) during the day (Mieusset et al. 1985).

Dr. Roger Mieusset of France, currently the chief proponent of artificial cryptorchidism, was the first to achieve effectiveness rates with artificial cryptorchidism that make it suitable for contraception (Mieusset et al. 1987). In Mieusset's method, a man wears an underbrief that holds the testes snug against the body but does not tightly enclose the penis. When some of the men in his study refined the retaining underwear by adding a circle of soft fabric to keep the testes from moving out of the inguinal canal, effectiveness rates shot up. Mieusset now uses this method in his research. The new method results in an average sperm count of 3 million/ml and average motility of 15 percent (Mieusset et al. 1991), as opposed to values with the old method of 12 million/ml and 22 to 30 percent (Mieusset et al. 1987). Since infertility is generally diagnosed as under 10 million/ml sperm count and 40 to 45 percent motility (Makler 1986), the desired result is clearly being achieved.

Artificial cryptorchidism meets the five criteria for an ideal male contraceptive. It also appears to be effective and relatively convenient. However, fertility return after long-term use has not been tested. This is the next crucial step. Short-term use (one to two years) appears to allow full return of fertility: the few tests in humans have all been favorable, as have tests of other heat methods in rats, dogs, and monkeys (Kandeel & Swerdloff 1988).

Many men fear that this method would cause "jock itch." However, Mieusset's volunteers showed no signs of jock itch. As for convenience, the only modification of habits required would be for men to wear slightly different underwear: jockey shorts with an inner layer for holding the testes (Mieusset et al. 1987). Since within the past ten years women have been convinced to wear both boxer shorts and jockey shorts, the task of creating this change seems within the capabilities of the advertising establishment!

Ultrasound

Considered on technical and practical merits alone, ultrasound is one of the most promising forms of new male contraception. It is technically simple and extremely convenient in that 15 minutes of ultrasound results in 6 months of sterility. However, as other researchers have shown (Wilmore 1988), the task of selling it to the public and convincing the public of its safety may be more difficult.

In ultrasound contraception, ultrasound waves (very short, inaudible sound waves) are used to heat the testes. To use the method, a man first sits in a special chair with his scrotum in a cup of water. In the bottom of the cup, shielded from the testes and scrotum, is an ultrasound element, which heats the water somewhat (not as hot as a hot tub) and also, it has recently been found, creates an ion transfer between the water and the testes that makes the environment in the testes inhospitable for sperm formation (Fahim et al. 1977). The method is painless. Some men even report the procedure to be pleasurable.

After 10 to 15 minutes of ultrasound, 6 months of infertility results. With two treatments 48 hours apart, 10 or more months of infertility will result

(Fahim 1980). As in all heat methods, fertility returns gradually once the infertile months are over, with a surge in fertility about 10 weeks later and then a gradual return to normal (Robinson & Rock 1967).

The most important priority for research is the question of whether, and how, fertility returns after multiple uses of the method (for example, after 5 to 15 years of use) (Kandeel & Swerdloff 1988). As was done with the pill trials, researchers should begin tests now so that longer and longer uses of ultrasound can gradually be approved (or not approved, as the case may be).

Once fertility returns after long-term use is shown, the remaining barrier for ultrasound will be psychological resistance. Although all the research so far on animals and humans has had excellent results, anything that sounds like radiation worries people, including those who determine funding (Wilmore 1988). And although ultrasound was tested as a treatment for herpes simplex in women (Corea 1985, Chap.9), has been used for years to view women's fetuses, and is even a regular part of chiropractic care for both sexes, fear and skepticism about male reproductive use prevail. Since a large and unequivocal body of information will be required to convince the public of the method's safety, the only way for ultrasound contraception to gain acceptance is for researchers, motivated by the overwhelmingly positive results so far, to put aside their skepticism and do the research.

Unfortunately, this is not happening. Apparently, the only researcher in the United States who has published on ultrasound contraception is Dr. Mostafa S. Fahim, director of the Center for Reproductive Science and Technology at the University of Missouri at Columbia. In a study of the comparative contraceptive effects of heat, ultrasound, infrared rays, and microwave rays, Fahim found ultrasound to be the safest and most effective (Fahim et al. 1975). He carried out the first definitive studies on the method of action of ultrasound and its genetic safety in future generations of animals (Fahim 1980). He holds patents on the concept of ultrasonic contraception (both for humans and for sterilizing pets) and the equipment used to accomplish it (Fahim 1988).

One would think that with so much investment in the idea, Fahim would be actively researching ultrasound and working to build the mass of data needed for its acceptance. Yet, although he is collaborating with the Chinese on using longer and higher doses of ultrasound for permanent sterilization, in 1980 Fahim stopped research on ultrasound as temporary contraception. One reason was the lack of available funding. (Apparently the United States government also will not fund his collaboration with China because of China's stand on the abortion issue.) A second reason is his university's requirement that he use men with prostate cancer (who will probably have their testes surgically removed anyway) in his first human trials (Corea 1985, Chap. 9). Since it is primarily the return of fertility and not the safety of ultrasound itself that is in question (as shown by long-term use in men and women), it seems that men who are planning vasectomies could also be used as subjects, but the university will not allow this. Due to other similar constraints and a lack of support from his institution and colleagues, Fahim has moved on to other areas of research. Thus, ultrasound contraception has lost its best supporter.

Conclusion

The five types of vas-based methods (no-scalpel vasectomy, chemical injection, injectable plugs, the Shug, and SMA) and three heat methods (simple wet heat, artificial cryptorchidism, and ultrasound) all would constitute significant advances for male contraception. Each has a clear advantage over current contraceptives (male and female) in one or more areas of safety, effectiveness, convenience, reversibility, and avoidance of surgery. These clearly promising methods merit more research attention and allocation of more resources. First priority for research should be SMA injection, followed by artificial cryptorchidism, permanent chemical injection, and ultrasound. However, the perfection and popularization of *any* of the methods discussed would significantly expand the contraceptive supermarket available to men (and thus also to women) in the years to come.

Acknowledgments

A previous version of this essay appeared in *WomenWise*, Spring 1991. I thank the Center for Communication Programs at Johns Hopkins University for permission to reproduce Figure 4–1 (Liskin et al. 1983) and Dr. Lourens J. D. Zaneveld and the American Fertility Society for permission to reproduce Figures 4–2 and 4–3 (Zaneveld et al. 1988). Special thanks go to the researchers mentioned and to everyone who supported me in this work, including Betsy Hartmann, Judy Norsigian, Barbara Wilson, and (indirectly) Kim Chernin for helping make this work possible.

References

Adams, F.I., translator. 1939. *The genuine works of Hippocrates*. Baltimore: Williams & Wilkins.

Corea, Gena. 1985. *The hidden malpractice*. Updated ed. New York: Harper & Row.

Davis, Joseph. 1980. New methods of vas occclusion. In *Research frontiers in fertility regulation*, ed. Gerald Zatuchni, Miriam Labbok, and John Sciarra. New York: Harper & Row.

Djerassi, Carl. 1981. *The politics of contraception*. 2nd ed. San Francisco: W.H. Freeman.

Djerassi, Carl. 1988. Personal communication with the author.

Droegemueller, William. 1978. Discussion summary. In *Reversal of sterilization*, ed. John Sciarra, Gerald Zatuchni, and J. Joseph Spiedel. New York: Harper & Row.

Engelmann, U.H., P. Schramek, G. Tomamichel, et al. 1990. Vasectomy reversal in central Europe: Results of questionnaire of urologists in Austria, Germany and Switzerland. *Journal of Urology* 143:64–67.

Fahim, Mostafa. 1980. Male fertility regulation by means of ultrasound. In *Regulation of male fertility*, ed. G. R. Cunningham, W. B. Schill, and E. S. E. Hafez. Boston: Martinus Nijhoff.

Fahim, Mostafa. 1985. Personal communication with the author.

Fahim, Mostafa, Zuhal Fahim, R. Der, et al. 1975. Heat in male contraception (hot water 60 degrees C., infrared, microwave, and ultrasound). *Contraception* 11:549–562.

Fahim, Mostafa, Zuhal Fahim, James Harman, et al. 1977. Ultrasound as a new method of male contraception. *Fertility and Sterility* 28:823–831.

Free, Michael. 1978. Reversible intravasal devices: State of the art. In *Reversal of sterilization*, ed. John Sciarra, Gerald Zatuchni, and J. Joseph Spiedel. New York: Harper & Row.

Fukui, N. 1923. On a hitherto unknown action of heat ray on testicles. *Japan Medical World* 3:27–28.

Goldsmith, A., D.A. Edelman, and G.I. Zatuchni. 1985a. Transcutaneous male sterilization. *Research Frontiers in Fertility Regulation* 3 (4):1–8.

Goldsmith, A., D.A. Edelman, and G.I. Zatuchni. 1985b. Transcutaneous procedures for male sterilization. *Advances in Contraception* 1:355–361.

Guha, Sujoy, Sneh Anand, Shirfuddin Ansari, et al. 1990. Time-controlled injectable occlusion of the vas deferens. *Contraception* 41:323–331.

Guha, Sujoy, Shirfuddin Ansari, Sneh Anand, et al. 1985. Contraception in male monkeys by intra-vas deferens injection of a pH lowering polymer. *Contraception* 32:109–118.

Hatcher, Robert, Felicia Guest, Felicia Stewart, et al. 1988. *Contraceptive technology 1988–1989*. New York: Irvington Publishers.

Hatcher, Robert, Deborah Kowal, Felicia Guest, et al. 1989. Reproductive health around the world. Wall chart. Watertown, MA: Pathfinder Fund.

Herr, J.C., S.S. Howards, D.R. Spell, et al. 1989. The influence of vasovasostomy on antisperm antibodies in rats. *Biological Reproduction* 40:353–360.

Huber, Douglas. 1987. The Chinese microvasectomy technique. *Advances in Contraception* 3:176.

Huber, Douglas. 1989. No-scalpel vasectomy: The transfer of a refined surgical technique from China to other countries. *Advances in Contraception* 5:217–218.

Kandeel, Fouad, and Ronald Swerdloff. 1988. Role of temperature in regulation of spermatogenesis and the use of heating as a method for contraception. *Fertility and Sterility* 49:1–23.

Liskin, Laurie, J. M. Pile, and W. F. Quillin. 1983. Vasectomy—safe and simple. Population Reports, Series D, No. 4. Baltimore, Johns Hopkins University, Population Information Program.

Lynne, Charles, and Victor Politano. 1978. Early experience with the bionyx control valve (Phaser). In *Reversal of sterilization*, ed. John Sciarra, Gerald Zatuchni, and J. Joseph Spiedel. New York: Harper & Row.

Makler, Amnon. 1986. Evaluation and treatment of the infertile male. In *Reproductive failure*, ed. A. H. DeCherney. New York: Churchill Livingstone.

Mieusset, Roger, Louis Bujan, Arlette Mansat, et al. 1987. Hyperthermia and human spermatogenesis: Enhancement of the inhibitory effect obtained by 'artificial cryptorchidism'. *International Journal of Andrology* 10:571–580.

Mieusset, Roger, Louis Bujan, Arlette Mansat, et al. 1991. Heat induced inhibition of spermatogenesis in man. In *Temperature and environmental effects on the testis*, ed. A. W. Zorgniotti. New York City: Plenum Press.

Mieusset, Roger, Hélène Grandjean, Arlette Mansat, and Francis Pontonnier. 1985. Inhibiting effect of artificial cryptorchidism on spermatogenesis. *Fertility and Sterility* 43:589–594.

Misro, Manmohan, Sujoy Guha, Harpal Singh, et al. 1979. Injectable non-occlusive chemical contraception in the male–I. *Contraception* 20:467–473.

Nirapathpongporn, Apichart, Douglas Huber, and John Krieger. 1990. No-scalpel vasectomy at the King's birthday vasectomy festival. *Lancet* 335:894–895.

Nistal, Manuel, and Ricardo Paniagua. 1984. Infertility in adult males with retractile testes. *Fertility and Sterility* 41:395–403.

Nullis, Clare. 1991. Hormonal, silicone contraceptives being tested. Associated Press release 27 June.

Population Crisis Committee. 1987. Access to birth control: A world assessment. *Population Briefing Papers* 19.

Robinson, Derek, and John Rock. 1967. Intrascrotal hyperthermia induced by scrotal insulation: Effect on spermatogenesis. *Obstetrics and Gynecology* 29:217–223.

Robinson, Derek, John Rock, and Miriam Menkin. 1968. Control of human spermatogenesis by induced changes of intrascrotal temperature. *Journal of the American Medical Association* 204:291–297.

Rock, John, and Derek Robinson. 1965. Effect of induced intrascrotal hyperthermia on testicular function in man. *American Journal of Obstetrics and Gynecology* 93:793–801.

Rubin, Lionel. 1983. Toxicologic update of dimethyl sulfoxide. *Annals of the New York Academy of Sciences* 411:6–10.

Segal, Sheldon. 1962. Report on research toward the control of fertility. In *Research in family planning*, ed. Clyde Kiser. Princeton, N.J.: Princeton University Press.

Segal, Sheldon. 1988. Personal communication with the author.

Sethi, N., R.K. Srivastava, and R.K. Singh. 1989. Safety evaluation of a male injectable antifertility agent, styrene maleic anhydride, in rats. *Contraception* 39:217–226.

Sethi, N., R.K. Srivastava, and R.K. Singh. 1990a. Histological changes in the vas deferens of rats after injection of a new male antifertility agent "SMA" and its reversibility. *Contraception* 41:333–339.

Sethi N., R.K. Srivastava, and R.K. Singh, 1990b. Male-mediated teratogenic potential evaluation of new antifertility compound SMA in rabbit (*Oryctolagus cuniculus*). *Contraception* 42:215–223.

Sethi, N., R.K. Srivastava, R.K. Singh, et al. 1990c. Chronic toxicity of styrene maleic anhydride, a male contraceptive, in rhesus monkeys (*Macca mulatta*). *Contraception* 42:337–347.

Shain, Rochelle. 1980. Objections to tubal sterilization: What reversibility can and cannot overcome. *Contraception* 22:213–225.

Shunqiang, L., and Z. Jinbo. 1986. Non-incisional sterilization with intravasal drug injection (10–year follow-up on control of blocking the length of the vas deferens). *Advances in Contraception* 2:241.

Thomas, Patricia. 1988. Male contraceptives remain elusive. *Medical World News* 14 March: 61.

Urry, Ronald, J. B. Heaton, Monty H. Moore, and Richard G. Middleton. 1990. A fifteen-year study of alterations in semen quality occurring after vasectomy reversal. *Fertility and Sterility* 53:341–345.

Wilmore, Laurie. 1988. The social biases affecting male contraceptive research. Unpublished paper, Program in Human Biology. Stanford, Calif.: Stanford University.

World Bank. 1984. *Population change and economic development*. New York: Oxford University Press.

Zaneveld, Lourens. 1990. Personal communication with the author.

Zaneveld, Lourens, Stan Beyler, Gail Prins, et al. 1978. Reversible vas deferens occlusion: A new device. In *Reversal of sterilization*, ed. John Sciarra, Gerald Zatuchni, and J. Joseph Spiedel. New York: Harper & Row.

Zaneveld, Lourens, James Burns, Stan Beyler, et al. 1988. Development of a potentially reversible vas deferens occlusion device and evaluation in primates. *Fertility and Sterility* 49:527–533.

Zaneveld, Lourens, M. de Castro, F. Derrick, et al. 1990. Clinical evaluation of a reversible vas deferens blocking device—the Shug. In *Proceedings of the Third International Symposium on Contraception*, 19–23 June, Heidelberg, West Germany.

Zhao, Sheng-cai. 1990. Vas deferens occlusion by percutaneous injection of polyurethane elastomer plugs: Clinical experience and reversibility. *Contraception* 41:453–459.

Chapter 5

CONDOM EFFECTIVENESS AND ACCEPTABILITY IN THE UNITED STATES

Susan Rubinstein, Kathleen Ford, and Elizabeth O'Dair

Background

Although the condom may have been used in ancient Egypt, the first indisputable evidence comes from several sixteenth-century European documents. By the eighteenth century condoms were widely used throughout Europe by the upper classes. These early condoms were usually made of cecum (part of the intestine) of sheep and were expensive, but with the vulcanization of rubber in the mid–nineteenth century came a drop in price, allowing for greater access. By the 1930s more than 300 million condoms were being sold annually in the United States (Goldsmith 1987). Although most of these condoms were used for family planning, they were also associated with illicit sexuality and the prevention of sexually transmitted diseases (STDs). This association was strengthened by the promotion of condoms for STD prevention during World War II (Williamson 1991). As other methods of birth control and cures for STDs were discovered, condom use declined drastically (Goldsmith 1987). Yet, the historical association of condoms with promiscuity, prostitution, and extramarital sex still influences people's perceptions (Solomon & DeJong 1989).

Financial support for this research has been provided by Grant Number 1 RO1 HD26250 from the National Institute of Child Health and Human Development.

Furthermore, the condom lost popularity when the diaphragm and the birth control pill, both coitus independent and under female control, became available; currently more women use the pill than any other method (Mosher & Pratt 1990). However, the acquired immunodeficiency syndrome (AIDS) epidemic has brought new attention to the condom. Between 1987 and 1989 sales of condoms increased 60 percent (Can you rely . . . 1989).

We shall examine condom efficacy, who is using condoms and how well they are using them, and barriers to use. Examples of trends and patterns of use among gay men, adolescents, and women of color illuminate the factors that help to shape behavior.

Properties and Efficacy of Condoms

Today condoms are still made of either latex or cecum of lamb (called natural or skin condoms), but they have many variations. For example, both types of condoms are available in different sizes. Among latex condoms, options include lubrication, either with spermicide or other substances, and a variety of shapes, textures, colors, and flavors. Although skin condoms vary in porosity and thickness, they are very strong and their pores are generally not large enough for sperm to penetrate (Hatcher et al. 1988, Chap. 18). On the other hand, latex condoms have no pores unless there has been a problem with the manufacture, storage, or use of those condoms (Feldblum & Fortney 1988). Thus, both latex and skin condoms are effective for contraception if used properly. Proper use of a condom means that it is placed on the penis before any contact with the vagina, that it is unrolled as far as possible, and that the rim of the condom is held while the penis is withdrawn from the vagina. Also, the penis should be withdrawn shortly after ejaculation, before it becomes flaccid.

The failure rate of a contraceptive is defined as the percentage of unintended pregnancies experienced during the first year of use of that method. For typical married couples during their first year of condom use, the failure rate is 12 percent. Comparable rates for the birth control pill and chance are 3 percent and 85 percent, respectively (Trussell et al. 1990). Most condom failure is user failure, not product failure (Centers for Disease Control 1988). The lowest expected failure rate for condoms is calculated by assuming that condoms are used consistently and correctly during an entire year, in effect eliminating user failure. Trussell et al. (1990) estimate the lowest expected failure rate to be 2 percent. Furthermore, people usually become better contraceptors over time—that is, they begin to use a method more correctly and more consistently as they become more experienced. For example, one study found that failure rates were higher for teenagers than for other groups because teenagers tend to use condoms incorrectly and carelessly (Condom use low . . . 1990).

Some condoms can also be effective in preventing the transmission of STDs if used properly (as described above). Although neither skin nor latex condoms allow sperm to pass through them, the pores in skin condoms do allow smaller organisms, such as viruses and some bacteria, to pass through. Some of these organisms can cause STDs; gonorrhea and chlamydia are two common STDs caused by bacteria. To survive, such bacteria require a supportive environment, such as the mucus from the genitals. Since these bacteria cannot penetrate latex, contact with genital mucus can be successfully avoided by using condoms (Hatcher et al. 1988, Chap. 2). Thus, if used correctly and consistently, latex condoms provide adequate protection from bacterial STDs.

Latex condoms can help protect against some viral STDs but do not offer complete protection. Some viruses can be shed from the skin near the genitals, such as the scrotum or vulva, areas not covered by a condom that may contact with a partner's genitals. For example, contact with lesions caused by either the herpes simplex virus or the human papillomavirus, which causes genital warts, may occur even if a condom is used (Hatcher et al. 1988, Chap. 2).

The human immunodeficiency virus (HIV) that causes AIDS cannot survive outside a fluid such as blood, semen, or vaginal secretions. Also, in vitro experiments demonstrate that HIV cannot penetrate latex condoms (van Griensven et al. 1988). Clinical studies have shown, however, that, although consistent condom use decreases risk of HIV transmission, it does not eliminate it (Hatcher et al. 1988, Chap. 1). "One working estimate suggests that condoms reduce risk by a factor of 10" (Stein 1990, 460). While it is recommended that individuals engaging in penile-oral sex use condoms to prevent the transmission of HIV and other STDs, we have found no reports of condom failure rates for this type of sex. It is also recommended that individuals use condoms if engaging in anal intercourse. One study of condom failure rates for anal sex is discussed below.

Spermicide and Condoms

The use of a spermicide with a condom decreases the risk of unintended pregnancy and of transmission of STDs. Some condoms contain spermicides, but condom users can also put spermicide in the reservoir of the condom. "Nonoxynol–9, the active ingredient in most over-the-counter spermicides, kills sperm cells through a detergent action that attacks the cell membrane" (Can you rely . . . 1989, 139). Even when ruptured, condoms that contain nonoxynol-9 are effective in preventing the transmission of HIV (Feldblum & Fortney 1988). Users can also place spermicides in the vagina for extra protection. In fact, this practice may provide more protection than spermicidally treated condoms because there is more spermicide and it is dispersed throughout the vagina (Centers for Disease Control 1988).

Certain lubricants also help to reduce condom breakage by reducing friction. Unfortunately, some frequently used lubricants contribute to condom breakage. Oil-based lubricants—such as baby oil, hand lotion, or mineral oil—damage the latex (Voeller et al. 1989). Lubricants that are safe to use with latex condoms include spermicidal creams and jellies and surgical jelly, such as KY jelly. Estimates are that one condom breaks for every 105 to 161 acts of vaginal intercourse (Can you rely . . . 1989; Hatcher et al. 1988, Chap. 18). During anal intercourse, in which there is not as much natural lubrication as in vaginal intercourse, condoms tend to break more frequently (Can you rely . . . 1989; van Griensven et al. 1988).

The concern about breakage motivated one small study on the failure rate of "qualified anal condoms," a stronger variety of condoms made specifically for anal intercourse by several manufacturers. These anal condoms were introduced in Holland in 1986 as part of a condom campaign for homosexual men and were then tested for safety and acceptability. The failure rate of these qualified condoms was 3 percent, with most failure resulting from slippage. Their failure rate was much lower than the rate for condoms originally developed for contraception (van Griensven et al. 1988). These special condoms, however, were distributed along with a sachet of lubricant during the information campaign, which may have helped reduce breakage.

Acceptability of and Barriers to Condom Use

Condom use behavior is extremely complex; it is determined by historical, cultural, social, and psychological factors as well as by the physical properties of the condom. Since the beginning of the AIDS epidemic in the early 1980s, many studies attempted to understand these factors and how they influence behavior. National data provide important information about which women are relying on condoms but do not explain why people do and do not use condoms, nor do they provide information about specific populations—such as gay men. We discuss results from some smaller studies of gay men, adolescents, and women of color in order to shed some light on this behavior and to emphasize how extremely complex condom use behavior is.

The best information on condom use among the general population in the United States comes from the 1988 cycle of the National Survey of Family Growth (NSFG), conducted by the National Center for Health Statistics (Mosher & Pratt 1990). NSFG provides information on family planning for a representative sample of noninstitutionalized United States women of reproductive age (i.e., between 15 and 44). According to these data, 60.3 percent of these women were using some method of contraception. Of these contraceptors, 14.6 percent were condom users. Including women who use the condom with other methods, the percentage increases to about 16.6 percent. These data indicate that older women (in the 25–34 and 35–44 age groups) are more likely to use some method of contraception than younger women (see Table 5–1). They are, however, less likely to rely on condoms. The NSFG data also indicate a slight overall increase in condom use between 1982 and 1988, with the biggest increase occurring in the 15–24 age group.

TABLE 5–1

Female Contraceptors Who Used Condoms, Broken Down into Age Groups and Race, in National Study of Family Growth: United States, 1988 (National Center for Health Statistics)

Age and race	% using any method	% of contraceptors using condom
All women	60.3	14.6
Age		
15–24	45.7	20.8
25–34	66.3	13.7
35–44	68.3	11.2
Race		
White	61.8	14.9
Black	56.7	10.3

Source: Excerpt from Table 4, Mosher & Pratt (1990, 5).

Condom acceptability and consistency of use are influenced heavily by barriers to their use. Barriers that transcend all populations include lack of access, failure to plan for sexual intercourse, use of alcohol/drugs before sex, the belief that condoms are unnatural or immoral, and a historical association of condoms with extramarital sex, prostitution, and promiscuity (Ford & Norris 1991; Hingson et al. 1990; Solomon & DeJong 1989; Valdiserri et al. 1989). Although condoms are increasingly available in drugstores, restrooms, health clinics, and elsewhere, embarrassment in purchasing them and/or their cost may prevent use. Many people cite interference with sexual spontaneity and decreased sexual pleasure as reasons for not using condoms (Baffi et al. 1989; Rickert et al. 1989; Valdiserri et al. 1989). In one study gay men who never used condoms were more likely than those who always used them to believe that condoms spoil sex (Valdiserri et al. 1988). Poor communication between partners may also prevent a couple from using them. Baffi et al. (1989) found that women with greater communication skills were more likely to use condoms for contraception. Communication skills may also relate to the belief that suggesting condom use with a partner is offensive or insulting. Another barrier is the belief that one is not at risk for contracting an STD or HIV. Both adolescents and gay men have expressed this belief (Kegeles et al. 1989; Valdiserri et al. 1988).

Furthermore, barriers to the proper and consistent use of condoms also exist. For example, individuals need to know the proper technique for using a condom and the importance of using it for every sexual encounter. However, Ledbetter et al. (1990) found that the readability levels on patient package inserts and generic instructions were above the comprehension level of many individuals at risk for transmission of AIDS, other STDs, and unintended pregnancy. Proper use of condoms includes using them not only for vaginal intercourse but also for oral and anal intercourse. Heterosexual couples are far more likely to use condoms for vaginal sex than for either oral or anal sex. Since some couples practice anal, rather than vaginal, sex to avoid pregnancy, they may not perceive the need for condoms except during vaginal intercourse. A widespread complaint about condom use for anal sex among both heterosexual and homosexual couples is that they tend to break (Can you rely . . . 1989; van Griensven et al. 1988). Complaints about condoms during oral sex include inconvenience, reduced feeling, and bad taste (Beaman & Strader 1989).

The condom is unique in that it can be used both to prevent pregnancy and to stop the transmission of STDs. Although it appears that these facts would positively influence condom use among people engaging in vaginal intercourse, this is not necessarily the case. In fact, individuals have very different reasons for choosing condoms for contraception than they have for STD prevention. Although adolescent contraceptive decision making is clearly influenced by peer norms, one study found that norms were not related to condom use for STD prevention (Catania et al. 1989). Another study of adolescent women found that the risk of contracting an STD did not play a role in their decision to use condoms (Weisman et al. 1991). And, of course, women who want to become pregnant cannot at the same time use condoms to protect themselves from STDs.

Gay Men

Although national data on the acceptability and use of condoms among gay men do not exist, examining the extent of and reasons for behavior change in this population is extremely instructive. These changes in the early 1980s were the result of the mobilization of the gay community in response to the AIDS epidemic (Becker & Joseph 1988; Stall et al. 1990). In a review of the literature, Becker and Joseph found that gay men are practicing risk-reduction behaviors throughout the United States. For example, among participants in the San Francisco Men's Health Study, unprotected insertive anal intercourse dropped from 37 percent to 2 percent between 1984 and 1988. During the same period unprotected receptive anal intercourse dropped from 34 percent to 4 percent (Ekstrand & Coates 1990). A sample of self-identified gay men in New York City reported that during episodes of receptive anal intercourse their partners' use of condoms increased from 2 percent to 19 percent over a period of one year (Martin study cited in Becker & Joseph 1988, 402).

Examining some variables associated with reductions in risky behaviors among gay men is useful because these changes have been so drastic. Valdiserri et al. (1988) found that knowledge about HIV seroprevalence and AIDS prevalence in the local gay community was associated with increased use of condoms during anal sex. These investigators also found that use for insertive anal sex was associated with knowing someone with AIDS personally. Those San Francisco Men's Health Study participants "who reported in 1985 that they had friends or lovers with AIDS were less likely to engage in unprotected anal sex in 1988 than were men who did not have this experience" (Ekstrand & Coates 1990, 975). In a Chicago study in which the use of condoms during receptive anal intercourse increased by about 10 percent over six months, the only consistent predictor of change was the perception of social norms that were supportive of behavioral change (Joseph et al. 1987). Membership in a gay community appears to influence risky sex behavior through indirect means: members are likely to know personally individuals with AIDS; have a reliable source of social support; have been exposed to AIDS education materials produced and distributed by gay-identified organizations; or belong to a community that, as a result of all of these factors, has established new norms for safer sexual behavior (Ekstrand & Coates 1990; Joseph et al. 1987).

The majority of gay men who changed their behavior continue to practice safer sex. Several studies, however, have reported relapse to risky sex behaviors following initial behavior change. In one of these studies 16 percent of the participants relapsed to unprotected insertive and 12 percent to unprotected receptive anal intercourse. In addition, among gay men in San Francisco occasional relapse is currently more prevalent than stable high-risk practices (Ekstrand & Coates 1990). Similarly, Stall et al. (1990) found that relapse from safer sex practices is more than four times more prevalent than is consistent high-risk sex throughout the epidemic. Those who continue to engage in high-risk sex are more likely to be young, report having less social support, and may have more difficulty changing their behavior (Ekstrand & Coates 1990). This group probably requires different interventions than those who have relapsed from safer behaviors. As with other health behaviors, maintaining change is often more difficult than an initial change in behavior (Stall et al. 1990).

Adolescents

Although condom use among adolescents has become more prevalent and more consistent in the past decade, significant barriers to use among this group remain. Evidence for this increase is found in the data from the National Survey of Adolescent Males (NSAM) (representative of the 15–19 year old noninstitutionalized never married U.S. male population) and in other smaller studies (Hingson et al. 1990; Mosher & Pratt 1990; Sonenstein et al. 1989). For example, NSAM data show that in 1988 almost 57 percent of the sexually active young men reported having used a condom at last intercourse. In contrast, comparable data show that only about 21 percent of the young men were using condoms in 1979 (Sonenstein et al. 1989). Adolescents use condoms mostly for pregnancy prevention, not STD prevention (Weisman et al. 1991). Rates of condom use for oral and anal intercourse, which are practiced less frequently, are significantly lower than the rates for vaginal intercourse (Catania et al. 1989; Jaffe et al. 1988).

Both the NSAM and a survey of Massachusetts adolescents found that about 30 percent of males report always using condoms during sex (Hingson et al. 1990; Pleck et al. 1990). However, 32 percent of the young men in the Massachusetts study reported using condoms only sometimes, and 37 percent reported never using them (Hingson et al. 1990). Variables associated with consistent use among both male and female adolescents include perceived susceptibility to AIDS, the belief that condoms are effective, few perceived barriers to condom use, and exposure to more cues to action, such as discussing condoms with a doctor (Hingson et al. 1990).

Of these four variables, Hingson et al. (1990) found that the strongest predictor of condom use among these adolescents was the perceived barriers to use. Such barriers include not carrying condoms, the belief that condoms are difficult and embarrassing to obtain, and the belief that it is embarrassing to be asked to use condoms by a partner. Adolescents also cite disruption of foreplay, decreased feeling, and the association of condoms with promiscuity or STDs as reasons (Rickert et al. 1989). Knowledge about AIDS per se does not appear to be associated with increased condom use (Jaffe et al. 1988; Strader & Beaman 1989; Weisman et al. 1989).

Other factors may also influence condom use among adolescents. For instance, evidence suggests that worry (not simple information) about AIDS influences changes in behavior (Jaffe et al. 1988). More specifically, Pleck et al. (1990) found that a significant predictor of condom use was the frequency of worry about AIDS. Kegeles et al. (1989) found that adolescents' intentions to use condoms are strongly associated with immediate, short-term consequences but are not associated with their beliefs about the effectiveness of condoms in preventing STDs or pregnancy. Also, some young women believe that women are likely to get pregnant while using condoms (Kegeles et al. 1989).

It is important to consider adolescent condom use in the context of birth control pill use among this group: 64.9 percent of sexually active contracepting 15–24 year old females are using the pill, whereas 20.8 percent are using condoms (Mosher & Pratt 1990). Adolescents tend to use condoms early in their sexual careers "before moving on to more effective prescriptive methods" (Kegeles et al. 1989, 912). For example, younger males (age 15–16) tend to use condoms more than their older counterparts (age 18–19) (Hingson et al. 1990; Sonenstein et al. 1989). Family planning providers believe that the pill is a very appropriate contraceptive for this age group because it does not require planning or a partner's cooperation and it is highly efficacious. Thus, "condoms typically have been provided as a backup method to the pill rather than as a primary contraceptive method" (Weisman et al. 1989, 217). Several studies have found that adolescent couples tend to use condoms if the female partner wishes to do so (Pleck et al. 1990; Weisman et al. 1989). The male partner's perceptions about his partner's use of the pill has a significant influence on condom use. In fact, consistency of condom use is negatively associated with partner's pill use (Pleck et al. 1990). Therefore an adolescent couple is not very likely to use condoms if the woman is using the pill, feels protected from pregnancy, and does not feel susceptible to AIDS and if her partner knows she is on the pill and does not himself feel susceptible to AIDS.

Women of Color

Barriers to condom use among low socioeconomic status women of color have more to do with cultural and social realities than with specific problems with the condom (Worth 1989). NSFG data show that condom use among white contraceptors is 14.9 percent and, among black contraceptors, 10.3 percent (Mosher & Pratt 1990). Marin (forthcoming) reports that Hispanics are also less likely than whites to use condoms for contraception. In fact, because of the high value placed on fertility and children in Hispanic culture, Hispanics are likely to cite pregnancy prevention as a disadvantage of condoms (Marin forthcoming). For low socioeconomic status women, "sex may function as a source of employment, a method for establishing ownership or proprietary rights in a relationship, or as a means of acquiring much needed tangible or emotional support" (Mays & Cochran 1988, 952). Other women may be physically or emotionally abused if they request that their partner use a condom (Mays & Cochran 1988). Also, in both black and Hispanic communities men are more likely to have sex outside of marriage than women; for Hispanic men, commonly with prostitutes (Fullilove et al. 1990; Marin forthcoming). Thus, women may not know that they are at risk of contracting HIV or other STDs.

For a Hispanic woman to suggest condom use is contrary to cultural norms. "In traditional Hispanic culture, the 'good' woman is not supposed to know about sex, so it is inappropriate for her to bring up subjects like AIDS and condoms" (Marin forthcoming). In the black community sexuality is discussed often in public but infrequently in intimate situations (Fullilove et al. 1990). Furthermore, there are significantly fewer marriageable men than women in the black community because of high mortality, high rates of incarceration, and high rates of unemployment among young black men. Because of this "community disintegration, in which men have been empowered to have greater sexual freedom, . . . women have lost ground in their ability to insist on protection from infection" (Fullilove et al. 1990, 62). Therefore, because of the imbalance of men to women, black women cannot insist on condom use.

Finally, black women are less likely to be using any type of contraception than their white counterparts (57 percent versus 62 percent). However, like all women, black women who do use contraception are more likely to be using the pill (38 percent) than the condom (10 percent) (Mosher & Pratt 1990). In these communities with high rates of HIV infection, women tend to rely on methods that they can control and that are available in public family planning clinics, but these methods cannot protect them from becoming infected with HIV or other STDs.

The Female Condom

The female condom is a polyurethane sheath that fits loosely in the vagina, with a flexible polyurethane ring at each end (see Figure 5–1). The ring at the closed end is used for insertion and serves as an internal anchor, although precise placement over the cervix is not required (Leeper & Conrardy 1989). "The other ring forms the external edge of the sheath and remains outside the vagina after insertion, protecting the labia and the base of the penis during intercourse" (Ruminjo et al. 1991). This device is designed for one-time use and can be inserted well before intercourse. It also requires lubrication; lubricated as well as unlubricated brands may become available.

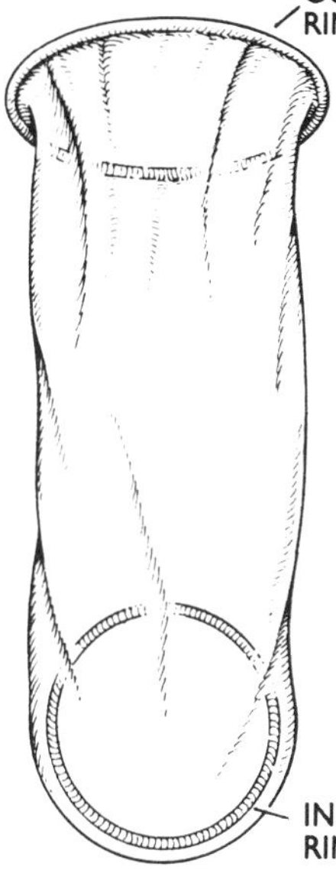

Figure 5–1
REALITY™ vaginal pouch. Source: *REALITY™ Intravaginal Pouch Instruction Manual* (1989), p. 1.

Although the female condom has undergone both in vitro and clinical trials, it is not currently on the market. In vitro studies indicate that it is impermeable to HIV and cytomegalovirus (Drew et al. 1990). Clinical studies of the female condom in several countries have had varying results. For instance, in the United States the participants wanted the condom to be longer (Bounds et al. 1988), whereas Thai participants thought it was too long and too wide (Sakondhavat 1989). Other complaints include that the outer ring can get pushed into the vagina, that the penis can go between the outer ring and the vagina, and that it does not stay in place (Leeper & Conrardy 1989; Ruminjo et al. 1991). Despite these complaints, most women in the trials found the female condom to be acceptable (Bounds et al. 1988; Ruminjo et al. 1991; Sakondhavat 1989; Users approve . . . 1991).

In these clinical trials the biggest barrier to use has been objections by male partners (Ruminjo et al. 1991; Sakondhavat 1989). Although use of the female condom is controlled by women, male cooperation is still necessary. If this new method is less objectionable to men than the male condom, it could have a large influence on slowing the spread of HIV and other STDs. Data on the effectiveness of the female condom in preventing pregnancy and STDs, however, are not yet available.

Conclusions

Condoms are effective for preventing pregnancy and the transmission of STDs when used properly; yet many factors prevent them from being used more widely. Experiences with family planning and with responses to the AIDS epidemic help illuminate why condoms are underused. Such experiences provide insight about developing appropriate interventions for behavior change as well as suggest areas for future research.

The condom lost popularity when female-controlled methods, such as the diaphragm and the pill, became available; currently, more women use the birth control pill than any other method. These facts indicate that female control of contraception is important for acceptance. If the female condom proves to be effective and if the objections of men are overcome, it may provide women with a method that would protect both against HIV and other STD transmission and against unintentional pregnancy and would allow female control. However, heterosexual men, including adolescents, must also be targeted for interventions that encourage condom use and emphasize male responsibility.

Although the gay male community differs significantly from other communities, knowledge of its response to AIDS is invaluable for research and program development in other communities. Knowledge of the role of social support and social norms is especially important. The experience with relapse to risky behaviors among this population indicates that relapse is likely to occur in other populations when behavior changes. The experiences of this community also indicate that interventions targeting populations that are hard to reach must be developed.

It is clear that most people in the United States are aware of AIDS; yet many continue to engage in behavior that puts them at risk for contracting HIV. Evidence for this consists of high unintentional pregnancy rates (about 6 in 10 pregnancies each year are unintentional) and the increasing incidence of syphilis and gonorrhea (Forrest & Singh 1990; Fullilove et al. 1990). These trends continue despite increased attention to condom use and other risk-reduction behaviors. Previous experience with underutilization of condoms, for both pregnancy and STD prevention, needs to be explored further to develop interventions for relapse prevention and for facilitating behavior change among those who are hard to reach in all segments of the population. Finally, more research is needed on new methods for STD prevention, especially methods that women can control.

References

Baffi, Charles R., Kelli Kenison Schroeder, Kerry J. Redican, and Lawrence McCluskey. 1989. Factors influencing selected heterosexual male college students' condom use. *Journal of College Health* 38:137–141.

Beaman, Margaret L., and Marlene Strader. 1989. STD patients' knowledge about AIDS and attitudes toward condom use. *Journal of Community Health Nursing* 6(3):155–164.

Becker, Marshall H., and Jill Joseph. 1988. AIDS and behavioral change to reduce risk: A review. *American Journal of Public Health* 78(4):394–410.

Bounds, Walli, John Guillebaud, Laura Stewart, and Stuart Steele. 1988. A female condom: A study of its user-acceptability. *British Journal of Family Planning* 14:83–87.

Can you rely on condoms? 1989. *Consumer Reports* March:135–142.

Catania, Joseph A., Thomas J. Coates, Ruth M. Greenblatt, et al. 1989. Predictors of condom use and multiple partnered sex among sexually active adolescent women: Implications for AIDS-related health interventions. *Journal of Sex Research* 26(4):514–524.

Centers for Disease Control. 1988. Condoms for prevention of sexually transmitted diseases. *Morbidity and Mortality Weekly Report* 37(9):133–137.

Condom use low despite increase. 1990. *American Pharmacy* NS30(6):14–15.

Drew, W. Lawrence, Margaret Blair, Richard C. Miner, and Marcus Conant. 1990. Evaluation of the virus permeability of a new condom for women. *Sexually Transmitted Diseases* 17(2):110–112.

Ekstrand, Maria L., and Thomas J. Coates. 1990. Maintenance of safer sexual behaviors and predictors of risky sex: The San Francisco Men's Health Study. *American Journal of Public Health* 80(8):973–977.

Feldblum, Paul J., and Judith A. Fortney. 1988. Condoms, spermicides, and the transmission of human immunodeficiency virus: A review of the literature. *American Journal of Public Health* 78(1):52–53.

Ford, Kathleen, and Anne Norris. 1991. Urban African American and Hispanic adolescents and young adults: Who do they talk to about AIDS and condoms? What are they learning? *AIDS Education and Prevention: An Interdisciplinary Journal* 3(3):197–206.

Forrest, Jacqueline Darroch, and Susheela Singh. 1990. The sexual and reproductive behavior of American women, 1982–1988. *Family Planning Perspectives* 22(5):206–214.

Fullilove, Mindy Thompson, Robert E. Fullilove, Katherine Haynes, and Shirley Gross. 1990. Black women and AIDS prevention: A view towards understanding the gender rules. *Journal of Sex Research* 27(1):47–64.

Goldsmith, Marsha F. 1987. Sex in the age of AIDS calls for common sense and 'condom sense.' *Medical News and Perspectives* 257(17):2261–2266.

Hatcher, Robert A., Felicia Guest, Felicia Stewart, et al. 1988. *Contraceptive Technology 1988–1989*. New York: Irvington.

Hingson, Ralph W., Lee Strunin, Beth Berlin, and Timothy Heeren. 1990. Beliefs about AIDS, use of alcohol and drugs, and unprotected sex among Massachusetts adolescents. *American Journal of Public Health* 80(3):295–299.

Jaffe, Leslie R., Mavis Seehaus, Claudia Wagner, and Bonnie J. Leadbeater. 1988. Anal intercourse and knowledge of acquired immunodeficiency syndrome among minority-group female adolescents. *Journal of Pediatrics* 112(6):1005–1007.

Joseph, Jill G., Susanne Montgomery, Carol-Ann Emmons, et al. 1987. Magnitude and determinants of behavioral risk reduction: Longitudinal analysis of a cohort at risk for AIDS. *Psychology and Health* 1:73–96.

Kegeles, Susan M., Nancy E. Adler, and Charles E. Irwin. 1989. Adolescents and condoms: Associations of beliefs with intentions to use. *American Journal of Diseases of Children* 143:911–915.

Ledbetter, Carol, Susan Hall, Janice M. Swanson, and Katherine Forrest. 1990. Readability of commercial versus generic health instructions for condoms. *Health Care for Women International* 11:295–304.

Leeper, M.A., and M. Conrardy. 1989. Preliminary evaluation of REALITY, a condom for women to wear. *Advances in Contraception* 5:229–235.

Marin, Barbara. Forthcoming. Hispanic culture: Implications for AIDS prevention. In *Sexuality and disease: Metaphors, perceptions and behavior in the AIDS era*, ed. J. Boswell, R. Hexter, and J. Reinisch. New York: Oxford University Press.

Mays, Vickie M., and Susan D. Cochran. 1988. Issues in the perception of AIDS risk and risk reduction activities by Black and Hispanic/Latina women. *American Psychologist* 43:949–957.

Mosher, William D., and William F. Pratt. 1990. Contraceptive use in the United States, 1973–88. *Advance Data* March(182):1–7.

Pleck, Joseph H., Freya L. Sonenstein, and Leighton C. Ku. 1990. Adolescent males' contraceptive attitudes and consistency of condom use. Paper presented at the 98th Annual Convention of the American Psychological Association, 12 August, Boston.

REALITY™ Intravaginal pouch instruction manual. 1989. Jackson, WI: Wisconsin Pharmacal Co.

Rickert, Vaughn I., M. Susan Jay, Anita Gottlieb, and Christie Bridges. 1989. Female's [sic] attitudes and behaviors toward condom purchase and use. *Journal of Adolescent Health Care* 10:313–316.

Ruminjo, J., E.G. Mwathe, N. Thagana, et al. 1991. Consumer preference and functionality study of the Reality™ female condom in a low risk population in Kenya. Manuscript, Family Health International. March.

Sakondhavat, Chuanchom. 1989. Consumer preference study of the female condom in a sexually active population at risk of contracting AIDS, Khon Kaen, Thailand. Final Report, Family Health International. August.

Solomon, Mildred Z., and William DeJong. 1989. Preventing AIDS and other STDs through condom promotion: A patient education intervention. *American Journal of Public Health* 79:453–458.

Sonenstein, Freya L., Joseph H. Pleck, and Leighton C. Ku. 1989. Sexual activity, condom use and AIDS awareness among adolescent males. *Family Planning Perspectives* 21(4):152–158.

Stall, Ron, Maria Ekstrand, Lance Pollack, et al. 1990. Relapse from safer sex: The next challenge for AIDS prevention efforts. *Journal of Acquired Immune Deficiency Syndromes* 3(12): 1181–1187.

Stein, Zena A. 1990. HIV prevention: The need for methods women can use. *American Journal of Public Health* 80:460–462.

Strader, Marlene K., and Margaret L. Beaman. 1989. College students' knowledge about AIDS and attitudes toward condom use. *Public Health Nursing* 6(2):62–66.

Trussell, James, Robert A. Hatcher, Willard Cates, Jr., et al. 1990. Contraceptive failure in the United States: An update. *Studies in Family Planning* 21(1):51–54.

Users approve of female condom. 1991. *Family Planning Perspectives* 23(1):5.

Valdiserri, Ronald O., Vincent C. Arena, Donna Proctor, and Frank A. Bonati. 1989. The relationship between women's attitudes about condoms and their use: Implications for condom promotion programs. *American Journal of Public Health* 79:499–501.

Valdiserri, Ronald O., David Lyter, Laura C. Leviton, et al. 1988. Variables influencing condom use in a cohort of gay and bisexual men. *American Journal of Public Health* 78:801–805.

van Griensven, Godfried J.P., E.M.M. de Vroome, et al. 1988. Failure rate of condoms during anogenital intercourse in homosexual men. *Genitourinary Medicine* 64:344–346.

Voeller, Bruce, Anne H. Coulson, Gerald S. Bernstein, and Robert M. Nakamura. 1989. Mineral oil lubricants cause rapid deterioration of latex condoms. *Contraception* 39(1):95–102.

Weisman, Carol S., Constance A. Nathanson, Margaret Ensminger, et al. 1989. AIDS knowledge, perceived risk and prevention among adolescent clients of a family planning clinic. *Family Planning Perspectives* 21(5):213–217.

Weisman, Carol S., Stacey Plichta, Constance A. Nathanson, et al. 1991. Consistency of condom use for disease prevention among adolescent users of oral contraceptives. *Family Planning Perspectives* 23(2):71–74.

Williamson, Nancy E. 1991. Barriers to the use of condoms. Unpublished manuscript, Family Health International, April.

Worth, Dooley. 1989. Sexual decision-making and AIDS: Why condom promotion among vulnerable women is likely to fail. *Studies in Family Planning* 20(6):297–307.

Chapter 6

CERVICAL CAPS AND THE WOMEN'S HEALTH MOVEMENT: FEMINISTS AS "ADVOCATE RESEARCHERS"

Dana Gallagher

In May 1988, the Prentif Cavity Rim cervical cap, a barrier method of contraception, was approved by the Food and Drug Administration (FDA) for contraceptive purposes in the United States. The cap, a thimble-shaped rubber device, holds spermicide against a woman's cervix and is held in place by suction and the vaginal walls.

While variations on the cervical cap have been in use since ancient times, the contemporary rubber cap was not developed until the mid-1800s, about the same time as the diaphragm (Hatcher et al. 1990). The cervical cap enjoyed decades of popularity in Europe and the United States but fell from favor with the advent of oral contraceptives and intrauterine devices in the 1960s. During the late 1970s, feminist health clinics became extremely interested in increasing the number of contraceptive methods available to women. This dovetailed with growing consumer concern about potentially serious side effects of available contraceptives (particularly oral contraceptives and intrauterine devices) and the desire for more convenient barrier methods.

Three types of cervical caps—the Prentif Rim, the Vimule, and the Dumas Vault—were reintroduced into the United States in the late 1970s; their manufacturer is Lamberts (Dalston) Ltd. of London. From that time until May 1988, the FDA approved cervical caps only for purposes of menses collection and aiding in artificial insemination. At this writing, the Vimule and Vault caps are not FDA approved.[1]

The cap's odyssey from obscurity to approval began in the late 1970s with the introduction of the method in feminist clinics throughout the United States, predominantly on the East and West coasts. Clinic staff trained themselves to fit caps, using each other and willing patients as models. By 1979, general interest in caps had developed, and demand for the cervical cap began to rise. During this period the cervical cap was imported directly from the manufacturer, simply by placing orders with the company. This changed in fall 1979, when cap shipments were seized at United States entry ports. These seizures were portents of the regulatory upheaval that was about to occur.

Device Classification and Investigational Exemption

Several months prior to the shipment seizures, the FDA had proposed a regulation classifying the cervical cap as a Class II device for the two approved uses—menses collection and aiding artificial insemination (U.S. Department of Health, Education & Welfare 1979). A Class II designation mandates the establishment of a performance standard for a device; a Class III is assigned to those devices posing "significant risk" to their users and "requiring premarket approval." The FDA issued a request for comment on the proposed classification of the cervical cap for contraceptive use.

Shortly thereafter, in early 1980, two FDA rulings were issued clarifying the cervical cap's status. First, the Investigational Device Exemption (IDE) Regulation mandated that providers obtain an IDE number from the FDA in order to continue fitting cervical caps for contraceptive purposes. Second, a ruling on the classification of cervical caps was issued, giving it a Class III designation for contraceptive use. This classification triggered an uproar within the cervical cap providing medical community. Practitioners found the classification arguable since they deemed the cervical cap more comparable to the diaphragm (Class II) than the IUD (Class III). By way of explanation for its classification, the FDA issued the statement that pregnancy was the "significant risk" requiring the cervical cap's (but not the diaphragm's) Class III designation.

Initially, the FDA stated that a United States sponsor, along with the manufacturer, would submit an IDE application that would cover all clinicians. This did not occur. Consequently, by January 1981, cap providers were expected to comply with the IDE regulation by submitting a locally approved study protocol to the FDA. Noncompliance would force the FDA to obtain a court order halting cap fitting, to conduct searches and seizures, and to impose fines and seek imprisonment. During the time that this compliance was expected (1981–1988), providers were compliant, thus avoiding such action.

As the January 1981 implementation of the Class III designation drew near, the women's health movement made a concerted effort to raise a national voice of dissension. Led by the National Women's Health Network and the New Hampshire Feminist Health Center, representatives of this movement began to talk with the FDA about the regulations. Feminists argued that the IDE regulations were prohibitive to grass-roots and feminist providers, who were unable to conduct research at that time. Major areas of concern included continuity of care to women already using caps, the cost to clinics of conducting research, and the clinics' lack of resources to design, implement, and maintain an approved study protocol. Although feminist providers repeatedly articulated these issues, the FDA could not be persuaded to reclassify the cap.

Perhaps the largest obstacle for cap providers was either access to or creation of the FDA-required Institutional Review Board (IRB). An IRB's tasks include reviewing and approving study protocols in its geographical area prior to submission for FDA approval, and providing postapproval study monitoring (U.S. Department of Health & Human Services 1983). Institutions with research branches for human subjects, e.g., many hospitals, have IRBs, but feminist health centers do not. In some cases the local IRB and the feminist health centers had a history of enmity on past issues, and in other cases the IRB saw no compelling reason to review the proposed protocol. This created deep concern in many communities about trying to enlist the help of IRBs. If an existing IRB would not cooperate, the cap provider had to create its own IRB to comply with FDA guidelines. However, if the IRB approved the study protocols, the FDA would likely follow suit.

Feminist Cap Providers: Researchers or Advocates?

Despite the initial obstacles that the cervical cap providers encountered, successful procurement of an IDE number through the IRB was what ultimately gave women access to the device while it was still under investigation. This was unprecedented: the FDA had never allowed access to a contraceptive method outside the arena of tightly controlled clinical trials.

Other interesting circumstances surrounded the cap. The foray into the realm of cap approval was the first involvement of the feminist health movement in extensive contraceptive research from the "inside." Usually in a position of questioning safety and efficacy of experimental contraceptives, feminist health workers found themselves straddling the consumer advocacy versus research "fence." Feminist providers believed that their expertise in fitting cervical caps in a women-controlled environment uniquely qualified them to conduct consumer-centered research and to play a role in distribution of the device after its approval. However, their long years of playing "watchdog" over pharmaceutical companies created a difficult irony.

This was particularly evident when it came time to choose a U.S. distributor of the cervical cap. Because of their decade of effort invested in the cap, members of the women's health movement were understandably interested in and involved with the decision of whom the manufacturer would designate. Cervical Cap Ltd. (CxC) was chosen to be the United States and Canadian distributor.[2] Issues of interest included distributor intentions as to cost of cap, as to curriculum and strategy for training new cap fitters, as well as to marketing and availability of the approved cap.

For the first time, feminist health providers were presented an opportunity to take leadership roles within a distribution company. However, many were concerned that formal affiliation with the cervical cap's distributor had the potential to dilute their credibility as advocates of women's health issues. Ultimately, CxC named a group of cervical cap researchers and long-time cap providers to its medical advisory board, one of whom serves as liaison between the company and the women's health movement.

Dispensation of Cervical Caps by Lay Health Workers

Yet another unusual occurrence during the cap's investigation was the dispensation of caps by lay health workers, under the supervision of licensed practitioners. Such health workers are trained, unlicensed paraprofessionals, not to be confused with licensed mid-level practitioners, i.e., nurse practitioners and physician assistants.

Carol Downer (1988) has estimated that 50 percent of preapproval cervical caps were fitted by lay health workers in their capacities as facilitators of self-help groups and employees of feminist health centers. Cap-fitting personnel were FDA approved when their cervical cap study protocols were submitted. Since lay health workers had been fitting caps before the caps became experimental devices, the mandated FDA studies did not interrupt cap availability to women seeking them from lay fitters.

Never before had the FDA permitted dispensation of experimental devices by lay health workers. Regardless of the FDA rationale for doing so on this occasion, women's access to the cap was clearly enhanced.

Just prior to cap approval, feminist cap fitters debated the advisability of arguing against a prescriptive designation (versus over-the-counter) for the postapproval cap. The benefit of an over-the-counter device was that it could be fitted by lay health workers, thereby ensuring continued, broad access. Unfortunately, it would also then be available to the public at large, with greater potential for poor outcome during usage. But designating the cap as a prescriptive device eliminated a large cadre of experienced fitters, at least temporarily decreasing the availability and, potentially, the efficacy of the method.

The question evaporated as feminist providers learned that the prescriptive designation was inevitable and that counterarguments could jeopardize the cap's FDA approval. Since the cervical cap is now regulated as a prescription device, direct dispensation of caps by lay fitters is not allowed.

Premarket Approval

After the clinical investigation of cervical caps was complete, the next step in the process prior to FDA approval was successful completion of a Premarket Approval Application (PMA) (U.S. Department of Health & Human Services, 1980). Components of the PMA that must be furnished for successful application include:

1. Comprehensive summary of all safety and efficacy data
2. Sections on clinical, animal, and laboratory data
3. A section describing device characteristics
4. A reference to performance standards
5. Labeling specifications
6. Bibliography with copies of significant articles
7. A manufacturing section
8. A sample of completed patient report forms
9. Sample of device to be approved

Ordinarily, the PMA process is completed and financed by the device's manufacturer. In this instance the manufacturer initially was reluctant to participate in the PMA process. Moreover, my 1986 survey (Gallagher 1986) showed that virtually no cervical cap providers were aware of the PMA process until their studies were well underway. When informed of this next step in the FDA approval process, providers reacted with surprise and anger. Many providers indicated that they would not have conducted their cap studies had they known in advance about the PMA process. Although providers did become resigned to the process, they clearly were unable to meet this additional challenge. Fortunately, at this juncture the manufacturer agreed to cooperate in submitting the application (Jordan 1986).

While the women's health movement was critical of the Class III investigational designation of the cap, overall they heralded the option of the Investigational Device Exemption. In 1988, when the feminist health movement collectively called for FDA approval of the cervical cap, they made an additional request that the FDA consider exercising the IDE option prior to approval of new contraceptives in the future (National Women's Health Network 1988).

As distributor of the cervical cap, CxC determined from the beginning that it would provide the cap only to practitioners who had been properly trained to fit it. Since those who had provided caps as investigational devices were "grandfathered in" as trained providers, the company expected that this cadre of experienced fitters would train a new generation of clinicians. The training was to include a mandatory didactic session and a "hands-on" session using live models; generally, training took a minimum of four hours.

As could be expected, this unconventional policy was fairly unpopular among physicians. While many clinicians considered themselves adequate cap providers by virtue of their medical training and argued for unfettered access, CxC held that the cap's success relied on its contraceptive efficacy, which, in turn, rested on its being fitted properly by experienced practitioners.

From 1988 to 1991, the company held to this policy. Guidelines about what constituted acceptable training were circulated by the company to trainers and prospective providers. Training was facilitated by the company's circulation of rosters of trainers to providers who made inquiry about the cap. CxC went the rounds of the major medical conferences offering a combination didactic/hands-on training session that entitled its attendees to become certified cap fitters. When individuals made training requests to the company, CxC forwarded their inquiries to trainers in their area for follow-up. This system should have worked.

However, the overall distribution of cap fitters nationally left many areas of the United States underserved at the outset, posing significant geographic obstacles to training. In addition, after years of advocacy, many cap providers that the company relied on felt that training new fitters was not their priority.

Moreover, there was no standardized training fee: trainers charged what they deemed reasonable for their expertise and costs. Fees might range from a few to several hundred dollars and were sometimes quite prohibitive. The lack of standardized training fee schedules created ill will.

Many practitioners, irate about this state of affairs, complained to CxC. Undaunted, the company maintained its position in the belief that quality assurance was the point on which cap popularity pivoted. Access to caps, however, did not rise in the exponential fashion the company had projected. After request for input on this policy from cap providers and months of discussion, Cervical Cap Ltd. rescinded its policy in early 1991 (Summerhayes 1991).

Currently, it is strongly recommended that potential cap providers receive training from experienced providers. However, the cap can be purchased without documentation of training if the clinician signs a waiver stating she or he has read fitting instructions and the patient package insert (Summerhayes 1991). It remains to be seen what effect this policy change will have on cervical cap accessibility nationwide.

Conclusion

The FDA approval process for the Prentif Rim cervical cap took nearly one decade to complete. Precedent setting in its participation of feminist providers and lay health workers, the process is a blueprint for contraceptive research and development in the future.

The need for a variety of safe, accessible contraceptive methods will continue. Health activists should continue strenuously to evaluate efficacy and safety of new methods and communicate consumer concerns to the Food and Drug Administration. Whether the women's health movement will ever again be so involved in the "birthing" of an approved contraceptive method remains to be seen. If a similar investigational process is required, along with similar logistic and ethical challenges, such involvement seems unlikely. However, the women's health movement will continue its efforts to have an impact on the research, development, and approval processes of new contraceptives, working in critical concert with regulatory agencies and pharmaceutical firms to expand women's contraceptive choices.

Notes

1. From 1980 to 1984, the Vimule cap was available in the United States. Its design and range of sizes offered more opportunity for successful fitting. However, in 1983, Bernstein et al. reported vaginal abrasions, lacerations, and mucosal thickening in 8 out of 12 Vimule users. In February 1984, the FDA withdrew approval of the investigation of Vimule caps, which many regard as an unwarranted move (Gallagher and Richwald, 1989).
2. The U.S. distributor of cervical caps is Cervical Cap Ltd. (CxC), 430 Monterey Avenue, Suite 1B, Los Gatos, CA 95030.

Acknowledgments

Many thanks to Sue Schemel, M.D., for her careful review and comments.

References

Bernstein, Gerald, L.H. Kilzer, A.H. Coulson, et al. 1983. Studies of cervical caps: I. Vaginal lesions associated with use of the Vimule cap. *Contraception* 5:443–446.

Downer, Carol. 1988. Personal communication with author.

Gallagher, Dana. 1986. The cervical cap: Issues in the Food and Drug Administration's regulatory approval system. Unpublished masters thesis, University of California at Los Angeles.

Gallagher, Dana, and Gary Richwald. 1989. Feminism and regulation collide: The Food and Drug Administration's approval of the cervical cap. *Women & Health* 15(2):87–96.

Hatcher, Robert A., Felicia Stewart, and James Trussell. 1990. *Contraceptive technology 1990–1992*. New York: Irvington.

Jordan, Susan. 1986. Personal communication with the author.

National Women's Health Network. 1988. Testimony presented to the Food and Drug Administration, Obstetric and Gynecological Devices Advisory Panel. Washington, D.C. February.

Summerhayes, Elizabeth. 1991. Personal communication with the author.

U.S. Department of Health, Education and Welfare. Food and Drug Administration. 1979. *Federal Register* Part VII: 19894–19899. Washington, D.C.: U.S. Government Printing Office.

U.S. Department of Health and Human Services. Food and Drug Administration. 1980. *Guidelines for the arrangement and content of a premarket approval application*. November. Washington, D.C.: U.S. Government Printing Office.

U.S. Department of Health and Human Services. Food and Drug Administration. 1983. *Code of Federal Regulations*, Title 21, Part 812. Washington, D.C.: U.S. Government Printing Office.

Chapter 7

PERSPECTIVES ON SEXUALITY, CONTRACEPTION, AND PREGNANCY AMONG BLACK TEENAGED WOMEN

Susan Shaw

As teenage pregnancy rates continue to escalate, sexuality, contraception, and pregnancy among teenagers has come under increasing scrutiny from policy makers and service providers alike. Current issues of cultural sensitivity have made people who work with adolescent pregnancy more aware of racial/cultural variations in the practice and meaning of contraception and childbearing for different women. As a consequence of this greater awareness of "difference,"[1] contraception use by black teenagers has become particularly important to service providers who operate in a system still dominated by white, middle-class goals. I ground my discussion in an historical context, beginning with the view originated by Daniel Patrick Moynihan of adolescent pregnancy as a symptom of a "crisis" in the black family. Moynihan, in his report *The Negro Family: The Case for National Action* (1965), argues that the crisis stemming from the combined forces of poverty, female-headed families, poor education, and unemployment that faced blacks in the 1960s was a consequence of the pathological "matriarchy" characterizing the black social structure. To Moynihan, the prevalence and apparent social acceptability of adolescent pregnancy among poor blacks in particular was just one manifestation of this matriarchal family structure.

In the 1990s, teenage pregnancy among blacks is still viewed as a product of the same economic problems, and "matriarchy" is still hotly debated as a cultural factor. While I cannot make a detailed analysis here of the Moynihan doctrine and its sexist/racist analysis, I will examine the continuation of his theories through current literature by presenting some responses by black women to the Moynihan report and to other social science literature on adolescent pregnancy and contraception.

I believe it is important to analyze academic writing on social issues such as adolescent pregnancy and contraception for two reasons: (1) the discourse of "experts" on social issues sets the terms of debate and (2) expert analysis determines what steps are taken to deal with the "problem." In general, however, little evaluation takes place of the experts' own biases relative to the subject at hand. The report "The Primary Prevention of Adolescent Pregnancy: New Yorkers Speak" (Mayor's Office . . . 1990) illustrates the great reliance by policy makers and service providers on scientific evaluation as the only valid means of judging a program's effectiveness. Likewise, sex education programs are evaluated by measuring and comparing contraception use before and after a program is conducted. Yet behavior change *as a consequence* of education is difficult to discern from such studies (Furstenberg et al. 1989).

In this chapter, I frame contraception and adolescent pregnancy (1) as a feminist issue through a brief presentation and analysis of a white feminist's perspective and (2) as a racial issue through an examination of the view that adolescent pregnancy among black teenagers is a consequence of black matriarchy. In addition, I regard adolescent pregnancy and contraception as a useful window through which to examine the failure of white feminism to fully address or include the experiences of black women in its analyses. (For a more complete history of this exclusion, see hooks 1981, 1984.) I will begin by discussing the mainstream social science literature on adolescent pregnancy with a focus on how these writings represent and affect black women. This process is necessary because too often black women are not the generators of discourse but are only represented through European-American stereotypes of black women's experiences. I shall begin with the bias or assumption that black women become subsumed under generalizations based on white experiences unless the specific realities of their experiences are attended to. One of the goals of this essay is to include writings by black women that contravene such stereotypes and to provide an alternative, or complement, to the views provided by the experts.

Statistics in the Debate

Teenage pregnancy rates, sexual activity rates, and sexually transmitted diseases continue to increase among teenagers (Zelnik & Kantner 1980). However, Forrest and Singh (1990) in their analysis of 1982 and 1988 data from the National Survey of Family Growth show that the increase in sexual activity among women age 15–19 is primarily accounted for by the increase in the number of white, *nonpoor* teenagers who are becoming sexually active. The current demography of adolescent pregnancy is in contrast to traditional ideas about pregnant teenagers, who are stereotypically black, unmarried, and on welfare; this contradiction has been cited as a primary cause for the media attention given to the issue of adolescent pregnancy (Furstenberg et al. 1989).

In the social science literature, teen pregnancy is often viewed as a greater problem among blacks than whites, in part because a greater proportion of black girls become pregnant as teenagers than whites. Beginning with the rate of sexual activity and the age at first intercourse, studies by the Alan Guttmacher Institute (AGI) found that, in 1982, 59 percent of black teenaged women age 15–19 had had intercourse, as opposed to 45 percent of white teens in the same age range. By 1988, 61 percent of black teenaged women age 15–19 had had intercourse (Forrest & Singh 1990). Another study by AGI, on condom use by high school students, found that 44 percent of black students had had more than two partners in the previous year (increasing their risk for HIV and, presumably, pregnancy), while 27 percent of white students did so; 28 percent of black students said they always used condoms, while 36 percent of white students said the same (Anderson et al. 1990). More partners presumably represents a greater risk for pregnancy since regular contraceptive use is generally associated with more stable, long-term relationships.

Different rates of sexual activity are amplified by pregnancy and varying abortion rates. For example, an unmarried black teenager is five times more likely to give birth before age 20 than an unmarried white teenager. One statistic states that 94.6 black teens per 1000 as opposed to 44.7 white teens per 1000 become pregnant each year (Fried 1990). However, the Select Committee on Children, Youth and Families (1986) put those figures at 86.4 for black teens and only 18.5 for white teens for 1983. Proportionally, more adolescent pregnancies among blacks end in birth because more whites have and utilize the option of abortion. For instance, 60 percent of white adolescent pregnancies end in abortion, while only 20 percent of black adolescents abort (Fried 1990). A study of 31,000 teenagers in New York City found that "at every age, White adolescents are the most likely to abort . . . " (Joyce 1988, 629). Fewer blacks who have children as teenagers marry the fathers of their babies; thus more black teenagers become a female family head at a young age. In 1980–1981, an estimated 28 percent of white adolescents married to legitimate their first pregnancies, while only 8 percent of blacks did (Joyce 1988).

Female-headed families are associated with poverty and AFDC (Aid to Families with Dependent Children); the Alliance against Women's Oppression (1988) reported that in 1985, 74 percent of families headed by a woman under age 25 were living in poverty. In Moynihan's argument, female-headed families are responsible for reproducing poverty among blacks (Moynihan 1965). In addition, children of female-headed families or adolescent mothers are more likely to have adolescent pregnancies themselves (Meriwether 1984).

Through this sequence of assumptions created and supported by statistical "facts," social science research on teen pregnancy links adolescent pregnancy with the pathology of female-headed families that is condemned in the Moynihan report. Indeed, by focusing on female-headed families and welfare dependency, social scientists come to view noncontraception and adolescent pregnancy among blacks as symptomatic of larger problems associated with black families and poverty (e.g., Darity & Myers 1984; Dietrich 1975; Hanley et al. 1975). These particular events become reified in the course of statistical or theoretical analysis and are made icons for the disadvantaged position of blacks as a group in the United States. When adolescent pregnancy is reduced to certain acts or non-acts by black women (such as contraception use or nonuse), the political context and power structure within which black women operate is disregarded.

The Social Science Approach

One premise of the social science approach to adolescent pregnancy appears to be the belief that if only the right variable could be isolated, we could understand "the" cause of adolescent pregnancy, address that cause, and have the key to the prevention of future adolescent pregnancies. The operational assumption is that adolescent pregnancy is a "social problem" that must be understood. This assumption itself stems from the perceived consequences of teen pregnancy. When studies focus on higher rates of adolescent pregnancy among blacks, the "problem" tends to get isolated to that community, somehow attributing adolescent pregnancy to race, ethnicity, or poverty. At the same time, adolescent pregnancy is thought to *cause* poverty because, for example, families headed by teen mothers are seven times more likely to be living below the poverty level than other families (Select Committee . . . 1986).

These perceived negative consequences, however, are themselves social in nature.[2] That is, it may be true that women who have children as teenagers are poorer and less educated than women who delay childbearing, but regarding these consequences as automatically following from a birth at age 16 is to presume a direct line of causation that has been a major issue in psychological literature. In other words, "Are they pregnant because they're different or are they different because they are pregnant?" Many of the circumstances (poverty, lack of education, or growing up in a female-headed family) that are said to be consequences of early pregnancy can also be considered causes or predisposing factors. As discussed in the introduction to New Yorkers Speak:

> In poor neighborhoods, the problems associated with teen pregnancy and parenting are magnified by the alienation, lack of hope and self-confidence, and even despair that result from grinding poverty and limited options. Indeed, some studies suggest, *it is these very problems that lead many teenagers to seek parenthood* as a form of "instant adulthood" (Mayor's Office . . . 1990, 6, emphasis added).

The issue here, however, is not causation but the constant association between poverty and adolescent pregnancy. For black women, the causation argument perpetuates the kinds of racist assumptions that were first legitimized by the Moynihan report. As a result of this fusion of class and race, certain other realities are ignored, such as how the welfare system functions to "keep down" women who have children nonmaritally or punishes them for being "unfit" to have children.

Some women (both white women and women of color) have described *non*contraception use as a healthy, adaptive response to the circumstances of poverty and dearth of opportunities experienced by many adolescents who "fail" to use contraception or who have children premaritally. As Zelnik, Kantner, and Ford (1981) conclude in their study, most policy recommendations do not "recognize the variety of tastes, interests, motivation, experiences, and moral values of the actors involved—the young women and their partners" (169). Kristin Luker (1975) provides an alternative theory of contraceptive decision making by studying the complex cost/benefit analyses made by women of all ages. In her view, the nonuse of contraception is an *action*, the product of reasoned consideration of alternatives and consequences. Luker's perspective is important because often judgments about teenagers' failure to use contraception are compounded with all the other ways these young people have failed, resulting in a deterministic dismissal of their capacity for decision making and action.

Black Responses to Moynihan

Several black women have articulated clear responses to the assumptions about black women in the Moynihan report and in current social science literature. They continue to respond to Moynihan's doctrine today because he created the context for academic discussion of black families by bringing the concept of "matriarchy" into widespread use. Moynihan has indirectly influenced every other author who has written about issues relating to the formation or function of black families, insofar as he was a foremost author on the subject. For examples that refute Moynihan's arguments, I will look to June Dobb Butts's reframing of the issue of adolescent pregnancy from a black perspective (1987), Louise Meriwether's popular article in *Essence* magazine (1984), and Bettina Aptheker's response published in 1982. My framework is provided by Rosalind Petchesky's chapter on adolescent sexuality and pregnancy because of her emphasis on the *cultural construction* of pregnancy and sexuality (Petchesky 1984, Chap. 6).

June Dobb Butts, in her article on adolescent pregnancy from a black perspective, defines adolescent pregnancy as a symptom not of the pathology of black families but of a larger societal illness called racism. Identifying the type that automatically comes to mind with the phrase "teenage pregnancy," Butts argues that the black teenage mother "epitomizes the crux of the problem, for it is in regard to her undeveloped, but emerging body that we find the culmination of all those abstract ideas—racism, sexism, and the stamp of despair—that are bred by grinding poverty" (Butts 1987, 308).

She enumerates several principles of the black community that characterize the black experience of teenage pregnancy, including a "sex-positive view of life," the extended family, and the historical value of fecundity to the black community. The first is perhaps most intriguing: Butts identifies a sex-positive view of life among blacks, in contrast to that of white society, which she calls sex-negative. In the process, she points out an important contradiction in mainstream discourse on adolescent pregnancy. One reason we give for teenagers' failure to use contraception is their supposed "inability to accept their own sexuality"—as we simultaneously proclaim that "the only respectable outlet for sexual expression is heterosexual coitus performed by legally married couples. The difference, she says, "between what we practice and what we preach is more than a charming little deceit—it borders on the psychopathic . . . " (Butts 1987, 309).

Butts reaches back to the "African roots" of today's teenagers for an explanation of this sex-positive view of life. She extends this to the present through references to the history of oppression in slavery and shows its current effects on black teenagers' use of contraception. She makes a defense of black sexuality based on an "instinctive" theory of sexuality that originates from black teenagers' historical connections to Africa. She cites a fondness for touch within black families that is part of the experience of sensuousness. She says it is "natural" for black teenagers to "accept and to glorify their sexual feelings . . . [for] socialization is always facilitated by the healthy expression of one's innate sensuality" (Butts 1987, 312). Butts points out that white teens engage more often in "nonprocreative" sex than black teenagers, which explains the higher rates of pregnancy among blacks even when compared to sexually active white teenagers. She says it is "a maladroit combination of ignorance and of innocence . . . that encourage[s] them to use coital patterns for 'natural' sexual expression and to eschew contraceptive measures" (Butts 1987, 316).

Butts believes the extended family, a "bulwark of the black experience," is based on "African tribalism."[3] The extended family is an important aspect of black identity and, according to Butts, is grounded on the egalitarian relationship between men and women. The extended family was threatened and nearly destroyed by slavery, which leads Butts to her third principle—the value of fecundity to the black community. This is summed up by the old adage, "a baby is the future." A consequence of this principle is the belief that "one proves one's worth through demonstrated fecundity," another cause for the higher birthrates among blacks (Butts, 1987, 315).

This simplistic portrayal of black adolescent sexuality mirrors Petchesky's idealized view of black female sexuality, as discussed below. Butts creates this image through an opposition to a white society she calls "sex-negative." Butts's defense of black adolescent sexuality is a response to the creation of an "epidemic" of adolescent pregnancy by white society. In other words, Butts, like Washington (1982), believes that the popular notion of an epidemic is a creation of racist media and the fear that teen pregnancy was "spreading" into white society. Butts argues that in strict epidemiological terms, however, and when we consider it within the context of black extended families, adolescent pregnancy is not an epidemic at all but a product of certain cultural beliefs and values specific to blacks.

Another black author, Louise Meriwether (1984), offers an analysis of adolescent pregnancy from a very different point of view, one more similar to that of the Moynihan report. I discuss her view here to provide a contrast to Butts's construction of a unitary "black experience" and to show how the Moynihan ideology has been absorbed by other members of the black community. Meriwether affirms that "teen pregnancy is one of the major problems confronting the black community today" (Meriwether 1984, 96). The lead paragraph of her article in *Essence* magazine states, "Pregnancy among Black teenagers has reached staggering proportions . . . and threatens . . . the very survival of the Black race" (45). That teen pregnancy is seen as symptomatic of the larger problems of the black family is evidenced by its inclusion in the *Essence* series on The Black Family in Crisis.

Meriwether justifies the moral outrage that seeps through her objective tone by listing the ways in which teen mothers are inadequate (e.g., poor mothering skills, lack of prenatal care, toxemia, high miscarriage rates, and low birth-weight rates) and the negative effects that can be seen in their children (who are less healthy, achieve less academically, and are more likely to continue the "cycle of poverty" by becoming teen parents themselves).[4] She links these problems to poverty through welfare, implying as Moynihan does that welfare is an indicator of pathology: the fastest growing population on welfare, she notes, is teen mothers. Also like Moynihan, Meriwether links female-headed families to the unemployment of black males, which prevents them from assuming their proper role of head of the family.

In contrast to the defense of black teen sexuality seen in Butt's naturalistic appeal to African roots, Meriwether definitely does *not* portray sexual activity among adolescents as the norm. She attributes sexual activity in teens to the influence of the media, sexism in the American culture, depression following emotional loss, alienation, dropping out of school or academic problems, and lack of ego strength (Meriwether 1984, 144). However, she refers infrequently to the male half of the "problem," perpetuating stereotypes about pregnancy and contraception as female responsibilities. Her only comment on teen fathers is that, while "some" take their role seriously, "many are a total failure at fatherhood . . . and must be made to understand that they are producing children who are in great danger of becoming emotional cripples." According to Meriwether, the prevalence of pregnancy among blacks is due to teenagers who know nothing about their bodies, believe popular myths about sex and pregnancy, do not contracept until nine months after they become sexually active, and once they do, use less effective birth control methods.

Black labor organizer Bettina Aptheker (1982) criticizes another aspect of what she labels the "Moynihan doctrine." She demonstrates the impact of the Moynihan report on black women through the story of Angela Davis's trial for murder in 1972. Aptheker cites the ideological themes in the Moynihan report as an integral part of the prosecution's case against Davis, as they tried to condemn Davis by casting her as a "Moynihan matriarch." She argues that the Moynihan doctrine was ideologically motivated in its call for the introduction of patriarchal relations to the black community. Aptheker focuses on this document as a weapon used at the time of the civil rights movement by white sociologists and the government against all blacks, but especially against black women. She recognizes Moynihan's victim-blaming tendencies, but she attributes a more malicious intent than mere ignorance or denial of the roots of the problem (i.e., white racism). She states that the Moynihan report "sought to turn the Black community in on itself by introducing a sexual battle that had not previously characterized the Black experience" (Aptheker 1982, 134). Aptheker sees Moynihan's patriarchal agenda as a direct response to the increased political and economic power gained by black women (of all classes) as they entered the work force in the 1960s in greater numbers than ever before. "The Moynihan Report . . . represented a necessary adjustment in racist/male supremacist ideology to correspond to the actual shift in the position of Black women in society" (132).

Aptheker attempts to disprove the matriarchy theory by drawing a distinction between *strength* and *dominance*. The experience of slave women providing for their broken families, she says, was a great trial of strength, yet it cannot be argued that they dominated their men. It is possible to be strong yet not dominant, though white men have a tendency to confuse the two. "Much of the misconception," she quotes Joyce Ladner (1972), "comes from the fact that women are held [by white men] to be the passive sex, but the majority of Black women have, perhaps, never fit this model, and have been liberated from many of the constraints the [white] society had traditionally imposed on women."[5]

A fundamental, almost instinctive, response to accusations of matriarchy is the argument that black men do in fact rule their families—or as Aptheker would have it, that black women, while strong, do not dominate. Cerullo and Erlien (1986) point out that, in the case of divisive sexism in a racist system, "The [only] defense against Moynihan was to accept the presumption of male leadership, and argue that it was intact in the Black community" (257). Aptheker cites statistics on the percentage of two-parent families among blacks to support her assertion that matriarchy does not in fact exist in black families. It is one thing, she says, to assert that female headship occurs in a greater proportion of black families than whites, but quite another to draw from that the conclusion that black women as heads of households are "characteristic" of black families. It is a testimony to the strength of Moynihan's argument and of the two-parent, patriarchal model that even as she recognizes the strength of black women through history, Aptheker will go to great lengths to preserve dominating-male imagery in the face of what she perceives as a racist attack.

Aptheker's argument was made in defense against what was perceived as a *racist* attack: to argue effectively against it, and to achieve legitimacy in a patriarchal system, Aptheker had to accept Moynihan's sexist terms in order to confront his racism. Indeed, the two isms are effectively fused together when a sexist, patriarchal agenda is directed against black women. Such is the difficulty in discussing adolescent pregnancy among blacks, for just as it has primarily been white feminists who criticize the Moynihan doctrine as sexist, white feminists (e.g., Petchesky 1984; Thomson 1984; Willis 1987) have responded to adolescent pregnancy as a feminist issue.

Rosalind Petchesky, a white feminist, devotes Chapter 6 of her book, *Abortion and Women's Choice: The State, Sexuality and Reproduction* (1984) to teenage sexuality, contraception, and abortion. Because she focuses on the power relationships both within teenage sexual relationships and in the dominant, heterosexual culture's efforts to regulate such relationships, she is crucial to my framework for this discussion of black teenaged women. Petchesky uses the events of sexual activity, pregnancy, and abortion as windows through which to examine heterosexual patriarchal culture because "getting pregnant . . . has no intrinsic social or political meaning; it receives its meaning from the historical and political context in which it occurs and the circumstances of the woman involved" (Petchesky 1984, 207). Sexuality takes its meaning from its context of social relations; insofar as women and teenagers exist in a patriarchal society, these social relations automatically become *power* relations in which gender, class, race, and adulthood are negotiated. In particular, I will focus on contraceptive use by black teens as practices within which power relations are embodied.

Petchesky views teenagers as a locus of political controversy, and contraception as a "crucial signifier of female adolescent sexuality." Pregnancy and/or abortion make sex visible, in great contrast to recent history, when various methods were employed primarily by white teenagers to hide adolescent sexuality. Insofar as pregnancy makes sex visible, it is seen as a "sexual event," which then must be "measured, scaled off, studied, categorized, organized, regulated and contained" (Petchesky 1984, 210). She notes that teen sexual activity (narrowly defined as heterosexual intercourse) is perceived as problematic in the above context because it occurs in age groups for which sex in general is not considered appropriate.

For my purposes, the most important aspect of Petchesky's work is her analysis of the different "sexual moralities" within race and class groups that are created, she theorizes, by their different social and economic realities. Petchesky begins with an historical analysis of the petting culture of the 1940s and 1950s, in which the "dominant [white, middle-class] morality" forbade sexual intercourse per se but created permissible alternatives (such as petting in your parents' car alone at night), as long as absolute secrecy was maintained. However, class differences often would not allow this, as working-class and lower-class kids generally did not have cars, the primary tool for concealment of sex. Also, living in more crowded and less private conditions made sex unavoidably more visible. Petchesky asserts that heterosexual intercourse was more frequently part of the sexual activity of youth in the lower and working classes, an interesting assertion that is also made by Butts (1987) about black teenagers.

I find it useful that Petchesky specifically comments on the construction of black women's sexuality, for throughout most of her analysis the "dominant heterosexual norms" to which she refers are products of *white* heterosexual culture, just as "middle- and working-class youth" are usually white youth. Her class analysis of teenage sexuality, necessary though it is, does not consider race or culture as crucial factors in the experience of class oppression. For example, she refers to one study of rural black teenagers to show the "freedom, versatility and self-assertion" with which they organize their sexual lives. These are not the passive, self-effacing teenagers of the white norm. Though poor, they are instead portrayed as somehow outside the same constraints experienced by lower-class white teenagers. Petchesky uses black female kinship and male unemployment (characteristics that she attributes to the "matrifocal" structure of black households) as an explanation for black teens' attitudes toward both sex and men. The values of this culture, she says, "emphasize women's sexual self-reliance as well as the communal value of babies and motherhood, . . . reinforc[ing] the general support among black kin networks for out-of-wedlock childbearing . . . " (Petchesky 1984, 229). She seems to use this stereotypical view of black female kinship to create a foil for white female sexuality, which is generally passive, as well as male-dominated and -controlled.

As Petchesky points out, the present political controversy about abortion and adolescent pregnancy is caused by applying a stereotypically self-assertive "sexual code" to white middle-class teenagers. The changes in the public discourse about sex (as white women become the subjects of discourse as well) "break down some of the entrenched cultural divisions between white women and women of color, between middle and working-class and poor women, that have long been rooted in sexual stereotypes" (Petchesky 1984, 230–231). The current crisis about teen pregnancy is a consequence of a new stereotype, "the promiscuous white teenager," whose sexuality used to be concealed. Petchesky states, "As long as it was black or poor white women who were having sex or showing up in the hospital wards with complications from illegal abortions, *these events were perceived not as sexual but as the 'natural' consequences of poverty and race*" (230, emphasis added).

This is an important point in the analysis of black women's representations in adolescent pregnancy literature. Petchesky argues that when relegated only to "other groups" such as black women, pregnancy and sexuality were part of the definition of their place in white-dominated society; I would further argue that this stereotyping contributes to their objectification in the literature. However, as the trends change and white teenagers no longer collude in the concealment of sex and pregnancy, Petchesky holds that "the *visibility* of those sexual changes through *white* teenage pregnancy and abortion rates challenge not only patriarchy but the sexual bases of racism and class domination" (Petchesky 1984, 232, emphasis in text). Petchesky appears to prioritize sexist discrimination above racism or classism, as gender is the basis for most of her discussion. Though she acknowledges the social construction of race, class, and gender, her conclusions imply that gender is essentially at the root of *all* forms of discrimination that are a consequence of heterosexual patriarchy.

Conclusion

This analysis exposes the interlocking effects of racism and sexism in the discourse that surrounds adolescent pregnancy. My critique shows the pervasiveness of the Moynihan doctrine throughout social science literature and provides some arguments by black women against his theories. Meriwether accepts the doctrine that pregnant teenagers are harmful to the black community and the nation; Butts denies much of the conservatism inherent in the views of Meriwether and (to an extent) Aptheker, but she does so only through an essentialist view of "the" black experience and an appeal to the "African roots" of today's teenagers. Aptheker illustrates the point that the dominance of patriarchy must be recognized and/or eventually acceded to in the fight against racism; Petchesky, a white woman, illustrates that fighting against sexism neglects the experience of racism if only white teenagers are referred to in her discussion of adolescent pregnancy.

These perspectives of different women put adolescent pregnancy and contraception among blacks into the context of the different forms of social relations attributed to or experienced by black women. Both the Moynihan report and contemporary social science literature reproduce the dominant culture's prejudices about black women and have established the framework within which discourse about black women's sexuality or adolescent pregnancy takes place. I have provided a critique of the social science posture toward black women and its construction of their sexuality to show how social science research becomes a tool of the dominant culture. The dominant culture is made up of the middle-class, patriarchal norm that is integral to the structure of our society.

Feminists and postmodernists tend to regard race, gender, and class as fragmented aspects of our identity, separating racial oppression from sex oppression from class oppression. The awareness is growing, however, that if feminists as a constituency are to accomplish anything worthwhile, feminist objectives must be recognized as nothing but self-aggrandizement unless they are for ALL women—not just for economically privileged white women. For feminists to work for the empowerment of ALL women means *actively embracing* an antiracist agenda because some women are discriminated against on the basis of their race or ethnicity, just as some women are discriminated against because they are lesbians. To be ethically acceptable and true to the basic principles of feminism, then, oppressions must not be hierarchized into orders of priority, and we must recognize the enmeshment of gender discrimination with racial discrimination.

Notes

1. In this essay I use quotation marks to indicate terms that have contested meanings or that suffer from overuse (e.g., "matriarchy," "difference"). I use quotes around the first occurrence of a term in question, but not in subsequent instances. In reviewing literature, quotes show my inherent skepticism of any analysis, study, or information source that does *not* take political realities such as race/class/gender and power disparities into account when discussing a stigmatized phenomenon such as "teenage pregnancy." "Mainstream literature" is that vast majority of literature that does not provide such analysis.
2. Most literature does not attribute negative consequences of adolescent motherhood to the biological age of the mother. "The disadvantaged situation of the teenage mother is most often attributed to the social, financial and psychological restraints associated with the *social position* of the adolescent." (McGonagle 1989, 18–19, emphasis added).
3. Another example of the "African tribalism" argument is seen in Washington (1982): she cites the significance of procreation to African clans as an important explanation for adolescent pregnancy among blacks. She argues that the black extended family provides for pregnancy at any age and that adolescent pregnancy as a "problem" exists only among whites, for whom it represents the decay of the nuclear family ideal.
4. This view assumes it is because children of teen parents are somehow defective that the cycle of poverty perpetuates itself. It fails to recognize how the system functions to maintain people in certain class positions in society.
5. At one time, a common response by black women to white feminism was that black women were already "liberated" and feminism was merely another ploy by the dominant culture to "divide and rule" blacks by introducing a gender division

that would prevent them from more effectively struggling against white racism. See, for example, Cade (1974); hooks (1981); Rodgers-Rose (1980).

Acknowledgments

Many thanks to my thesis committee members, Barbara Yngvesson and Stephanie Schamess at Hampshire College, and Lynn Morgan at Mt. Holyoke College, for their help with the work from which this paper grew. Thanks to Meredith Michaels for being my mentor.

References

Alliance Against Women's Oppression. 1988. Teenage mothers: Setting the record straight. Discussion paper.

Anderson, John, Laura Kann, Deborah Holtzman, et al. 1990. HIV/AIDS knowledge and sexual behavior among high school students. *Family Planning Perspectives* 22(6): 252–255.

Aptheker, Bettina. 1982. *Woman's legacy: Essays on race, sex and class in American history.* Amherst: University of Massachusetts Press.

Butts, June Dobb. 1987. Adolescent sexuality and teenage pregnancy from a Black perspective. In *The Black adolescent parent*, ed. Stanley Battle. New York: Haworth Press.

Cade, Toni. 1974. *The Black woman.* New York: Mentor.

Cerullo, Margaret, and Marla Erlien. 1986. Beyond the "normal family": A cultural critique of women's poverty. In *For crying out loud: Women and poverty in the U.S.*, ed. R. Lefkowitz and A. Withorn. New York: Pilgrim Press.

Darity, William, and Samuel Myers. 1984. Does welfare dependency cause female headship? The case of the black family. *Journal of Marriage and the Family* 46:765–778.

Dietrich, Kathryn. 1975. A reexamination of the myth of black matriarchy. *Journal of Marriage and the Family* 37:367–373.

Forrest, Jacqueline Darroch, and Susheela Singh. 1990. The sexual and reproductive behavior of American women, 1982–1988. *Family Planning Perspectives* 22(5): 206–214.

Fried, Marlene. 1990. *From abortion to reproductive freedom.* Boston: South End Press.

Furstenberg, Frank, Jeanne Brooks-Gunn, and Lindsay Chase-Lansdale. 1989. Teenaged pregnancy and childbearing. *American Psychologist* 44(2): 313–320.

Hanley, C. Allen, Robert Michielutte, Carl Cochrane, et al. 1975. Some consequences of illegitimacy in a sample of Black women. *Journal of Marriage and the Family* 37: 359–366.

hooks, bell. 1981. *Ain't I a woman?* Boston: South End Press.

hooks, bell. 1984. *Feminist theory from margin to center.* Boston: South End Press.

Joyce, Theodore. 1988. The social and economic correlates of pregnancy resolution among adolescents in New York City, by race and ethnicity . . . *American Journal of Public Health* 78(6): 626–631.

Luker, Kristin. 1975. *Taking chances: Abortion and the decision not to contracept.* Berkeley: University of California Press.

McGonagle, Christine. 1989. Social service networks of teen mothers in Holyoke, Massachusetts. Division III thesis, Hampshire College, Amherst, Mass.

Mayor's Office for Children and Families, City of New York. 1990. The primary prevention of adolescent pregnancy: New Yorkers speak. Unpublished manuscript.

Meriwether, Louise. 1984. Teenage pregnancy. *Essence* 14(12): 94–86, 144–151.

Moynihan, Daniel Patrick. 1965. *The Negro family: The case for national action.* Washington DC: U.S. Department of Labor.

Petchesky, Rosalind. 1984. *Abortion and women's choice: The state, sexuality and reproductive freedom.* New York: Longman Press.

Rodgers-Rose, La Frances. 1980. *The Black woman.* London: SAGE.

Select Committee on Children, Youth and Families. 1986. *Teen pregnancy: What is being done? A state by state look.* Washington D.C.: U.S. Government Printing Office.

Thomson, Sharon. 1984. Search for tomorrow: On feminism and the reconstruction of teen romance. In *Pleasure and danger: Reconstructing female sexuality*, ed. Carol S. Vance, 350–384. Boston: Routledge and Kegan Paul.

Washington, A.C. 1982. A cultural and historical perspective on pregnancy-related activity among U.S. teenagers. *Journal of Black Psychology* 9(2): 1–28.

Willis, Sharon. 1987. Teen lust . . . *Ms.* July/August: 68–70, 193–194.

Zelnik, Melvin, and John F. Kantner. 1980. Sexual activity, contraceptive use and pregnancy among metropolitan-area teenagers: 1971–1979. *Family Planning Perspectives* 12(5):230–237.

Zelnik, Melvin, John F. Kantner, and Kathleen Ford. 1981. *Sex and pregnancy in adolescence.* London: SAGE.

PART II

NEW FACETS TO THE ABORTION DEBATE

Chapter 8

ABORTION: NEW COMPLEXITIES

Mary Anne Warren

The issues surrounding abortion have never been simple, but they were once *relatively* simple. Feminists and civil libertarians wanted women to have safe, legal, and affordable abortion services. Opponents of abortion wanted all or most abortions prohibited by law, as was the case in the majority of American states prior to 1973. While that basic schism remains, the legal and moral complexities have multiplied in the past two decades.

Roe v Wade, the 1973 Supreme Court case that established women's constitutional right to abortion in the first two trimesters of pregnancy, looked for a time like a lasting (though incomplete) victory for reproductive freedom. But the appointment to the Court of conservative justices, chosen on the basis of an antiabortion litmus test, has produced subsequent decisions that have undermined the protection afforded by *Roe*. The 1989 case of *Webster v Reproductive Health Services* not only broadened the power of state and federal governments to limit women's access to abortion, but signaled the willingness of at least four justices to overturn *Roe* entirely. Many states now have laws requiring parental consent or notification for teenagers seeking abortion, spousal consent for married women, medically unnecessary tests for signs of fetal viability, or laws prohibiting abortion—or any *mention* of abortion—in facilities receiving government funding. The appointment of Justice

Clarence Thomas presages a likely return to the states of the power to prohibit all or most abortions. Several states already have legislation in place that will have the effect of outlawing abortion the moment that *Roe* falls.

At the same time that the legal status of abortion in the United States been growing more perilous, the emergence of new reproductive technologies has generated new ethical issues. These issues have sometimes divided feminists and occasionally placed them in awkward alliances with conservative opponents of abortion and reproductive technologies. Most of these new bioethical issues involve, in one way or another, the rights or moral status of embryos or fetuses, as well as the rights and obligations of women, couples, physicians, and biomedical researchers. There are, for instance, issues involving (1) the selective abortion of genetically or developmentally abnormal fetuses, (2) sex-selective abortion (usually meaning the abortion of female fetuses), (3) selective termination (the destruction of one or more fetuses in a multiple pregnancy), (4) in vitro fertilization (IVF) as a treatment for infertility, (5) experimental uses of IVF embryos, (6) experimental or therapeutic uses of tissues from aborted fetuses, e.g., in the treatment of Parkinson's Disease, (7) court-ordered cesareans, and other cases involving so-called maternal-fetal conflicts, and (8) the possible introduction of RU486, the new abortifacient developed in France.

The papers in this section address just three of these abortion-related issues. They do so, however, in ways that illustrate more widely applicable feminist approaches to the medical and ethical evaluation of new reproductive technologies.

In "Inducing a Miscarriage: RU486 and Prostaglandin for Early Abortion," Marge Berer explains how this new method of abortion works, and describes its clinical use in France. Berer analyzes the respective advantages and disadvantages of RU486 in comparison to surgical methods such as vacuum aspiration both from a medical perspective and from the perspective of the woman having the abortion. In her view, RU486 can help to "demedicalize" the experience of abortion. Rather than submitting to a surgical invasion of her body, the woman takes the pill herself—and receives an injection of prostaglandin two days later—after which "her body makes the abortion happen."

Some feminists have been more skeptical about the potential benefits of RU486. They argue that a method that requires four (sometimes five) clinic visits, plus the use of two powerful drugs that are known sometimes to have dangerous side effects, can scarcely be described as a *demedicalization* of abortion. As Berer herself is quick to point out, the introduction of RU486 poses significant medical hazards in impoverished nations that may lack the facilities to administer the treatment safely and effectively and with the needed follow-up care. There are contraindications for the use of RU486 (such as being over 35 and smoking), and the risk that women will not always be properly screened for those contraindications. For Third-World women in particular, the need to return to the clinic after exactly two days for the prostaglandin injection can also pose a serious problem.

Berer argues, however, that even where medical facilities are far from ideal, RU486 could provide a safer alternative to the often clandestine methods that are currently in use. In much of the world—and increasingly in the United States—although it is legal, many women have little or no access to abortion. The high cost of legal abortion, the bureaucratic red tape and waiting often required, and the difficulty of traveling to one of the centers where it is offered can all require women to rely upon unsafe illegal abortions. RU486 might eventually provide a lower-cost and more widely available abortion method, thus saving many lives. Where abortion is illegal, the development of a controlled black market in RU486 presents an intriguing possibility. However, given the tight controls on distribution maintained by the manufacturer, that possibility appears remote.

Where safe and affordable surgical abortion is already available, RU486 may be important not so much for the lives it would save (if any), as for the difference it could make to the experience of abortion. RU486 cannot, under any circumstances, be regarded as a comprehensive alternative to surgical abortion, since it can safely be used only up to eight weeks of pregnancy and is not considered safe for all women. Some women will probably continue to prefer vacuum aspiration as a faster and surer method of early abortion. Yet the French experience suggests that, given the choice, a significant proportion of women would strongly prefer this nonsurgical method of early abortion to more invasive surgical methods. If so, that is a powerful argument for proceeding with testing and possible eventual approval of RU486 for use in the United States. Another argument for proceeding is that RU486 is thought by some researchers to have potential value for the treatment of breast cancer and other diseases.

In "Selective Termination in Pregnancy," Christine Overall examines ethical questions raised by the selective destruction of some but not all of the fetuses in a multiple pregnancy. This may be done because there are more fetuses than can be safely brought to term or because one or more have been found to be at risk for a disability—or both reasons may apply. Overall argues that it would be inconsistent to permit ordinary abortion (i.e., termination of pregnancy) while prohibiting women from making decisions about how *many* fetuses will occupy their womb at the same time. She emphasizes, however, that the need for selective termination is in part iatrogenic.

Overall points out that in discussions of selective termination the impression is sometimes given that this is an option that women demand for "selfish" reasons, e.g., not wanting to raise both of a (perfectly healthy) set of twins. In fact, most of the multiple pregnancies in which selective termination is considered involve more than two fetuses and there is usually little chance that all of them could be born alive and healthy and without great risk to the woman's own life and health. Moreover, some of these multiple pregnancies are the result of prior medical interventions, particularly the use of fertility drugs, and the practice in some IVF programs of placing as many as 12 embryos in the uterus at the same time. To reduce the need for selective termination, greater care needs to be taken in the administration of therapies that can cause multiple pregnancies.

Finally, in "How Parents of Affected Children View Selective Abortion," Dorothy Wertz presents an overview of studies of the attitudes of prospective parents toward the abortion of fetuses found to be abnormal and reports on her own study of a group of parents of children with cystic fibrosis. These parents were asked whether they would abort a future pregnancy if the fetus were affected by cystic fibrosis or one of several other conditions. Most of them said that they would abort an otherwise wanted pregnancy only to avoid the birth of a child with *very serious* mental or physical disabilities. Very few would abort because the fetus was of the "wrong" sex, or because of a treatable physical defect, or the prospect of a severe disorder at age 60. On the other hand, over half would abort if the child would be severely mentally retarded and about a third if the degree of mental retardation would be moderate. The women, in particular, gave reasons that reflected a consideration of many complex factors. These included the child's predicted quality of life and their own, effects on other children and family members, effects on the marriage and family finances, and the strength of their own and their spouse's desire to have a child.

Wertz finds some causes for concern in the attitudes of prospective parents toward selective abortion. For one thing, the apparent greater willingness of couples with higher levels of education and income to consider abortion for (certain) fetal abnormalities—in addition to the economic and other obstacles to early prenatal care and testing faced by poor women—creates the danger that certain disabilities will become relatively more common among the children of the poor. Such a trend, as Wertz notes, would not bode well for the opportunities and quality of life of disabled persons in the future.

Wertz also finds it problematic that a significant minority (about 12 percent) of her group would consider abortion if the child would suffer from "severe untreatable obesity." (Obesity, it should be noted, is not a problem that can be prenatally predicted at the present time.) Such a finding might be taken to establish that some parents would abort for relatively minor or predominantly aesthetic reasons. In my view, however, it does not. It is at least as likely that these parents had, or thought they had, reasons for regarding extreme obesity as more than a minor or aesthetic problem.

Be that as it may, Wertz concludes that it is "probably better to allow some parents to make what some would consider 'frivolous' decisions...than to interfere legally and thereby jeopardize the entire structure of patient autonomy." Most of her subjects evidently agree: with the significant exception of sex-selective abortion, the majority favored legal access to abortion even for conditions for which *they* would not consider abortion.

These essays illustrate, in diverse ways, elements that I think have been of central importance in feminist ethical analyses of the new reproductive technologies. Respectful attention is paid to the situations, needs, motivations, and experiences of women who have used or considered using the procedures in question. The moral issues raised by these technologies are considered within their wider medical, social, economic, and political contexts rather than narrowly construed as conflicts between fetal and maternal rights. There is a recognition that new biomedical and reproductive technologies have a dual potential: either to expand individual reproductive freedom, and responsibility or to be used as means or excuses for imposing increasingly harsh controls. Despite the medical and moral uncertainties, each author concludes that women need legally and—to the extent possible—economically unimpeded access to these relatively new abortion-related procedures.

On that point, some feminist critics of reproductive technologies might disagree. Since the advent of prenatal testing and selective abortion, there have been feminist critics who have feared that the detection and elimination of "imperfect" fetuses will become socially if not legally mandatory (e.g., Rothman 1986, 12). Some predict that parents will come to demand more and more "perfect" children, and will thus abort for more and more minor (or merely imagined) fetal defects. Advocates for the disabled worry that the abortion of fetuses with abnormalities such as Down syndrome or spina bifida will lead to a loss of support and concern for persons born with similar disabilities (e.g., Asch 1987). The selective abortion of female fetuses may contribute to further loss of status and rights for women, particularly in nations such as India and China where sex-selective abortion is not uncommon (Warren 1985). Hormonal contraceptives, IVF, and most recently nonsurgical abortion have all been criticized by some feminist analysts as medically risky interventions that may do more to extend the power and wealth of the male-dominated medical profession than to enable women to make authentic decisions about their own reproductive lives.[1]

Sometimes feminists have argued that when women "choose" to make use of such new reproductive technologies, that choice is illusory, shaped not by their own priorities and deliberations but by coercive social pressures and ideologies. Some claim, for instance, that the social pressure upon married women to have children is such that it can be all but impossible for infertile women (i.e., those who can afford high-tech medical care) to say no to innovative techniques such as IVF, regardless of the risks to their own health or the actual efficacy of the treatment (Corea 1985, 169). Similarly, it is said that the social expectation that women will do everything possible to make sure that the children they have are healthy (or male) can make it difficult for women to reject prenatal testing and selective abortion.

I think that it is important to listen to such warnings, coming as they often do from women who have an extensive knowledge of the history of gynecological and obstetric medicine and of the dubious value of many of the treatments offered to women in the past. Nevertheless, I remain convinced that women who have accurate and adequate information, and affordable, legal, voluntary access to a wide range of reproductive technologies, for the most part will make reasonably sound decisions about the use of those technologies—and that in any case they have the right to make those decisions themselves. Of course, mistakes will be made, and some procedures that at first seemed beneficial will turn out on balance not to be. But I see no reason to believe that providing voluntary access to innovative reproductive or abortion-related procedures will inevitably lead to any of the dystopian consequences envisioned by feminist or conservative critics.

Wertz's article, in particular, lends some support to this view. It does not reveal strong tendencies on the part of (these) prospective parents to make decisions about selective abortion on the basis of pernicious eugenic standards. Fewer than half of one percent said they would consider abortion for sex selection. They do not appear to take the attitude that a child is a "product" that ought to be "perfect." Instead they appear to (at least try) to take due account of a wide range of morally relevant factors, not least of which is the potential child's own expected quality of life. Nor do their choices seem dictated by social pressures or internal compulsions to make use of whatever reproductive interventions they might be offered. On the contrary, the diversity of their attitudes toward abortion for various fetal conditions, and the thoughtfulness of the reasons given, strongly suggest that these people were drawing their own conclusions about when abortion would be an appropriate choice for them.

The feminist focus on how women make decisions about abortion—and why it is they who are entitled to make them—will seem question begging to the advocates of fetal rights. Abortion opponents maintain that fetuses are human beings with a right to life from conception onward and that therefore *no one* is entitled even to consider destroying them. But this argument appears compelling only to the extent that it successfully obscures precisely what feminist analysts have insisted upon: women's moral agency.

The claim that fetuses are persons or human beings from conception on is false on straightforward conceptual and empirical grounds (Warren 1973, 1992). Fetuses, particularly in the earlier stages, have none of the emotional, perceptual, social, or mental capacities that make people *people*. They are not yet *beings*, or centers of experience, let alone *persons*, or beings with a degree of social and self-awareness. They are, to be sure, living things that may (or may not) be on the way to becoming people. The decision to end that developmental process has moral significance; but it is radically different from deciding to kill a child or an adult human being.

Yet the fact that fetuses are not people is only half of the moral story. The other half is that women *are* people and that they are not only entitled but morally compelled to play an active role in the shaping of their own reproductive lives (Harding 1984; Whitbeck 1983). It requires an enormous commitment of a woman's self, of her life energy, to transform a zygote or embryo into an infant. She is the only one who can make that commitment—and the only one who can determine whether she *ought* to make it, under the circumstances. To attempt to coerce that commitment by limiting access to abortion is to turn pregnancy and birth into a form of involuntary servitude and to treat women as something less than persons.

The claim that a human being comes into existence at conception not only obscures women's moral agency, but it also erases, in a curious way, women's *biological* role in human reproduction. Aristotle belittled women's reproductive role, holding that only the male's semen contributes form and spirit to the offspring; the woman contributes nothing but (grossly inferior) matter (Aristotle 1943, 103, 175, 191). An analogous belittlement of the significance of pregnancy and birth occurs when abortion opponents insist that the newly fertilized ovum is already a human being, with exactly the same value and rights as a child who has already been born.

The erasure of women and women's agency that occurs in so much moral theorizing about abortion undoubtedly has a great deal to do with the fact that, until quite recently, nearly all of that theorizing was done by men. When women philosophers began to write about abortion, they questioned the presumption that all of the moral issues involving abortion can be settled on the basis of some highly abstract claim about the moral or metaphysical nature of the fetus. They saw at once that one must also consider the pregnant woman, and the situation in which she finds herself (e.g., Thomson 1971). That point remains sound; but now, with the advent of prenatal testing, it is sometimes necessary also to consider the genetic or developmental condition of the fetus(es), and/or how many of them there are.

The ease with which women's agency can still be obscured in debates about abortion adds to the dangers women face in turning to the medical profession for new methods or uses of abortion. For that very reason, I think that feminists need to reject the argument that the possible abuses or misuses of new reproductive technologies are so alarming that individual woman cannot be trusted to make appropriate choices about their use. We need to work for legal and affordable access for all women not only to basic reproductive health care (including abortion), but also to those new abortion-related technologies that have proven medical value and that society can reasonably pay for—and to education and information about all of them. We in the United States urgently need a national health care system to make reproductive and other essential health care universally available. Toward that end, we need patiently to insist upon what should have been clear from the beginning—that women make decisions about abortion not on the basis of whim, or disrespect for human life, but out of compelling need and right.

Notes

1. Various of these reproductive technologies are discussed from critical feminist perspectives in such anthologies as Arditti et al. (1984), Callahan and Callahan (1984), and Stanworth (1987). See also Overall (1987), Spallone (1989), Donchin (1989), and Warren (1988).

References

Arditti, Rita, Renate Klein, and Shelley Minden, eds. 1984. *Test tube women: What future for motherhood?* Boston: Pandora Press.

Aristotle. 1943. *The generation of animals*. Trans. A.L. Peck. Cambridge: Harvard University Press.

Asch, Adrienne. 1987. Can aborting "imperfect" children be immoral? In *Ethical issues in medicine*, ed. John Arras and Nancy Rhoden. Mountain View, Calif.: Mayfield.

Callahan, Sydney, and Daniel Callahan, eds. 1984. *Abortion: Understanding differences*. New York and London: Plenum Press.

Corea, Gena. 1985. *The mother machine: Reproductive technologies from artificial insemination to artificial wombs*. New York: Harper & Row.

Donchin, Anne. 1989. The growing feminist debate over the new reproductive technologies. *Hypatia* 4(3):136–149.

Harding, Sandra. 1984. Beneath the surface of the abortion debate: Are women fully human? In *Abortion: Understanding differences*, ed. Sydney Callahan and Daniel Callahan, 203–224. New York and London: Plenum Press.

Overall, Christine. 1987. *Ethics and human reproduction: A feminist analysis*. Boston: Allen & Unwin.

Rothman, Barbara Katz. 1986. *The tentative pregnancy: Prenatal diagnosis and the future of motherhood*. New York: Viking.

Spallone, Patricia. 1989. *Beyond conception: The new politics of reproduction*. Granby, Mass.: Bergin and Garvey.

Stanworth, Michelle, ed. 1987. *Reproductive technologies: Gender, motherhood and medicine*. Minneapolis: University of Minnesota Press.

Thomson, Judith Jarvis. 1971. A defense of abortion. *Philosophy and Public Affairs* 1(1): 47–66.

Warren, Mary Anne. 1973. On the moral and legal status of abortion. *The Monist* 57(1): 43–61.

Warren, Mary Anne. 1985. *Gendercide: The implications of sex selection*. Totowa, N.J.: Rowman and Allenheld.

Warren, Mary Anne. 1988. IVF and women's interests: An analysis of feminist concerns. *Bioethics* 2(1): 37-57.

Warren, Mary Anne. 1992. The moral significance of birth. In *Feminist perspectives in medical ethics*, ed. Helen Bequaert Holmes and Laura M. Purdy. Bloomington: Indiana University Press.

Whitbeck, Caroline. 1983. The moral implications of regarding women as people: New perspectives on pregnancy and personhood. In *Abortion and the status of the fetus*, ed. William B. Bondeson, H. Tristram Engelhardt, Jr., Stuart F. Spicker, and Daniel H. Winship, 247-272. Dordrecht, Neth.: Reidel.

Chapter 9

INDUCING A MISCARRIAGE: RU486 AND PROSTAGLANDIN FOR EARLY ABORTION

Marge Berer

> When I swallowed the tablets, it seemed as if something was released in my head. I felt as if there were a lump in my heart. But no physical symptoms, or pain. [The next day] my "period" came, just like normal. I continued working as usual. The [next] morning I went back to the clinic to have the prostaglandin pessaries inserted. . . . People looked after me and talked to me. After a few slight contractions I lost some large clots . . . I felt as if I was having a miscarriage, me, on my own, almost naturally. It was different from a normal abortion where someone removes the egg from you.
>
> A week has passed. I am still losing a lot of blood, but I no longer have any symptoms of pregnancy. I feel a bit shaken up, a bit on edge, but I don't find the method aggressive. There is a very difficult moment to go through morally, when you have to take responsibility for swallowing the drug. From then on, you know that you have to go through with it . . . I was lucky. My check-up showed that everything was all right. The whole thing lasted two weeks. In my opinion, it's important that you don't have to wait for weeks with a child in your womb. Because that leaves scars. . . . (I tested . . . 1988)

Throughout known history, women have swallowed many types of substances and inserted others into their uterus in hopes of ending their unwanted pregnancies. Too many of these substances were and are not effective for terminating pregnancy. Those that work are usually toxic and threaten the woman's health and life. Many women have died and continue to die or suffer serious effects from such substances, because access to a safe abortion is denied them.

In the increasing number of countries where abortion is performed safely, up to several generations of women have had abortions using dilatation and curettage (D&C) or vacuum aspiration and, in the case of second trimester abortions, by dilatation and evacuation (D&E). All of these are surgical techniques. The only safe nonsurgical techniques in use until recently have been saline, urea, or prostaglandin for second trimester abortions.

The vast majority of women have come to identify abortion as a surgical experience—whether on an inpatient or outpatient basis, whether with local or general anesthetic, whether in a freestanding clinic, a doctor's office, a hospital, or a back room. Surgery means that the abortion itself is done to them, while they lie still and often asleep until it is over. There will be short-lived pain or cramps, bleeding, perhaps some weakness for a day or two, and then it is over. The majority will have been pregnant for 7 to 12 weeks, and a minority for longer. They will typically make up to three visits to the abortion provider—to arrange the abortion, have counseling, and have a pelvic examination; to have the abortion; and for follow-up. Where facilities are limited or clandestine, counseling, an examination, and/or follow-up may not take place.

A small number of these women will have failed or incomplete abortions and will need to have a repeat procedure of some kind. Some will get infections that require treatment. A very few will have more serious complications, such as cervical damage, perforation of the uterus, or hemorrhage, and will need longer treatment. In clandestine conditions, the numbers of women adversely affected in these ways will be much higher, since a much lower quality of skill and care generally prevails.

In this context, and because new methods of abortion have not come on the scene nearly as often as new methods of contraception, the appearance of RU486 + prostaglandin (PG) as an alternative method of abortion has received a great deal of attention and acclaim. Where surgical abortion is the norm, its widespread use will once more alter women's experience of abortion. One woman described this new experience as having a premeditated miscarriage (Birman 1989).

The term "inducing a miscarriage," once used in criminal law to describe abortion, fell out of use because it was not appropriate as a description of surgical abortion. Today it takes on a new relevance. The major difference from clandestine methods of inducing a miscarriage is that this method is not toxic and works about 96 percent of the time.

It is unfortunate that RU486 + PG is being called a "medical" abortion technique, in order to distinguish it from surgical techniques, when from women's point of view, this method actually demedicalizes the abortion experience in certain ways. A different label would be preferable. Whatever the label, there is no longer much doubt that the combination of RU486 + PG could be introduced safely into clinical practice in many countries.

RU486 was approved in China in September 1988, though it is not generally available there. It has been licensed and available in France since January 1989. A licensing application was made in Britain in September 1990 and was granted in mid-1991. At this writing, the Department of Health has published guidelines, but the method is not in actual use. There are plans to make similar licensing applications in the Netherlands and the Scandinavian countries soon (Baulieu 1990), and this will probably lead to applications in other European countries in the following several years.

Other countries where abortion is legally available, especially those where RU486 + PG has been used in clinical trials, may follow suit. By 1990, clinical trials and/or pilot studies had taken place in France, China, Britain, Cuba, Hong Kong, India, Hungary, Italy, Sweden, Yugoslavia, and Singapore (Oppewal 1990; RU486 continued 1990). Very limited trials were done in the Netherlands and Switzerland. In addition, trials of RU486 alone were done in the United States, USSR, and Spain.

This chapter will describe the RU486 + PG method and how it is used, explore women's experiences with it and how they compare it to surgical abortion, and then look at how its introduction would affect women, taking into account the widely differing conditions under which women currently have abortions internationally.

The Method

RU486 or mifepristone is the generic name of a steroid hormone related in structure to the natural hormone progesterone. It was developed at Roussel Uclaf (a subsidiary of Hoechst Pharmaceuticals) in France. Their brand name for RU486 is Mifegyne. It is most commonly known as "the abortion pill."

Progesterone is necessary to the maintenance of a pregnancy. RU486 works by blocking the effect of progesterone, and this makes it impossible for a pregnancy to develop. RU486 also seems to lead to the production of prostaglandin by the lining of the uterus. As yet no one fully understands how this works (Baird 1990, 12).

Sufficient prostaglandin, whether produced by the body or used in drug form, causes the uterus to contract and to expel the embryo or fetus. The more advanced the pregnancy, the more prostaglandin is needed to do this completely.

RU486 used alone causes the embryo to be expelled without additional prostaglandin in very early pregnancy in the majority of women, but it becomes less effective every day that pregnancy continues. A series of studies has shown that at 38 days of pregnancy RU486 causes a complete abortion about 85 percent of the time. By 42 days of pregnancy it works only 60 percent of the time, and by 60 days of pregnancy, only 40 percent of the time (Van Look & Bygdeman 1989).[1]

Most women are not even sure they are pregnant, much less know if they want an abortion, at a point when RU486 might be worth trying alone. The rapidly rising rate of failure does not justify a policy of using RU486 alone for abortion, when vacuum aspiration at a slightly later stage is safe and almost 100 percent effective. Instead, RU486 may end up being developed as a postcoital method (Baird 1990).

Prostaglandin used alone in early pregnancy also causes an abortion, but the dose and type of prostaglandin needed when it is used by itself leads to more severe side effects than women are willing to tolerate.

However, the combination of RU486 and a small dose of a prostaglandin does provide an effective and tolerable method of abortion, up to eight weeks of pregnancy, for 94–96 percent of the women who use it. Recent research shows that this can be extended to nine weeks of pregnancy.

How the Method Is Used: A Model Clinic

In France, having an early abortion with RU486 + PG at the family planning center at the Hospital Broussais in Paris is as follows (Aubeny 1990a, 1990b). This center, run by Dr. Elizabeth Aubeny, has been in the forefront of RU486 + PG research and use and is one of the most experienced with this method.

First Visit

> A woman requests an abortion, has a pregnancy test, counseling, and a pelvic examination. She is told about alternative abortion methods and can choose RU486 + PG if she is six weeks pregnant or less.

Six weeks is the limit in France because French guidelines currently allow this method only up to seven weeks of pregnancy (although this will probably be extended). French law also requires a period of reflection of one week before any abortion. Gynecologist David Paintin's experience in Britain is that 5–10 percent of women do not go through with an abortion they have arranged. He believes that a waiting period of three to five days should be built into the procedure to allow for this (Paintin 1990). However, it would be unfair if women on the borderline were prevented from using the method because of a reflection period. Flexibility should prevail.

> If RU486 + PG is the woman's choice, she is checked for contraindications to both drugs.

The contraindications to RU486 are blood clotting disorder, chronic adrenal gland failure, long-term corticosteroid therapy, and kidney or liver failure.

The contraindications to PG are asthma, fibroid tumors, a pregnancy with an IUD in place, a cesarean in the previous year, or risk of cardio-vascular disease, including regular cigarette smoking in the past two years in women over age 35.

Psychological contraindications are wanting a one-day method of abortion and not wanting to be involved in the process of abortion (Aubeny 1990a; Baird 1990).

> If there are no contraindications, the woman receives an information leaflet and a consent form.

Second Visit

> The woman returns one week later and signs the consent form. She is given 600mg of RU486 (three tablets) to take by mouth and can leave the clinic. She has addresses where she can go at any time if she needs support or help.

In a few women, bleeding begins within 24 hours, but for most, within 48 hours. Out of 100 women, 3 or 4 will abort completely before the third clinic visit.

Third Visit

> The woman returns to the clinic 36–48 hours later. If she has already completely aborted, no further treatment is needed and she will have to return only for follow-up.
>
> If not, she is given a prostaglandin. She stays at the clinic in an informal lounge area, dressed and able to sit or walk round or lie down if she wishes. An analgesic (not aspirin, as it may reduce effectiveness) is given if required.
>
> Within about four hours, about 9 out of 10 women will have aborted and can leave when they feel ready.

RU486 causes bleeding even if there is not a complete abortion, but it has no secondary side effects. Recent studies suggest that a lower dose than the 600 mg currently being used may be as effective (Van Look 1990).

Prostaglandin can have short-term secondary effects of diarrhea, vomiting, and abdominal pain from uterine contractions. The higher the dose of prostaglandin, the greater these effects tend to be. Women who have never given birth tend to experience more pain than those who have.

During the actual expulsion of the embryo, bleeding is less than that of menstruation or spontaneous miscarriage. The bleeding following the expulsion usually lasts 8 to 15 days and is equivalent to a heavy menstrual period or slightly heavier for most women. Aubeny emphasizes that the bleeding is comparable to that following vacuum aspiration or a few days longer. "However, pilot studies carried out among Chinese women in Hong Kong and Singapore suggest that the blood loss associated with the abortion may be greater than that observed in European women. Further studies are needed to determine whether this is a true or a chance finding, and if true, how important it is" (Van Look 1990).

There is a slight risk of immediate or delayed hemorrhage, as with vacuum aspiration. The Broussais center has never encountered "any significant bleeding" (Aubeny 1990). However, hemorrhage has occurred in other centers, and emergency facilities need to be available, including blood transfusion.

> If the woman has not yet aborted, she can wait longer or leave. If she leaves before the abortion occurs, an ultrasound examination is arranged for three days later to check that complete abortion has taken place.

The need to use ultrasound to check that the abortion is complete may eventually disappear as practitioners become more experienced with this method.

> All RH negative women are given RH antibodies. Contraceptive counseling is given on this or the next visit.
>
> The procedure will not have worked for about 1 in 100 women, and the pregnancy will be in place. For about 3 in 100 women, the pregnancy will have ended but the embryo and/or other products of conception remain in the uterus. In either case, a vacuum aspiration is done within eight days of this visit.

Fourth Visit

> All women return for a checkup 8 to 12 days later. For 96 out of 100 women for whom the abortion was complete, this checkup is to ensure that there are no adverse effects needing treatment.

Unresolved Issues

In France, two types of prostaglandin were in use until 1991. One was sulprestone, in the form of an injection. A dosage of 0.500 mg, 0.375 mg,

0.250 mg, or 0.125 mg was used. The lowest dose of 0.125 mg, which was used in the Broussais center, was only one-quarter of the dose used originally. It was found that side effects with this lower dose were considerably lessened and also that the success rate of the procedure was not affected using this dose (Aubeny 1990a), although a multicenter trial in France showed that it took somewhat longer for the abortion to take place (Silvestre et al. 1990).

Sulprestone was used in France for 85 to 90 percent of women having this type of abortion. An ampule of 0.500 mg was easily divided in half or a quarter and used for two to four women, making it possible to use a lower dose.

Sulprestone was also cheaper than gemeprost, the other type of prostaglandin used. Gemeprost comes in a vaginal pessary with a dose of 1 mg. This dose probably need not be that high, but a pessary cannot be cut into pieces so easily. The manufacturer has shown no interest in producing pessaries with a lower dose. The injection worked faster than the pessary, which made the abortion occur more quickly. On the negative side, side effects are more likely, since there is a peak in circulation almost immediately with the injection, whereas the drug in the pessary is absorbed more slowly.

In April 1991, for the first time, a French woman died of heart failure an hour after having the injection of prostaglandin during this procedure. She was 31, a heavy smoker, and in her thirteenth pregnancy. This woman should never have been permitted to use RU486 + PG, as this method was medically contraindicated for her (Riding 1991). Her death, which need never have happened, serves as a stark reminder that maternal mortality, though rare in Western countries, still occurs and, as in this instance, is often due to medical misjudgment.

Two other French women had previously had cardiac problems, one requiring hospitalization, soon after having the prostaglandin injection following RU486. Both were over 35 and regular smokers. After this happened, the clinic at the Broussais hospital decided not to allow women smokers over age 35 to use the method.

French guidelines have now been amended similarly. In addition, the guidelines recommend that younger smokers not smoke several days before and during the procedure. Although one death in 60,000 uses is a very low figure, it occurred. Clearly, the use of prostaglandin needs monitoring, and as low a dose as possible should be used.

Sulprestone is no longer the prostaglandin of choice for use in this procedure in France, but the higher dose of PG with the pessary also remains a problem. In Britain, the pessary is the only PG that will be used for the moment. Researchers are now looking into the alternative of using an oral prostaglandin. Ironically, an oral PG (brand name Cytotec), which is available over the counter in Brazil as an anti-ulcer drug, is being clandestinely used by many Brazilian women as an abortifacient. Trials with this form of PG have been started to determine whether it can safely replace the other two PGs with RU486. This may, in turn, influence pessary manufacturers to reduce the dose in the pessary. The situation remains fluid at this writing.

Meanwhile, researchers are also still working out the lowest optimum dose of RU486 that can be used with the prostaglandin in this combined method.

Possible Long-Term Effects

It is too early for any possible long-term adverse effects of this method in women to have been assessed.

One question that apparently has not even been asked by research is whether RU486 and/or prostaglandin might have any adverse effects for women with HIV/AIDS (Carrasco 1991). Since both drugs are given as single doses, it seems unlikely that the natural course of HIV infection would be influenced (Fathalla 1991). Other advantages and disadvantages appear to be the same.

Studies in rabbits, though not in other animals, have indicated a theoretical risk of fetal abnormality from RU486. Hence, the French consent form says that the woman understands the possibility of fetal abnormality if the procedure fails and the pregnancy is allowed to continue. As a condition of their participation, during clinical trials women had to agree to vacuum aspiration if the drugs failed. Since the drug came on the market, only a few women have taken the RU486 with or without the PG, have not aborted, and have continued their pregnancies to term. Their babies have been fine. Further information on this issue is still needed but will take time to gather because so few babies fall into this category.

Advantages and Disadvantages of RU486 + PG as Women Have Experienced It in France

Advantages

1. Many women feel the abortion is more under their control, and they find this important. It is the woman who takes the drugs, and her body makes the abortion happen. No one else does the abortion for her. The role of medical staff is reduced to giving her the drugs, monitoring her progress, and giving her support. This is the "demedicalization" women experience with this method.

2. For the 96 percent of women who have a complete abortion with this method, the invasiveness of a surgical method, even of a simple method like vacuum aspiration, is eliminated. Women who prefer this method name this as an important issue for them psychologically and physically. Medically, the chance of infection may be reduced, and cervical or uterine damage that can be caused by instruments is eliminated.
3. No anesthetic is needed, so the after effects and the risks of anesthetic are eliminated. Analgesics are almost always enough to deal with pain from contractions with the lower dose of PG.
4. Most practitioners prefer not to do vacuum aspiration until after seven weeks of pregnancy. With RU486 + PG, the pregnancy can be terminated earlier.[2] This reduces the period of time the woman is actually pregnant and therefore how long she is anxious and upset at having an unwanted pregnancy.
5. Because the abortion occurs over a period of several days, the woman has time to disengage herself emotionally from the pregnancy as it ends.

Disadvantages

1. Some women prefer to have the abortion done for them as quickly as possible, and even to be asleep while it is happening. They dislike the various delays and the feeling of being more in control with this method. A vacuum aspiration is preferable for these women.
2. The time limit of eight to nine weeks of pregnancy means that women who do not recognize early enough that they are pregnant, or cannot decide quickly enough whether they definitely want an abortion, will not be able to use this method.
3. The procedure involves at least one more clinic visit than vacuum aspiration. Extra clinic visits can be a problem, even if the total time spent at the clinic is similar to that with vacuum aspiration. It complicates child care arrangements and/or taking time off from work.
4. The fact of and the experience of miscarrying, even when it is chosen, are difficult. Waiting for it to happen, from the point when the RU486 tablets are taken, and not knowing when the bleeding will begin, can cause anxiety. Seeing the embryo and blood clots when it does happen can be upsetting. If it happens somewhere where the woman has no privacy, it can create problems.

5. A small number of women may decide in the time between taking the RU486 tablets and having the prostaglandin that they cannot cope with the waiting. Ideally, clinics should be prepared to provide a vacuum aspiration at short notice; in reality, they may not.
6. If the procedure fails or is incomplete, the woman has to have a vacuum aspiration or D&C. A repeat procedure may also be necessary with surgical methods, but much less frequently.

Some of the disadvantages are due to the time lag of 36–48 hours required before using the prostaglandin and the resulting added visit. Getting both drugs at the same time would help to reduce some of the disadvantages. Pharmacologically, the prostaglandin would probably have to be put into a delayed-release injection form. This has been considered but not developed.

Such a change would have its consequences. Would women still want to return to the clinic to abort, for example? Would clinicians or policy makers give them a choice? In fact, such an injection may not be developed, since the injectable form of PG has gone out of favor.

Many of the women who participated in clinical trials with RU486 were initially sent home to abort. When asked about this experience, many said they felt isolated at having to abort alone. Yet some preferred it to happen at home. At present it is standard practice for women to stay in the clinic for the third visit, where any adverse effects can be dealt with immediately and where support is available until the abortion takes place (Aubeny 1990a).

Chantal Birman, a French midwife who has done trials with this method and interviewed women about their experience with it, believes that this method has advantages, as long as the procedure is *socialized* (Birman 1989). By this, she means that being able to have the abortion in a clinic ensures not only that the procedure is safe, but also that it can be provided in a caring and sympathetic way and the experience acknowledged and shared. Consideration could even be given to allowing a woman to have a "support person" with her during the abortion, to enhance this.

Of course, not all clinic doctors/staff are caring and sympathetic. But the shame, fear, guilt, secrecy, and isolation, which are common elements of the clandestine abortion experience, have been vastly reduced with clinic-based abortions.

From this point of view, it would be a major step backward for women to *have* to take this method home and deal with all the negative aspects and emotions alone. On the other hand, some women have considered it an advantage to be able to abort at home with this method. This preference has now been left out of the options, since it is not offered. Given the very low rate of complications, should this be possible? The advantages of demedicalization and increased autonomy felt by women as important with this procedure could be enhanced by such options. However, the 1991 death in France from the effects of prostaglandin will doubtless militate against anyone considering this possibility for some time.

Overall, in 1991, after two years of use in France, about 25 percent of women having abortions chose RU486 + PG over vacuum aspiration. Jany Rademakers, a researcher in the Netherlands, believes that the uptake of the method in the Netherlands may be very low because of the high quality of care available for vacuum aspiration, which is often done there earlier than seven weeks (Rademakers 1989). In Britain, the initial uptake of this method in one clinic was low until information about it had spread, and then it began to increase rapidly (Parsons 1990).

The large majority of French women for whom the method was successful say they have been satisfied with it and would use it again. Many who had also had a surgical abortion said they would choose the nonsurgical method again. Women's preferences in other countries remain to be seen.

Broad Structural Changes for the Inclusion of RU486 + PG in Countries Where Existing Services Are Good

If the method is approved for use, services for RU486 + PG would be added to existing facilities for vacuum aspiration and later abortion methods in countries where these already exist. This ought to entail a complete rethinking about how abortion services as a whole are provided in these national settings.

Certainly, all the bureaucratic obstacles and requirements that would prevent women from getting a very early abortion would have to be eliminated structurally for an RU486 + PG service to be worthwhile. For example, women should be able to contact the clinic directly for an appointment. In Britain, women must currently see their GP (general practitioner) for a referral first. Other delays are caused by having to get consent from parents or from more than one doctor or a committee, delays in getting pregnancy test results, and restrictions on public health information on where to get an abortion. A very early abortion method makes it even more imperative that all of this unnecessary detritus be removed from women's paths. Unfortunately, new technology is rarely sufficient in itself to bring about changes that are essentially political ones. Political campaigns would probably also be needed.

Women should be able to choose the surgical or the nonsurgical method, unless there are specific medical or psychological reasons to rule one of them out. This implies offering both methods in the same clinic. However, cost differentials could become a factor preventing equal access to both methods, and the consequences should be considered when prices and insurance coverage are determined.

There is no good reason why either vacuum aspiration or RU486 + PG services should necessarily be hospital-based, as long as emergency backup is available. But where vacuum aspiration is done in hospitals, the likelihood is that RU486 + PG will be offered there too, making its use more expensive than need be. It would be unfortunate if this were so.

With RU486 + PG, trained GPs or midwives, under the supervision of a gynecologist, could handle first visits, prescribing and administering the drugs, the follow-up visit, and any treatment needed for most side effects. Nursing and counseling staff could handle the rest. In countries where trained nurses or midwives are permitted to do abortions, they could handle the entire procedure.

Hence, this method could be provided in community-based clinics or in freestanding family planning and/or abortion clinics, making it widely and easily accessible.

If RU486 + PG were offered in these clinics, vacuum aspiration abortions should be offered there as well. This implies major changes in the structuring of abortion services in some countries, changes they may not be willing to make.

Once such issues are resolved, in countries where abortion statistics are collected, planning for the extent of services can be quite straightforward. To a large extent, pre-introductory trials can indicate how many women would opt for the method. Even if facilities were hospital-based, the more women who choose RU486 + PG, the more pressure off anesthesiologists' and gynecologists' time. A health service would very likely find that any additional initial expenditure would be offset by savings on these specialists' time, and on anesthetic and surgical procedures (MacKenzie 1990).

Although such services are much more likely to be possible in developed countries, countries like Cuba and China, where good abortion facilities also prevail, should be able to provide these as well.

Provision of RU486 + PG in Countries Where Abortion Services Are Inadequate and Underresourced

Countries like Turkey, Tunisia, India, and some in Eastern Europe will have much greater problems to overcome if they are to offer this method well. As clinical and pre-introductory trials of RU486 + PG move more and more move more and more to such countries, new information and problems to overcome will undoubtedly come to light.

Trying to integrate RU486 + PG into the poor quality of existing abortion services in the "Second World" will perhaps encourage badly needed rethinking about how all these services are offered. As in Third-World countries, the lack of resources for any and all health care will make this a very difficult situation to address.

Some of the more expensive technical requirements that accompany the provision of RU486 + PG are ultrasound for follow-up, deep-freeze facilities for storing some types of prostaglandin, HIV-tested blood supplies, facilities for treating hemorrhage, and procedures for controlling supplies of both drugs to keep them off the black market (Ulmann 1990).

The problem is even more difficult in countries like Turkey, Tunisia, Zambia, and India, where abortion has been legal for some time but where medical facilities are extremely limited and mainly confined to major urban areas, serving only a fraction of the women needing and having abortions. In these circumstances, few resources are being used for vacuum aspiration. To provide RU486 + PG, new services would need to be added at a time of debt crisis, economic recession, and public spending cuts.

In all these countries, if the political and professional will exists, providing this method would cost less than vacuum aspiration and would certainly solve some of the problems of maternal mortality and morbidity from the unsafe abortions that continue to occur because of inadequate services. If the will does not exist, the possibilities remain extremely limited.

Bangladesh permits menstrual regulation (MR) within a few weeks of a missed period, but not abortion as such, and the few existing services are hard pressed to cater to the number of women coming to them. Most women still have no access to a clinic at all, and as many as 30 percent who find their way to a clinic are turned away because their pregnancies are too advanced (Kabir 1991).

Morbidity and deaths from unsafe abortions are high. Would it be better to have a minimal procedure for supplying RU486 + PG to women in these overburdened clinics— and let them go home to take their chances?

Sandra Kabir, director of the Bangladesh Women's Health Coalition, whose clinics provide menstrual regulation, believes not. Women hear about MR facilities almost totally by word of mouth. She believes that if a campaign for RU486 + PG is feasible to encourage women to attend early, then so is a campaign for menstrual regulation. So far no such campaign has taken place. The absence of controversy over abortion probably exists because this anomalous situation has never had much publicity. A public campaign for either method might upset this balance. In addition, given the insufficient facilities for MR, a campaign encouraging women to use RU486 + PG would probably increase demand for both methods dramatically. Clinics could be flooded beyond their capacity to cope, and even larger numbers of women might end up being turned away, in the absence of greatly increased provision (Kabir 1991).

Kabir believes that the infrastructure for introducing RU486 + PG into Bangladesh's health services does not exist.[3] There are problems with provision of all health services in Bangladesh, and those with RU486 + PG would not in any way be unique. In her view, there is little point in adding new techniques, one on top of the other, in an already heavily overburdened service (Kabir 1991).

In India, if women want an abortion in a hospital, they attend without an appointment. If there is a bed, they get it and have the abortion the same day. If not, they have to come back whenever they can and try again. There may be no pelvic examination or medical history taken and no follow-up visit. Although abortion is supposed to be free, payment based on the number of weeks of pregnancy is often demanded by doctors. Not surprisingly, women may prefer to seek a clandestine abortion. Women's health activist and researcher T.K. Sundari believes that "choice" in such circumstances consists of women choosing the "mess" they are most prepared to accept. If women had information about the pros and cons of this new method, and were aware of the conditions under which it would be provided in India, they would know enough to be able to decide whether to use it or not. She thinks women's groups could put their efforts into mass media information campaigns to ensure that women would get this information.

One of the reasons why this method was seen as potentially inappropriate for settings like India is the problem of women having to return for the prostaglandin. Women in the rural women's group with whom Sundari works said that as it is necessary, they would return to the clinic for the PG, but they might not be able to return exactly two days later (Sundari 1991).

Before introduction of this method ought even to be considered, much more information like this from women themselves is crucial.

Where Abortion Is Clandestine/Illegal

Obviously, RU486 will not be approved or imported legally into any country where abortion is illegal. At the moment, because supplies of RU486 are available only under the strictest conditions, in France or for clinical trials, it would be almost impossible for this drug to get onto an international black market.

The extent of parent company Hoechst's unwillingness to let Roussel Uclaf supply RU486 became obvious in 1988 when the company attempted to withdraw its application for approval in France. In 1989 the Italian parliament announced that the government would invite Roussel Uclaf to apply for approval of RU486 in Italy. Roussel decided not to apply on the grounds that the Italian system of drug distribution would make tight control over supplies difficult (*Abortion Review* 1989). Such stringency on the part of a pharmaceutical company is almost unheard of since it results in a reduction in sales and therefore profits. The decision to allow at least one further licensing application in Europe in 1990 implies that Hoechst may slowly be loosening up in response to international encouragement to make this method available. In the long run, such tight controls over supplies would presumably become harder to maintain.

Would RU486 find its way onto the black market in drugs in Third-World countries eventually, where it would be used clandestinely? Because doctors and others providing clandestine abortions might well prefer to give drugs that would allow women to abort at home rather than do a suction abortion or D&C on their own premises, they may be eager to gain access to this method. If they thought women could get hold of it without their participation, this would be even more true, as otherwise it could be seen as competition with their own "services" (Carrasco 1991).

For the many women who are used to taking responsibility for their own abortions, and for those who are used to taking drugs to "bring on their periods," this method would seem more acceptable than a surgical method.

If women themselves got hold of RU486 and/or PG pessaries or injections, it is less likely that they could get them both, get the right doses, know which one to use first, or how much time to leave between the two. Even knowing the effective time limit might not stop practitioners or women from trying it at a later stage of pregnancy for want of an alternative.

Among women whose health is already poor, who might not know whether contraindications to this method apply to them, who might have no way to check whether they had had a complete abortion, who may be anemic, who may have been through more pregnancies, or who might be more prone to heavy bleeding, there would undoubtedly be more complications and deaths than in well-controlled clinical settings. But in the context of clandestine abortion today, where women have access to a range of drugs and procedures that either do not work or that send them to hospital with sepsis, incomplete abortions, hemorrhage, and much worse, this would just be another drug on the circuit. In fact, it would be marginally better, since it would work more often and probably harm or kill fewer women than some methods they currently use, particularly invasive ones.

With maternity hospitals all over the Third World packed with women suffering from complications of unsafe abortion techniques, and with at least 200,000 deaths per year worldwide among those whom the hospitals could not save or never saw, one must ask whether the lesser of two evils is not better. There is no substitute for safe abortion in good conditions, but meanwhile, women are dying.

A *controlled* black market can be an effective political tool. This is essentially what happened in the 1970s in a number of European countries when women and doctors set up an illegal abortion network and then announced publicly that they were doing abortions in defiance of the law. Such subversion pushed governments to legalize abortion in spite of themselves in order to assert political and medical control over de facto practice. In Europe in the 1970s, it was the doctors who had to be convinced to participate. Such subversion could still be tried today in other countries, with surgical abortion.

In order to try something similar using RU486 + PG, the problem would not only be getting doctors to participate, it would be getting the drugs. Roussel (Hoechst) would be unable to supply them legally; some other source would have to be found. This would be impossible, given the strict conditions under which supplies of RU486 are controlled at present. However, women are using the oral PG Cytotec in Brazil, and the practice is likely to spread in other countries where this drug is available on the open market, regardless of the law or the possible adverse effects. The use of RU486, let alone medical supervision, has simply been bypassed out of a greater necessity, making the need to decriminalize abortion all the more cogent.

The Future: Medical Issues

The scientific breakthrough in fertility control that RU486 represents is probably only a first step on the way to future discoveries and more changes.

RU486 has already been found to have many other potential uses. In addition to its possibilities as a postcoital contraceptive method, it has been tried as a pretreatment before first trimester vacuum aspiration abortion and before second trimester prostaglandin abortion.

With RU486 as a pretreatment before first trimester vacuum aspiration, one study found that 35 percent of women needed no mechanical cervical dilatation and the rest needed much less dilatation. If this pretreatment proves to be effective on a wide scale, it may reduce cervical damage in surgical abortion. Significantly less blood loss also occurred during the procedure in this study (Templeton 1990).

With RU486 as a pretreatment before second trimester prostaglandin abortion, the amount of prostaglandin required and the time between induction and abortion were significantly reduced. This in turn meant a reduction in the secondary effects of the prostaglandin for the women. These improvements would be welcome, since this type of abortion is currently a very unpleasant experience for women (Templeton 1990).

In one trial, RU486 was given to women whose babies had died before birth. Use of RU486 alone was sufficient to cause labor and expulsion of the dead baby, and meant that other forms of induction did not have to be used. No significant side effects were noted.

RU486 is also being tested as a possible therapy for such conditions as endometriosis, certain types of breast and other cancers, and certain forms of Cushing's syndrome (Ulmann 1990). Yet research on and possible approval for these varied uses may be held hostage as a result of opposition to its use for abortion.

The Future: Political Issues

As could be expected, antiabortionists have played their usual role in attempting to stop the development, licensing, and distribution of RU486. They have intimidated Hoechst with various forms of harassment, such as threatening to boycott their products, and dubbed this method of abortion "chemical warfare in the womb" in their ongoing propaganda war against women's right to decide whether and when to have children.

Such campaigns have been answered by the feminist abortion rights movement in a number of developed countries. Information and public campaigns by the Reproductive Health Technologies Project in the United States and the Union Suisse pour le Decriminalisation de l'Avortement in Switzerland are only two examples. Doctors and doctors' associations in many countries have also supported further studies and, more recently, licensing and availability of this method. The World Health Organization is sponsoring clinical and premarketing trials in a number of countries; the International Planned Parenthood Federation has also voiced its support.

Feminist opinion about this method diverges, however. A few have gone overboard in calling for this method to be made available to all women immediately, as if there were no problems with it at all. Others are far from convinced they should support its use. This latter group are showing a form of caution that could become dangerously close to being a knee-jerk response to whatever new method of reproductive technology is developed. This response says that we do not know what the long-term effects might be; we do not know if women will be fully informed of risks as well as benefits; we have been told before that a new method was safe for women and it turned out to be dangerous; problems with this method have not yet been solved; there are many reasons why we should not trust researchers or drug companies, let alone directly support them, if we are to maintain an autonomous, critical position.

This response grew out of a period (not so long ago) when we did not know where to find out about clinical trials, had fewer tools for assessing their results, did not hear the views of women participants in trials because no one asked them, and certainly did not have access to researchers to make our opinions as a movement heard. That time is becoming part of the past. We can and do have better access to both information and the researchers who produce it. It is our role to take a critical view. But we do women a disservice if we forget that all of us accept certain disadvantages and less than 100 percent safety and efficacy in pursuit of what we need and want.

Many members of the medical and research community, especially those who are trying to provide what women need, and those who are more and more open to dialogue with feminists about this, are displaying exactly the vigilance and caution we call for in relation to RU486. They themselves are on the line for supporting a new method of abortion and cannot afford to get it wrong either.

I believe the women's health movement should support and campaign for the introduction of RU486 + PG for early abortion in good conditions as part of the continuing campaign for safe abortion internationally.

At a policy level, approval of RU486 + PG in the United States would make a major difference, because of the influence that the U.S. Food and Drug Administration (FDA) approval has internationally. Given the longstanding antiabortion stance of the government, however, such approval is not imminent. Although the FDA has said that RU486 can be imported for clinical trial purposes, many people think the opposite is true. The American Medical Association, for example, passed a resolution in mid-1990 supporting its use in clinical trials because of this misunderstanding. Some doctors in California even suggested state-level approval in order to bypass the FDA (Hixson 1990). This may be unconstitutional, but it could be a potent political gesture.

For the moment, Europe seems to be the only region where we can expect this method to become available as part of abortion services. Elsewhere, for example in any national campaign for decriminalization of abortion, such as in Latin America, the RU486 + PG method will become one issue among many in the wider campaign for safe abortion and is bound to influence the terms of the debate.

It is quite remarkable that people are discussing "the abortion pill" all over the world, even though it is available in only one country so far and even though the method is actually far from being a simple pill.

> That there are such ramifications is both a consequence of how women are regarded in our society and a reflection of the fierceness of the moral debate about abortion. As Dr. Annie Bureau[4] says, RU486 is not a revolution, but in moving abortion from a surgical to a medical procedure, it could well be the first step along the path towards a future in which a woman can pop along to her local chemist for a completely safe early abortion pill. The "real" revolution will have happened when that news is greeted by universal rejoicing (Lloyd 1991).

Notes

1. Pregnancy in this paper is defined as starting from the first day of the last menstrual period. Thus, 38 days of pregnancy is about a week or 10 days after the date a woman's period is due, if she is regular.
2. Details of a comparison between RU486 + PG and vacuum aspiration can be found in Bureau 1989.
3. For an excellent overview of the conditions for menstrual regulation that prevailed in Bangladesh up to 1988, see Dixon-Mueller 1988.
4. Annie Bureau has done research on and provided RU486 + PG in France.

Acknowledgments

My thanks to the following for editorial and political comments on parts or all of this paper: T.K. Sundari, Sandra Kabir, Renee Holt, Frescia Carrasco. Special thanks to someone who does not wish to be named for many corrections and additions to the medical information. Any errors are the sole responsibility of the author.

References

Abortion Review 1989. No. 33–34.

Aubeny, Elizabeth. 1990a. New perspective for patients: Drug-induced abortion by RU486 and prostaglandins. Paper presented at From Abortion to Contraception: Public Health Approaches to Reducing Unwanted Pregnancy and Abortion through Improved Family Planning Services, 10–13 October, Tblisi, USSR.

Aubeny, Elizabeth. 1990b. Paper presented at RU486: The French Experience, 9–11 July, Washington, D.C., as reported by the Reproductive Health Technologies Project, organizers of the meeting.

Baird, David T. 1990. What it is, how it works and its development. In *The abortion pill: Widening the choice for women*, 11–15. London: Birth Control Trust.

Baulieu, Etienne. 1990. RU486 and the early nineties. Paper presented at From Abortion to Contraception: Public Health Approaches to Reducing Unwanted Pregnancy and Abortion through Improved Family Planning Services, 10–13 October, Tblisi, USSR.

Birman, Chantal. 1989. The experiences of women having an abortion with RU486. Paper included in a press packet on RU486 by the Union Suisse Pour le Decriminalisation de l'Avortement, Switzerland. April. Summarized in English in *WGNRR [Women's Global Network for Reproductive Rights] Newsletter* 31 (Oct.–Dec.):7–9.

Bureau, Annie. 1989. Clinical results of a trial with RU486 and a prostaglandin injection (Nalador). Paper included in a press packet on RU486 by the Union Suisse Pour le Decriminalisation de l'Avortement, Switzerland. April. Summarized in English in *WGNRR Newsletter* 31 (Oct.–Dec.):9–10.

Carrasco, Frescia. 1991. Personal communication with the author.

Dixon-Mueller, Ruth. 1988. Innovations in reproductive health care: Menstrual regulation policies and programs in Bangladesh. *Studies in Family Planning* 19(3):129–139.

Fathalla, M.R. 1991. Personal communication with the author.

Hixson, Joseph R. 1990. RU486: California seen as test site. *Medical Tribune* 5 April:21.

I tested the RU486 pill. 1988. *Medecine et Hygiene* 8 Nov.

Kabir, Sandra. 1991. Personal communication with the author.

Lloyd, Ann. 1991. RU ready? *The Guardian* 1 May.

MacKenzie, Ian. 1990. The potential effects on NHS resources. In *The abortion pill: Widening the choice for women*, 41–47. London: Birth Control Trust.

Oppewal, Jolke. 1990. The abortion pill debate. *Midweek* 18 July:31.

Paintin, David. 1990. The organisation of the use of mifepristone for pregnancy termination. In *The abortion pill: Widening the choice for women*, 36–40. London: Birth Control Trust.

Parsons, Tony. 1990. The potential for the private sector. In *The abortion pill: Widening the choice for women*, 48–51. London: Birth Control Trust.

Rademakers, Jany. 1989. Personal communication with the author.

Riding, Alan. 1991. Frenchwoman's death tied to use of abortion pill. *New York Times* 10 April: A4, A10.

RU486 continued. 1990. *Abortion Research Notes* 19(3–4):5.

Silvestre, Louise, Catherine Dubois, Naguy Renault, et al. 1990. Voluntary interruption of pregnancy with mifepristone (RU486) and a prostaglandin analogue: A large-scale French experience. *New England Journal of Medicine* 322(10):645–648.

Sundari, T.K. 1991. Personal communication with the author.

Templeton, Allan. 1990. How women respond to mifepristone: Results of the clinical trials. In *The abortion pill: Widening the choice for women*, 22–28. London: The Birth Control Trust.

Ulmann, Andre. 1990. RU486: Present and future uses. Paper presented at From Abortion to Contraception: Public Health Approaches to Reducing Unwanted Pregnancy and Abortion through Improved Family Planning Services, 10–13 October, Tblisi, USSR.

Van Look, Paul. 1990. The use of RU486 (mifepristone) as a medical abortifacient: Current and future research needs. Paper presented at Seminar on RU486: The Abortion Pill. Wemos Women and Pharmaceuticals Project, April.

Van Look, Paul, and M. Bygdeman. 1989. Anti-progestational steroids: A new dimension in human fertility regulation. In *Oxford Review of Reproductive Biology II*, ed. S.R. Milligan, 1–60. Oxford: Oxford University Press.

Chapter 10

SELECTIVE TERMINATION IN PREGNANCY AND WOMEN'S REPRODUCTIVE AUTONOMY

Christine Overall

The recent development of a new technological procedure has added additional questions to debates about women's reproductive self-determination. Variously called "selective termination in pregnancy," "selective reduction of multifetal pregnancy," or "selective fetal reduction," the process is performed during the first or second trimester in some instances of multiple pregnancy, either to eliminate a fetus found through prenatal diagnosis to be handicapped or at risk of a disability, or simply to reduce the number of fetuses in the uterus. More than 200 cases of selective termination are known to have been performed around the world (Lipovenko 1989).

There are several methods of selective termination, all of which first involve ultrasound imaging to locate the target fetus or fetuses. One method is the transcervical aspiration of amniotic fluid and fetal tissue (Berkowitz et al. 1988). Another is the placing of a needle into the fetal thorax until cardiac motion ceases. In the third method, a lethal dose of potassium chloride is injected into the fetal thorax to stop the heart (Evans et al. 1988). In the two latter methods the "terminated" fetus is reabsorbed into the woman's body

This essay first appeared in the May/June 1990 issue of *The Hastings Center Report* and is reprinted by permission.

during the course of pregnancy, and no further surgery is required to remove it from her uterus.

In recent news stories and journal articles some physicians and ethicists have expressed reservations about selective termination, both with respect to its moral justification and with respect to the formation of social policy governing access to and resource allocation for this procedure. Says Abbyann Lynch, former director of the Westminster Institute for Ethics and Human Values in London, Ontario: "It's like saying to a fetus you are good enough to come on the trip but not make the final voyage" (Lipovenko 1989, A4). Margaret Somerville, of the Centre for Medicine, Ethics and Law at McGill University, states:

> With abortion, a woman has the right to control over her own body. Selective reduction is different. Control over the body moves to the right to kill a fetus who is competing with another for space. I have a lot of problems with that (Multiple pregnancies . . . 1989, 3).

Some commentators are worried that the procedure establishes "precedents for infanticide or euthanasia." They are also concerned that it will be unjustifiably used by women pregnant with twins who wish to reduce their pregnancy to a singleton, and they therefore recommend restricting availability of the process to multiple pregnancies of three or more (Evans et al. 1988). In general, according to Walter Hannah, president of the Canadian Society of Obstetricians and Gynecologists, "There's no question there should be national guidelines [for selective pregnancy termination]" (Lipovenko 1989, A4).

Many discussions of selective termination appear to assume that the procedure is primarily a matter of acting against some fetus(es) on behalf of others. For example, Diana Brahams (1987, 1409) describes the issue as follows: "Is it ethical and legally appropriate to carry out a selective reduction of pregnancy—that is, to destroy one or more fetuses in order to give the remaining fetus or fetuses a better chance?" Richard L. Berkowitz et al. (1988, 1046) pose the problem in the following way: "Is it justifiable to lower the number of fetuses in the uterus in order to reduce an unspecified risk to all the fetuses?" Similarly, in their report on four selective pregnancy terminations Mark I. Evans et al. (1988) discuss the issue as if the primary choice is the killing or the preservation of the fetuses.

However, this construction of the problem is radically incomplete, since it omits attention to the women—their bodies and their lives—who should be at the center of any discussion of selective termination. In fact, selective termination vividly instantiates many of the central ethical and policy concerns that must be raised about the technological manipulation of women's reproductive capacities. When Margaret Somerville expresses concern about "the right to kill a fetus who is competing with another for space", what she neglects to mention is that the "space" in question is the pregnant woman's uterus.

According to Evans and colleagues (1988, 293), "the ethical issues [of selective termination] are the same in multiple pregnancies whether the cause is spontaneous conception or infertility treatment." Such a claim is typical of many discussions in contemporary bioethics; they abstract specific moral and social problems from the cultural context that produced them. But the issue of selective termination of pregnancy vividly demonstrates the necessity of examining the social and political environment in which issues in biomedical ethics arise.

Selective termination itself must be understood and evaluated with reference to its own particular context. The apparent need or demand for selective termination in fact is created and elaborated in response to prior technological interventions in women's reproductive processes, themselves the result of prevailing cultural interpretations of infertility.

Hence, it is essential to explore the significance of selective termination for women's reproductive autonomy. The issue acquires added urgency at this point in both Canada and the United States when abortion access and allocation are the focus of renewed controversy. Although not precisely the same as abortion, selective termination is similar insofar as in both cases one or more fetuses are destroyed. The difference is that in abortion pregnancy ends, whereas in selective termination, ideally, the pregnancy continues, with one or more fetuses still present. I will argue that, provided a permissive abortion policy is justified (that is, a policy that allows abortion until the end of the second trimester), a concern for women's reproductive autonomy precludes any general policy restricting access to selective termination in pregnancy, as well as clinical practices that discriminate on nonmedical grounds as to which women will be permitted to choose the procedure or how many fetuses they must retain.

The "Demand" for Selective Termination

In recent discussions of selective termination, women with multiple pregnancies are often represented as demanding the procedure—sometimes by threatening to abort the entire pregnancy if they are not allowed selective termination. One television interviewer who talked to me about this issue described women as "forcing" doctors to provide the procedure. Similarly, a case study of selective pregnancy termination (Holder & Henifin 1988, 21) presents a "Ms. Q" who is pregnant with triplets and asks her doctor to "terminate" two of the fetuses.

> She says she really wants to have a child and "be a good mother," but doesn't feel capable of caring for more than one child at a time. Even though all three fetuses appear healthy, her preference is to abort all rather than have triplets.

The assumption that individual women "demand" selective termination in pregnancy places all moral responsibility for the procedure on the women themselves. However, neither the multiple pregnancies nor the "demands" for selective termination originated *ex nihilo*. An examination of their sources suggests both that moral responsibility for selective termination cannot rest solely on individual women and that the "demand" for selective termination is not just a straightforward exercise of reproductive freedom.

Deliberate societal and medical responses to the perceived problem of female infertility generate much of the need for selective termination, which is but one result of a complex system of values and beliefs concerning fertility and infertility, maternity, and children. Infertility is not merely a physical condition; it is both interpreted and evaluated within cultural conditions that help to specify the appropriate beliefs about and responses to the condition of being unable to reproduce. According to the prevailing ideology of pronatalism, women must reproduce, men must acquire offspring, and both parents should be biologically related to their offspring. A climate of acquisition and commodification encourages and reinforces the notion of child as possession. Infertility is seen as a problem for which the solution must be acquiring a child of one's own, biologically related to oneself, at almost any emotional, physical, or economic costs (Overall 1987, Chap. 7).

The recent increase in numbers of multiple pregnancies comes largely from two steps taken in the treatment of infertility. The use of fertility drugs to prod women's bodies into ovulating and producing more than one ovum at a time results in an incidence of multiple gestation ranging from 16 to 39 percent (Hobbins 1988). Gamete intrafallopian transfer (GIFT) using several eggs and in vitro fertilization (IVF) with subsequent implantation of several embryos in the woman's uterus to increase the likelihood that the woman will become pregnant may also result in multiple gestation. "Pregnancy rate increments are about 8 percent for each pre-embryo replaced in IVF, giving expected pregnancy rates of 8, 16, 24, and 32 percent for 1, 2, 3, and 4 pre-embryos, respectively" (Selective fetal reduction 1988, 774).

A "try anything" mentality is fostered by the fact that prospective IVF patients are often not adequately informed about the very low clinical success rates ("failure rates" would be a more appropriate term) of the procedure

(Corea & Ince 1987; Ellis 1989). One physician implants as many as twelve embryos after IVF (Brahams 1987), and a woman who sought selective termination after use of a fertility drug was pregnant with octuplets (Evans et al. 1988). Another case reported by Evans and colleagues (1988, 291) dramatically illustrates the potential effects of these treatments: One woman's reproductive history includes three cesarean sections, a tubal ligation, a tuboplasty (after which she remained infertile), in vitro fertilization with subsequent implantation of four embryos, selective termination of two of the fetuses, revelation via ultrasound that one of the remaining twins had "severe oligohydramnios and no evidence of a bladder or kidneys," spontaneous miscarriage of the abnormal twin, and intrauterine death of the remaining fetus.

In a commentary critical of selective termination, Angela Holder (1988, 22) quotes Oscar Wilde's dictum: "In this world, there are only two tragedies. One is not getting what one wants, and the other is getting it." But this begs the question of what is meant by saying that women "want" multiple pregnancy or "want" selective termination in pregnancy. What factors led these women to take infertility drugs and/or to participate in an IVF program? How do they evaluate fertility, pregnancy, motherhood, children? How do they perceive themselves as women, as potential mothers, as infertile, and where do children fit into these visions? To what degree were they adequately informed of the likelihood that they would gestate more than one fetus? Were they provided with support systems to enable them to understand their own reasons and goals for seeking reproductive interventions and to provide assistance throughout the emotionally and physically demanding aspects of the treatment? Barbara Katz Rothman's appraisal of women who abort fetuses with genetic defects has more general applicability (1986, 189):

> They are the victims of a social system that fails to take collective responsibility for the needs of its members, and leaves individual women to make impossible choices. We are spared collective responsibility, because we individualize the problem. We make it the woman's own. She "chooses," and so we owe her nothing.

Uncritical use of the claim that certain women "demand" selective termination implies that they are just selfish, unable to extend their caring to more than one or two infants, particularly if one has a disability. For example, one physician (O'Reilly 1987, 575) speaks dismissively of women who are bothered by the "inconvenience" of a multiple pregnancy. But this interpretation is unjustified. In general, participants in IVF programs are extremely eager for a child. They are encouraged to be self-sacrificing, to be acquiescent in the medical system and in the manipulations the medical system requires their bodies to undergo. As John C. Hobbins notes (1988, 1063), these women "have often already volunteered for innovative treatmei ts and may be desperate to try another." The little evidence so far available suggests (Lorber 1988) that, if anything, these women are, by comparison to their male partners, somewhat passive in regard to the making of reproductive decisions. There is no evidence to suggest that most are not willing to assume the challenges of multiple pregnancy.

An additional cause of multiple pregnancy is the conflicting attitudes toward the embryo and fetus manifested in infertility research and clinical practice. One report suggests that multiple pregnancies resulting from IVF are generated not only because clinicians are driven by the motive to succeed—and implantation of large numbers of embryos appears to offer that prospect—but also because of "intimidation of medical practitioners by critics and authorities who insist that all fertilised eggs or pre-embryos be immediately returned to the patient" (Selective fetal reduction 1988, 774). Such "intimidation" does not, of course, excuse clinicians who may sacrifice their patients' well-being. Nevertheless, conservative beliefs in the necessity and inevitability of procreation and the sacredness and "personhood" of the embryo may contribute to the production of multiple pregnancies.

Thus, the technological "solutions" to some forms of female infertility create an additional problem of female hyperfertility—to which a further technological "solution" of selective termination is then offered. Women's so-called "demand" for selective termination in pregnancy is not a primordial expression of individual need, but a socially constructed response to prior medical interventions.

The debate over access to selective pregnancy termination exemplifies a classic no-win situation for women, in which medical technology generates a solution to a problem itself generated by medical technology—yet women are regarded as immoral for seeking that solution. While women have been, in part, victimized through the use of reproductive interventions that fail to respect and facilitate their reproductive autonomy, they are nevertheless unjustifiably held responsible for their attempts to cope with the outcomes of these interventions in the forms that are made available to them. From this perspective, selective termination is not so much an extension of women's reproductive choice as it is the extension of control over women's reproductive capacity—through the use of fertility drugs, GIFT, and IVF as "solutions" to infertility that often result, when successful, in multiple gestations; through the provision of a technology, selective termination, to respond to multiple gestation that may create much of the same ambivalence for women as is generated by abortion; and, finally, through the installation of limitations on women's access to the procedure.

In decisions about selective termination, women are not simply feckless, selfish, and irresponsible. Nor are they mere victims of their social conditioning and the machinations of the medical and scientific establishments. But they must make their choices in the face of extensive socialization for maternity, a limited range of options, and sometimes inadequate information about outcomes. When women "demand" selective termination in pregnancy, they are attempting to take action in response to a situation not of their own making, in the only way that seems available to them. Hence my argument is not that women are merely helpless victims and therefore must be permitted access to selective termination, but rather that it would be both socially irresponsible and also unjust for a health care system that contributes to the generation of problematic multiple pregnancies to withhold access to a potential, if flawed, response to the situation.

A Grim Option

There is reason to believe that women's attitudes toward selective termination may be similar to their attitudes toward abortion. Although abortion is a solution to the problem of unwanted pregnancy, and the general availability of abortion accords women significant and essential reproductive freedom, it is often an occasion for ambivalence and remains, as Caroline Whitbeck has pointed out, a "grim option" for most women (1984, 251–252). It is not something women straightforwardly seek, in the way that they may seek a rewarding career, supportive friends, healthy children, or freer sexuality; rather it is wanted "only because of a still greater aversion to the only available alternatives.... [W]omen do not want abortions, although under duress they may resort to them." Women who abort are, after all, undergoing a surgical invasion of their bodies, and some may also experience emotional distress (McDonnell 1984, 33–36). Moreover, for some women the death of the fetus can be a source of grief, particularly when the pregnancy is wanted and the abortion is sought because of severe fetal disabilities (Rothman 1986, Chap. 7).

Comparable factors may contribute to women's reservations about selective termination in pregnancy. Those who resort to this procedure surely do not desire the invasion of their uterus, nor do they make it their aim to kill fetuses. In fact, unlike women who request abortions because their pregnancy is unwanted, most of those who seek selective termination are originally pregnant by choice. Such pregnancies are "not only wanted but achieved at great psychological and economic cost after a lengthy struggle with infertility" (Evans et al. 1988, 292).

For such women a procedure that risks the loss of all fetuses, as selective termination does, may be especially troubling. The procedure is still experimental, and its short- and long-term outcomes are largely unknown. Evans et al. (1988, 292) state, "Many more cases will have to be observed to appreciate the true risks of the procedure to both the mother and the remaining fetuses," and Berkowitz et al. (1988, 1046) say, "Although the risks associated with selective reduction are known, the dearth of experience with the procedure to date makes it impossible to assess their likelihood." Evans et al. (1988, 290) add: "[A]ny attempt to reduce the number of fetuses [is] experimental and [can] result in miscarriage, and . . . infection, bleeding, and other unknown risks [are] possible. If successful, the attempt could theoretically damage the remaining fetuses."

Note that "success" in the latter case would be seriously limited, assuming that the pregnant woman's goal is to gestate and subsequently deliver one or more healthy infants. In fact, success in this more plausible sense is fairly low. The success rate for Evans et al. was 50 percent; for Berkowitz et al., 66 2/3 percent. As a consequence, in their study of first trimester selective terminations, Berkowitz et al. (1988, 1046) mention the "psychological difficulty of making the decision [to undergo selective termination]," a difficulty partly resulting from "emotional bonding" with the fetuses after repeated ultrasound examinations.

Thus, women undergoing selective termination, like those undergoing abortion, are choosing a grim option; they are ending the existence of one or more fetuses because the alternatives—aborting all the fetuses (and taking the risk that they will never again succeed in becoming pregnant) or attempting to maintain all the fetuses through pregnancy, delivery, and childrearing—are untenable. Women do not seek selective termination for its own sake, or even simply as a means to an end, but because, as the next section will show, their circumstances and the nature of the pregnancy make any other course of action or inaction unacceptable, morally, medically, or practically.

The Challenges of Multiple Gestation

Why do not women who seek selective termination simply continue their pregnancies? John Woods, a philosopher highly critical of abortion, makes the following claim (1978, 80):

> Pregnancy does not radically impede locomotion, does not necessarily entail a long-term loss of income, does not disrupt a wide range of social and personal relationships, is not a radical and continuous disturbance, is not a socially anomalous condition, and is not an invasion of privacy.

This quotation is extraordinary primarily because of its complete falsity in every clause. As any mother or pregnant woman could explain, pregnancy and its outcome can and do have all of these effects, if not in every case, then in many. Rosalind Hursthouse (1987, 300) remarks, "Most pregnancies and labours call for courage, fortitude and endurance, though most women make light of them—so why are women not praised and admired for going through them?" No matter how much it is taken for granted, the accomplishment of gestating and birthing even one child is an extraordinary event; perhaps even more credit is owed to the woman who births twins or triplets or quadruplets. Rather than setting policy limits on women who are not able or willing to gestate more than one or two fetuses, we should be recognizing and understanding the extraordinary challenges posed by multiple pregnancies.

There are good consequentialist reasons why a woman might choose to reduce the number of fetuses she carries. For the pregnant woman, continuation of a multiple pregnancy means "almost certain preterm delivery, prefaced by early and lengthy hospitalization, higher risks of pregnancy-induced hyptertension, polyhydramnios, severe anemia, preeclampsia, and postpartum blood transfusions" (Evans et al. 1988, 292). Another commentator (Hobbins 1988) describes the risks for the pregnant woman as including preeclampsia, serious postpartum hemorrhage, thrombophlebitis, embolic phenomena, and polyhydramnios. The so-called "minor discomforts" of pregnancy are increased in a multiple pregnancy, and women may suffer severe nausea and vomiting (MacLennan 1989) or become depressed or anxious (Scerbo et al. 1986). There is also an increased likelihood of cesarean delivery, entailing more pain and a longer recovery time after the birth (MacLennan 1989).

Infants born of multiple pregnancy risk "premature delivery, low infant birthweight, birth defects, and problems of infant immaturity, including physical and mental retardation" (Selective fetal reduction 1988, 773). There is a high likelihood that these infants "may be severely impaired or suffer a lengthy, costly process of dying in neonatal intensive care" (Evans et al. 1988, 295). Thus a woman carrying more than one fetus also faces the possibility of becoming a mother to infants who will be seriously physically impaired or will die (MacLennan 1989).

It is also important to count the social costs of bearing several children simultaneously, where the responsibilities, burdens, and lost opportunities occasioned by child rearing fall primarily if not exclusively upon the woman rather than upon her male partner (if any) or more equitably upon the society as a whole—particularly when the infants are disabled. An article on Canada's first set of "test-tube quintuplets" reported that the babies' mother, Mae Collier, changes diapers 50 times a day and goes through 12 liters of milk a day and 150 jars of baby food a week. Her husband works full time outside of the home and "spends much of his spare time building the family's new house" (Stevens 1989, A7).

Moreover, while North American culture is strongly pronatalist, it is simultaneously antichild. One of the most prevalent myths of the West is that North Americans love and spoil their children. In fact, however, a sensitive examination—perhaps from the perspective of a child or a loving parent—of the conditions in which many children grow up puts the lie to this myth (Pogrebin 1983). Children are among the most vulnerable victims of poverty and malnutrition. Subjected to physical and sexual abuse, educated in schools that more often aim for custody and confinement than growth and learning, exploited as opportunities for the mass marketing of useless and sometimes dangerous foods and toys, children, the weakest members of our society, are often the least protected. Children are virtually the last social group in North America for whom discrimination and segregation are routinely countenanced. In many residential areas, businesses, restaurants, hotels, and other "public" places, children are not welcome, and except in preschools and nurseries, there is usually little or no accommodation to their physical needs and capacities.

A society that is simultaneously pronatalist but antichild and only minimally supportive of mothering is unlikely to welcome quintuplets and other multiples—except for their novelty—any more than it welcomes single children. The issue, then, is not just how many fetuses a woman can be required to gestate, but also how many children she can be required to raise and under what sort of societal conditions.

To this argument it is no adequate rejoinder to say that such women should continue their pregnancy and then surrender some but not all of the infants for adoption by eager childless and infertile couples. It is one thing for a woman to have the choice of making this decision after careful thought and with full support throughout the pregnancy and afterward when the infants have been given up. Such a choice may be hard enough. It would be another matter, however, to advocate a policy that would restrict selective termination in such a way that gestating all the fetuses and surrendering some becomes a woman's only option.

First, the presence of each additional fetus places an additional demand on the woman's physical and emotional resources (MacLennan 1989); gestating triplets or quadruplets is not just the same as gestating twins. Second, to compel a woman to continue to gestate fetuses she does not want for the sake of others who do is to treat the woman as a mere breeder, a biological machine for the production of new human beings (Atwood 1985; Corea 1985). Finally, it would be callous indeed to underestimate the emotional turmoil and pain of the woman who must gestate and deliver a baby only to surrender it to others. In the case of a multiple gestation, an added distress would arise because of the necessity of somehow choosing which infant(s) to keep and which to give up.

For women who seek selective termination, then, it is both the physical stress of large multiple pregnancies and the social conditions for rearing several infants simultaneously that can contribute to making the continued gestation of all their fetuses an untenable possibility.

Reproductive Rights

Within the existing social context, therefore, access to selective termination must be understood as an essential component of women's reproductive rights. But in staking reproductive rights claims it is important to distinguish between the right to reproduce and the right not to reproduce. Entitlement to access to selective termination, like entitlement to access to abortion, falls within the right not to reproduce (Overall 1987).

Entitlement to choose how many fetuses to gestate, and of what sort, is in this context a limited and negative one. If women are entitled to choose to end their pregnancies altogether, then they are also entitled to choose how many fetuses and of what sort they will carry. If it is unjustified to deny a woman access to an abortion of all fetuses in her uterus, then it is also unjustified to deny her access to the termination of some of those fetuses. Furthermore, if abortion is legally permitted in cases where the fetus is seriously handicapped, it is inconsistent to refuse to permit the termination of one handicapped fetus in a multiple pregnancy.

One way of understanding abortion as an exercise of the right not to reproduce is to see it as the premature emptying of the uterus or the deliberate termination of the fetus's occupancy of the womb. If a woman has an entitlement to an abortion, that is, to the emptying of her uterus of all of its occupants, then there is no ground to compel her to maintain all the occupants of her uterus if she chooses to retain only some of them. While the risks of multiple pregnancy for both the fetuses and the pregnant woman increase with the number of fetuses involved (MacLennan 1989), it does not follow that restrictions on selective termination for pregnancies with smaller numbers of fetuses would be justified. Legal or medical policy cannot consistently say, "You may choose whether to be pregnant, that is, whether your uterus shall be occupied, but you may not choose how many shall occupy your uterus."

More generally, if abortion of a healthy singleton pregnancy is permitted for any reason, as a matter of the woman's choice, within the first five months or so of pregnancy, it is inconsistent to refuse to permit the termination of one or more healthy fetuses in a multiple pregnancy. To say otherwise is unjustifiably to accord the fetuses a right to occupancy of the woman's uterus. It is to say that two or more human entities, at an extremely immature stage in their development, have the right to use a human person's body. But no embryo or fetus has a right to the use of a pregnant woman's body—any more than any other human being, at whatever stage of development, has a right to use a person's body (Overall 1987; Thomson 1971). The absence of that right is recognized through state-sanctioned access to abortion. Fetuses do not acquire a right, either collectively or individually, to use a woman's uterus simply because there are several of them present simultaneously. If one fetus alone in a singleton pregnancy does not have such a right, there is no reason to give several fetuses together, either individually or jointly, such a right. Even if a woman is willingly and happily pregnant, she does not surrender her entitlement to bodily self-determination, and she does not, specifically, surrender her entitlement to determine how many human entities may occupy her uterus.

Making Changes

Although I defend a social policy that does not set limits on access to selective termination in pregnancy, there can be no denying that the procedure may raise serious moral problems. For example, as some disabled persons themselves have pointed out, there is a special moral significance to the termination of a fetus with a disability such as Down syndrome (Asch 1989; Kaplan 1989; Saxton 1988). The use of prenatal diagnosis followed by abortion or selective termination may have eugenic overtones (Hubbard 1988), when the presupposition is that we can ensure only high-quality babies are born and that "defective" fetuses can be eliminated before birth. The fetus is treated as a product for which "quality control" measures are appropriate. Moreover, since amniocentesis and chorionic villus sampling reveal the sex of offspring, there is also a possibility that selective termination in pregnancy could be used, as abortion already is, to eliminate fetuses of the "wrong" sex—in most cases, that is, those that are female (Holmes & Hoskins 1987; Kishwar 1987; Rowland 1987; Steinbacher & Holmes 1987).

These possibilities are distressing and potentially dangerous to disabled persons of both sexes and to women generally. But the way to deal with these and other moral reservations about selective termination is not to prohibit selective termination or to limit access to it on such grounds as fetal disability or fetal sex choice. Instead, part of the answer is to change the conditions that generate large numbers of embryos and fetuses. For example, since "[m]any of the currently known instances of grand multiple pregnancies should have never happened" (Evans et al. 1988, 296), the administration of fertility drugs to induce ovulation can be carefully monitored (Hobbins 1988), and for IVF and GIFT procedures, more use can be made of the "natural ovulatory cycle" and of cryopreservation of embryos (Selective fetal reduction 1988, 774). The number of eggs implanted through GIFT and the number of embryos implanted after IVF can be limited—not by unilateral decision of the physician, but after careful consultation with the woman about the chances of multiple pregnancy and her attitudes toward it (Brahams 1987). To that end, there is a need for further research on predicting the likelihood of multiple pregnancy (Craft et al. 1988). And, given the experimental nature of selective termination, genuinely informed choice should be mandatory for prospective patients, who need to know both the short- and long-term risks and outcomes of the procedure. Acquiring this information will necessitate the "long-term follow-up of parents and children...to assess the psychological and physical effects of fetal reduction" (Selective fetal reduction 1988, 775). By these means the numbers of selective terminations can be reduced, and the women who seek selective termination can be protected and empowered.

More generally, however, we should carefully reevaluate both the pronatalist ideology and the system of treatments of infertility that constitute the context in which selective termination in pregnancy comes to seem essential. There is also a need to improve social support for parenting and to transform the conditions that make it difficult or impossible to be the mother of triplets, quadruplets, etc., or of a baby with a severe disability. Only through the provision of committed care for children and support for women's self-determination will genuine reproductive freedom and responsibility be attained.

References

Asch, Adrienne. 1989. Reproductive technology and disability. In *Reproductive laws for the 1990s*, ed. Sherrill Cohen and Nadine Taub. Clifton, N.J.: Humana Press.

Atwood, Margaret. 1985. *The handmaid's tale*. Toronto: McClelland and Stewart.

Berkowitz, Richard L., Lauren Lynch, Usha Chitkara, et al. 1988. Selective reduction of multifetal pregnancies in the first trimester. *New England Journal of Medicine* 118(16):1043–1047.

Brahams, Diana. 1987. Assisted reproduction and selective reduction of pregnancy. *Lancet* (8572):1409–1410.

Corea, Gena. 1985. *The mother machine: Reproductive technologies from artificial insemination to artificial wombs*. New York: Harper & Row.

Corea, Gena, and Susan Ince. 1987. Report of a survey of IVF clinics in the U.S. In *Made to order: The myth of reproductive and genetic progress*, ed. Patricia Spallone and Deborah Lynn Steinberg. Oxford: Pergamon Press.

Craft, Ian, Peter Brinsden, Paul Lewis, et al. 1988. Multiple pregnancy, selective reduction, and flexible treatment (letter). *Lancet* (8619):1087.

Ellis, Gary B. 1989. Trends in medically assisted conception. Hearing before the Subcommittee on Regulation, Business Opportunities, and Energy of the Committee on Small Business, House of Representatives, 101st Congress, Washington, D.C., 9 March:246–248.

Evans, Mark I., John C. Fletcher, Evan E. Zador, et al. 1988. Selective first-trimester termination in octuplet and quadruplet pregnancies: Clinical and ethical issues. *Obstetrics and Gynecology* 71(3) pt. 1:289–296.

Hobbins, John C. 1988. Selective reduction—A perinatal necessity? *New England Journal of Medicine* 318(16):1062–1063.

Holder, Angela R., and Mary Sue Henifin. 1988. Case study: Selective termination of pregnancy. *Hastings Center Report* 18(1):21–22.

Holmes, Helen B., and Betty B. Hoskins. 1987. Prenatal and preconception sex choice technologies: A path to femicide? In *Man–made women: How new reproductive technologies affect women*, ed. Gena Corea et al. Bloomington: Indiana University Press.

Hubbard, Ruth. 1988. Eugenics: New tools, old ideas. In *Embryos, ethics, and women's rights: Exploring the new reproductive technologies*, ed. Elaine Hoffman Baruch, Amadeo F. D'Adamo, Jr., and Joni Seager. New York: Haworth Press.

Hursthouse, Rosalind. 1987. *Beginning lives*. Oxford: Basil Blackwell.

Kaplan, Deborah. 1989. Disability rights perspectives on reproductive technologies and public policy. In *Reproductive laws for the 1990s*, ed. Sherrill Cohen and Nadine Taub. Clifton, N.J.: Humana Press.

Kishwar, Madhu. 1987. The continuing deficit of women in India and the impact of amniocentesis. In *Man-made women: How new reproductive technologies affect women*, ed. Gena Corea et al. Bloomington: Indiana University Press.

Lipovenko, Dorothy. 1989. Infertility technology forces people to make life and death choices. *Globe and Mail* 21 January: A4.

Lorber, Judith. 1988. In vitro fertilization and gender politics. In *Embryos, ethics, and women's rights: Exploring the new reproductive technologies*, ed. Elaine Hoffman Baruch, Amadeo F. D'Adamo, Jr., and Joni Seager. New York: Haworth Press.

McDonnell, Kathleen. 1984. *Not an easy choice: A feminist re-examines abortion*. Toronto: Women's Press.

MacLennan, Alastair H. 1989. Multiple gestation: Clinical characteristics and management. In *Maternal-fetal medicine: Principles and practice*, 2nd ed., ed. Robert K. Creasy and Robert Resnick. Philadelphia: Saunders.

Multiple pregnancies create moral dilemma. 1989. *Kingston Whig-Standard* 21 January:3.

O'Reilly, Colum. 1987. Selective reduction in assisted pregnancies (letter). *Lancet* (8558):575.

Overall, Christine. 1987. *Ethics and human reproduction: A feminist analysis*. Boston: Allen & Unwin.

Pogrebin, Letty Cottin. 1983. *Family politics: Love and power on an intimate frontier*. New York: McGraw-Hill.

Rothman, Barbara Katz. 1986. *The tentative pregnancy: Prenatal diagnosis and the future of motherhood*. New York: Viking.

Rowland, Robyn. 1987. Motherhood, patriarchal power, alienation and the issue of "choice" in sex preselection. In *Man-made Women: How new reproductive technologies affect women*, ed. Gena Corea et al. Bloomington: Indiana University Press.

Saxton, Marsha. 1988. Prenatal screening and discriminatory attitudes about disability. In *Embryos, ethics, and women's rights: Exploring the new reproductive technologies*, ed. Elaine Hoffman Baruch, Amadeo F. D'Adamo, Jr., and Joni Seager. New York: Haworth Press.

Scerbo, Jose C., Powan Rattan, and Joan E. Drukker. 1986. Twins and other multiple gestations. In *High-risk pregnancy: A team approach*, ed. Robert A. Knuppel and Joan E. Drukker. Philadelphia: Saunders.

Selective fetal reduction (review article). 1988. *Lancet* (8614):773–775.

Steinbacher, Roberta, and Helen B. Holmes. 1987. Sex choice: survival and sisterhood. In *Man-made women: How new reproductive technologies affect women*, ed. Gena Corea et al. Bloomington: Indiana University Press.

Stevens, Victoria. 1989. Test-tube quints celebrate first birthday. *Toronto Star* 6 February:A7.

Thomson, Judith Jarvis. 1971. A defense of abortion. *Philosophy and Public Affairs* 1:47–66.

Whitbeck, Caroline. 1984. The moral implications of regarding women as people: New perspectives on pregnancy and personhood. In *Abortion and the status of the fetus*, ed. William B. Bondeson, H. Tristram Engelhardt, Jr., Stuart F. Spicker, and Daniel H. Winship. Boston: Reidel.

Woods, John. 1978. *Engineered death: Abortion, suicide, euthanasia and senecide*. Ottawa: University of Ottawa Press.

Chapter 11

HOW PARENTS OF AFFECTED CHILDREN VIEW SELECTIVE ABORTION

Dorothy C. Wertz

Introduction

Between 1972 and 1990 the National Opinion Research Center's yearly General Social Surveys (GSS) reported that about 79 percent of the U.S. population thought that legal abortion should be available "if there is a strong chance of serious defect in the baby" (University of Chicago 1990, 248–249, 277). In 1972, the last year that the survey asked about personal choices, 71 percent said that they themselves would have an abortion if the child would have a serious defect. The GSS did not define "serious defect" for its respondents, nor did it examine acceptance of abortion for particular disorders.

The literature indicates that the vast majority of women choose abortion for the most serious mental and physical conditions but are less willing to abort for less serious conditions. Families who have intimate experience with a disorder, as expressed in a child or other relative, are frequently ambivalent toward selective abortion, regarding it as a rejection of their affected child or relative. Some studies suggest that the majority of parents of affected children do not consider selective abortion acceptable for the disorder in question (Elkins et al. 1986). After reviewing the literature on selective abortion, I shall describe a study of attitudes of parents of children with cystic fibrosis, a common genetic disorder, toward abortion under various circumstances and shall discuss some of the factors that parents weigh in making their decisions.

Prenatal Diagnosis and Screening

Prenatal diagnosis is now available for over 300 genetic conditions. These range from disorders with profound mental retardation and death in infancy (e.g., trisomies 13 and 18, Tay-Sachs) to disorders that usually shorten the life span but do not cause mental or physical disability (e.g., hemophilia) or disorders that cause disastrous mental deterioration but do not begin until middle age (e.g., Huntington disease, Alzheimer disease in some families).

Many people think that by having a prenatal diagnostic "checkup" they can be assured about *everything* that will happen to their child. In other words, they believe that prenatal diagnosis can insure the "perfect" baby. This is not the case. Thousands of disorders, including some fairly common ones such as congenital heart disease, cannot be diagnosed prenatally. Furthermore, although several hundred disorders *can* be diagnosed prenatally, to test for all these would be prohibitively expensive, clinically impossible, and also unwarranted. Most disorders are extremely rare. What standard prenatal diagnosis reveals is (1) whether the fetus has the correct number of chromosomes and (2) whether there is an opening in the neural tube that forms the brain and spinal column. This information will reveal some of the most commonly occurring types of intrauterine birth defects, which are Down syndrome (an extra chromosome 21), sex chromosome abnormalities (extra X or Y chromosome or a missing Y chromosome), anencephaly (missing brain), and spina bifida (a damaged spinal column, with moderate to severe physical disability). Tests for other types of disorders are done only if there is a family history of a particular disease or a risk factor that would increase the likelihood that the parents carry genes for that disease. Thus it is possible to have a standard prenatal test that shows all the chromosomes in good order and still have a baby with Tay-Sachs, cystic fibrosis, or hemophilia, unless specific tests are done for these disorders.

Women over age 35 are at increased risk for Down syndrome and other chromosomal abnormalities. Prenatal diagnosis is part of the medical "standard of care" for these women, meaning that a woman can sue her doctor if the procedure is not offered. Another test that is becoming routine for all pregnant women is a simple maternal blood test (MSAFP) that screens for neural tube defects such as anencephaly and spina bifida. Health departments in several states, and government health departments in other countries, have mounted campaigns to do such screening at low or no cost to the woman.

Some health departments have special screening programs for ethnic groups at high risk for particular disorders, such as African-Americans for sickle cell anemia or Greeks and Italians for thalassemia (a blood disorder). Although all programs are voluntary, some rest on the premise of "informed refusal" rather than "informed consent," meaning that a woman who does not wish to be screened must make a specific request that the test not be done (Holtzman 1989).[1]

Abortion Decisions: A Review of the Literature

Responses to routine screening programs are perhaps the best indications of the general public's views on abortion for fetal defects. Most women accept prenatal screening, if offered at no cost (Frets & Niermeijer 1990; Richwald et al. 1990). In public health screening programs abroad, 60 to 90 percent of pregnant women receive prenatal diagnosis (Cao et al. 1987; Swerts 1987). The most common reason for not having prenatal diagnosis is arrival for prenatal care too late in pregnancy to have an elective abortion. In Britain, only 7 percent of pregnant women now decline testing on moral grounds (Cuckle & Wald 1987). A California study reported a similar figure (Richwald et al. 1990).

Table 11–1 shows the percent of women who have actually chosen abortion for some common genetic disorders after receiving positive results (bad news) from prenatal diagnosis. For the most part, these are women who *do not* have children with genetic disorders. Most chose abortion for severe mental retardation, death in early childhood, or substantial physical disability. For example, among the first 7000 women receiving prenatal diagnosis under a public health program in New York City, 97 percent of those whose fetuses were diagnosed with Down syndrome and two other disorders with even more severe retardation had abortions, and 100 percent whose fetuses were diagnosed with anencephaly or spina bifida had abortions, regardless of race or income (Benn et al. 1985).

In some cases, the cumulative effects have been so great as to reduce dramatically the incidence of some common birth defects. Thus geneticists report a 94 percent decline in births of children with anencephaly in England and Wales between 1964 and 1972 and a 68 percent decline in spina bifida (Cuckle et al. 1989). Geneticists attribute most of this decline to prenatal diagnosis and termination of pregnancy (Carstairs & Cole 1984; Great Britain . . . 1988; Laurence 1985). The longer a screening program has been in place, the greater the acceptance of both prenatal diagnosis and selective abortion. For example, in Scotland the percent of women choosing abortion for spina

TABLE 11–1

Abortion Choices After Prenatal Diagnosis

Disorder	Effects
Chromosome abnormality: trisomy 13, 18 or 21 (Down syndrome)	severe mental retardation; for 13 and 18, death in infancy
Metabolic disorders accompanied by severe mental retardation (e.g. Tay-Sachs)	profound mental retardation; death before age 5
Anencephaly	no higher brain function; brain stem only; death soon after birth
Spina bifida	open spinal column with nerve damage; usually some paraplegia; sometimes mild retardation
Thalassemia	blood disorder usually leading to death by age 20 after increasing pain & disability; found among Greeks, Italians, other Mediterranean people
Sickle cell anemia	blood disorder; decreased life expectancy; painful crises; found in persons of African descent, also some Greeks and South Asians. Prognosis considerably better than for thalassemia
Sex chromosome abnormality (47, XXY; 47, XXX; 47, XXY 45, X; etc.)	various; possible infertility, failure to mature sexually, extremes in height (unusually tall or short), sometimes learning disorders

% choosing abortion	Geographic area	Source
100	Switzerland	Engel & DeLozier-Blanchet 1989
94	U.S.A	Golbus et al. 1979
97	New York City	Benn et al. 1985
73	Atlanta	Priest et al. 1988
79	Maryland	Faden et al. 1987
100	Australia	Rogers & Taylor 1989
close to 100	U.S.A.	President's Commission 1983
100	Wales	Cuckle et al. 1989
100	New York City	Benn et al. 1985
74	Scotland	Ferguson-Smith 1983
close to 100	Wales	Cuckle et al. 1989
100	New York City	Benn et al. 1985
95	Australia	Rogers & Taylor 1989
90	United Kingdom	Modell & Petrou 1988
close to 100	Sardinia	Cao et al. 1987
100	U.S.A.	Pearson et al. 1987
99	Ferrara, Italy	Lalatta & Tognoni 1989
39	U.S.A.	Rowley 1989
54	U.S.A. (NYC)	Driscoll et al. 1987
79	Switzerland	Engel & DeLozier-Blanchet 1989
62	New York City	Benn et al. 1985
38	Denver	Robinson et al. 1989
63	England & Finland	Holmes-Siedle et al. 1987
67	24 published studies	Verp et al. 1988

bifida rose from 21 percent in 1976 to 74 percent in 1985 (Ferguson-Smith 1983; Harris & Wertz 1989).

For thalassemia, a blood disorder that leads to death in adolescence or early adulthood after years of increasing pain and disability, the birth incidence declined by 90 percent in 10 years in the Ferrara region of Italy; only about four families a year did not choose abortion (Lalatta & Tognoni 1989). In Sardinia and in Greek Cypriot communities in England close to 100 percent of women have accepted screening, and about 90 percent with affected fetuses chose abortion (Cao et al. 1987; Modell & Mouzouras 1982; Modell & Petrou 1988).

Although there are no nationwide figures for reductions in birth defects in the United States, a study in metropolitan Atlanta estimates that in 1986 prenatal diagnosis and "genetic elective interruption" led to a 63 percent reduction in births of children with Down syndrome to women over 35 and to a 26 percent reduction in Down syndrome births to women of all ages (Priest et al. 1988).

The President's Commission for the Study of Ethical Problems in Medicine and Biomedical and Behavioral Research (1983, 18–20) has estimated that as a result of screening in Ashkenazi Jewish populations in the United States, the incidence of Tay-Sachs (a disorder that leads to profound mental retardation and death before age five) was reduced from 50–100 births per year in 1970 to about 13 in 1980. Almost all women with Tay-Sachs fetuses have chosen abortion.

Although the primary reason for initiating genetic screening programs is to prevent human suffering, cost-benefit analyses play a role. In order to justify providing free procedures to poor women, public health departments must convince state or federal legislatures that the program will save money (Duster 1990, 67–68). Thus they weigh the cost of lifetime care for an affected child against the cost of detecting the presence of that child in the womb. Cost-benefit analyses usually assume that 100 percent of affected fetuses will be aborted. Such arguments have a similar ring throughout the world. Some examples:

Israel

> The total cost of the program for the detection and prevention of birth defects for the fiscal year 1985/86 was approximately $370,000. . . . Among the interrupted pregnancies there were 37 cases of Down syndrome. The calculated cost of their management was almost $5,000,000 (Chemke & Steinberg 1989, 274–275).

Switzerland

> The cost of thousands of prenatal tests, of which fewer than 2% will result in the detection of abnormalities, is only a fraction of the money that would necessarily be spent if these methods of prenatal detection were not available. . . . The bill for institutionalization of a child in Switzerland is about $4,000 per month, which represents an annual sum of some $48,000; if this figure is multiplied over 30 years (a common lifespan figure in Down syndrome), it easily reaches one-and-a-half million dollars for each individual. In economic terms, then, the sums of money invested to permit this type of prenatal testing are quite justified (Engel & DeLozier-Blanchet 1989, 362).

Denmark

> Prenatal chromosome investigation of women ≥ 35 years of age for Down syndrome alone would give a benefit of around . . . $555,000 per year. Adding the benefit caused by the concomitant diagnosis of other chromosome abnormalities and neural tube defects, prenatal investigations are very attractive from the economic point of view (Therkelsen et al. 1989, 146).

The health policy planners and economists making the above statements clearly expect most women to abort for Down syndrome or spina bifida, and in fact, most do. Parents make their own "cost-benefit" calculations, using social and emotional costs and benefits, and come to the same conclusion as the economists, namely, that prenatal diagnosis and selective abortion offer the "least-lose" options. At least this is so for people who are not already the parents of a disabled child. Most people who have to make decisions about aborting a fetus with mental retardation or physical disability have not experienced, and have no wish to experience, the profound changes in family life that the births of such children occasion.

Many genetic disorders, however, are not accompanied by severe mental retardation or physical disability. For some sex chromosome abnormalities (XYY, XXY, 45,X, XXX, etc.), some of the major disabilities are social: the child may not reach puberty without hormonal treatment, may be infertile, may be too tall or too short, or may have a learning disorder. In these cases, fewer families choose abortion: 62 percent in one U.S. study (Benn et al. 1985), 79 percent in a Swiss study (Engel & DeLozier-Blanchet 1989, 363). The sex chromosome disorders most likely to be aborted involve infertility.[2] These are XXY (Klinefelter syndrome) and 45,X (Turner syndrome) (Verp et al. 1988). Often parents fear that children with these disorders, especially boys, will be homosexual (Robinson et al. 1989). Parents are more accepting of disorders involving possible learning disorders but no sexual dysfunction (XYY or XXX).

TABLE 11–2

Attitudes Toward Abortion Among Families with Members Affected by This Disorder

Disorder	Effects
Cystic fibrosis*	Enzyme deficiency affects lungs and digestive system. Median life expectancy now 26.
Hemophilia A*	"Bleeder's disease" Absence of blood clotting factor requires frequent medical treatment. Risk of HIV from transfusions and blood products
Huntington disease***	Severe mental and motor deterioration ending in death; first symptoms appear at about age 40

* Respondents are parents of affected children.
** Study represents actual decisions after a positive prenatal diagnosis rather than attitudes.
*** Respondents are adult children of affected parents.

Parents of affected children (Elkins et al. 1986) and parents who are themselves affected (Czeizel 1988, 51–53) sometimes regard a disorder as less disabling than do persons with no experience of the disorder. Table 11–2 describes attitudes toward abortion among the parents of affected children. (For Huntington disease, which appears in middle age, the table shows the attitudes of the adult children of affected parents, who may pass the disease on to their own children). A comparison between Tables 11–1 and 11–2 may suggest that people with experience of a genetic disorder in the family are less willing to use selective abortion than are members of the general population. Direct comparison between the tables is misleading, however. Most disorders in Table 11–2 are not comparable in severity to those in Table 11–1. Huntington disease, although severe and incurable, appears only after 40 or more years of healthy, productive life. Cystic fibrosis and hemophilia involve neither mental retardation nor serious limitations on physical activity. Most of the conditions listed in Table 11–1, on the other hand, involve retardation, early death, or profound physical disability.

The two tables are also based on different kinds of studies. Table 11–1 reports the actual behavior of women who have had prenatal diagnosis, while

% who say they would abort	Area	Source
95**	France	Boue et al. 1986
52	Wales	Al-Jader et al. 1990
20	New England	Wertz et al. 1991
42	Belgium	Evers-Kiebooms 1987
65	Belgium	Denayer et al. 1990
46	Australia	Rogers & Taylor 1989
100	U.S.A.	Miller et al. 1987
43	England	Evans & Shaw 1979
40	Scotland	Markova et al. 1984
43	Canada	Markova et al. 1984
71	U.S.A.	Kessler et al. 1987
43	U.S.A.	Markel et al. 1987
33	U.S.A.	Schoenfeld et al. 1984
35	England	Craufurd & Harris 1988
30	U.S.A.	Meissen & Berchek 1987

Table 11–2 (with one exception) reports the *attitudes* of *all* parents at risk, including those who have *not* had prenatal diagnosis. Many parents who object to aborting a fetus with their child's disorder simply do not have prenatal diagnosis. An interest in prenatal diagnosis usually implies a willingness to consider abortion. Studies reporting attitudes of *all* parents usually show less approval of abortion than studies of women who have (1) chosen prenatal diagnosis and (2) found out that they are carrying an affected fetus.

The few studies that make scientifically valid comparisons suggest that for some disorders the parents of affected children are actually more receptive to prenatal diagnosis and selective abortion than are families without affected children. Parents of boys with fragile-X syndrome (moderate to severe retardation) or Duchenne muscular dystrophy (a severe physical disorder that puts the boy in a wheelchair by the age of 12) are more likely to favor abortion than are people with no personal experience of the condition (Beeson & Golbus 1985; Meryash 1989; Meryash & Abuelo 1988). One study found the perceptions of women who had lived with affected children "clear and concrete," full of "intimate detail about the realities of care and the experience of those affected," while the perceptions of women without affected children were "vague and abstract" (Beeson & Golbus 1985, 110).

The demographics of abortion suggest that women with less income and education are less likely to have prenatal diagnosis than women who are better off. Rayna Rapp, in her excellent anthropological studies of genetic counseling among New York City minority groups, observes that about half of minority women do not keep their appointments for counseling or prenatal diagnosis, as compared to 10 percent for white, private patients (Rapp 1988a, 1988b, 1991). She attributes this to failures in communication between hospital (or counselor) and patient, to patients' logistical problems (transportation, babysitting, etc.), and to out-of-pocket costs, rather than to moral objections. Even a small amount of money can be an insurmountable barrier to poor women; in California, a $49 payment for spina bifida screening (which included ultrasound and amniocentesis, if necessary) deterred one-quarter of clinic patients from screening (Richwald et al. 1990).

Some studies have found college-educated, upper-income career women less willing to risk having a disabled child than women with less education and income (Beeson & Golbus 1985; Luker 1984). In Wales, however, neither education nor social class were related to attitudes toward abortion among parents of children with cystic fibrosis (Al-Jader et al. 1990), possibly because of greater acceptance of selective abortion among all social classes in the U.K. than in the U.S.A.

Table 11–1 raises other questions. Thalassemia is a blood disorder affecting mostly whites; sickle cell anemia affects mostly African-Americans. Why are the abortion rates so different? First, thalassemia is a more severe disorder than sickle cell anemia and has fewer treatments. Children suffer more and die earlier. Second, about 60 percent of African-American women (as compared to 20 percent of white women) receive prenatal care too late to have prenatal diagnosis (National Center for Health Statistics 1990). Third, failures in communication occur more frequently in counseling minority women (Rapp 1988a, 1988b, 1991). Fourth, some clinics offer prenatal diagnosis for sickle cell only to women whose partners agree to be tested and who are found to be positive.[3] In about 45 percent of cases, the partners of women who carry the sickle cell gene are unavailable or unwilling to be tested (Rowley et al. 1991).

Long-Term Follow-Up Studies

No one knows how many parents subsequently regret their decisions. The impact of the decision to abort is usually short term. The decision to carry a fetus to term, however, has a permanent impact on the parents' lives. It is easier for parents to conclude that abortion was the "wrong" decision and then to go on with their lives than it is for parents of an affected child to admit that they may have made the wrong decision. There are studies of depression and other "psychological sequelae" of abortion for fetal defects (Blumberg et al. 1975; Donnai et al. 1981) and support groups for families who have made the abortion decision, but there is a lack of long-term studies of families who have carried affected fetuses to term. The possibility of prenatal diagnosis and selective abortion is almost never mentioned in support groups for families with disabled children; it is too threatening to parents who are in the process of coping with a disorder.

The studies described above give a general overview of families' responses in specific situations. In what follows, we examine how the parents of children with a particular genetic disorder, cystic fibrosis, look at abortion for a wide range of conditions and where they place their own child's disorder on the overall spectrum.

A Study of Parents of Children with Cystic Fibrosis

In 1989, we studied the psychosocial factors affecting parents' decisions about using prenatal diagnosis for cystic fibrosis (Wertz et al. 1991). Cystic fibrosis (CF) is the most common recessive disorder (see note 3) affecting white populations, with an incidence of 1 in 2000 to 3000 births. If affects the lungs and digestive system; death usually results from lung collapse, after a period of increasing disability. Improved treatment has extended life expectancy and generally improved quality of life. In 1988, 75 percent of patients survived into their late teens, half reached the age of 26, and about 40 percent reached the age of 30, though few survived to their fifth decade (Boat et al. 1989). Since late 1985, accurate prenatal diagnosis has been possible for families who have a living family member with CF. The availability of this technique has presented parents with the possibility of new and potentially troubling decisions about selective abortion. As part of this larger study, we asked parents of children with CF about attitudes toward abortion in 23 situations, including 12 maternal or family situations and 11 conditions affecting the child. We presented these situations in random order. For each situation and for each of the first two trimesters of pregnancy, respondents were asked to respond "I would have an abortion," or "I would not have an abortion, but it should not be prohibited for others," or "I think abortion should be prohibited by law."

In developing questions, we tried to include situations frequently described in opinion polls (e.g., mother's life, rape, incest) or used as rationales for abortion (e.g., low maternal age, mother's career, financial burden, family completed). In describing characteristics of the potential child, we avoided listing names of specific disorders and instead briefly described the child's condition (e.g., instead of trisomy 18, we indicated "severe mental retardation: child unable to speak or understand"; instead of Tay-Sachs, we indicated a "severe genetic disorder leading to death before age 5"; instead of Huntington disease, we indicated a "severe painful disorder starting at age 40, incurable"). We also included several disorders or susceptibilities that are not presently diagnosable prenatally, such as susceptibility to alcoholism, "severe, incurable disorder at age 60" (Alzheimer disease), and "severe, untreatable obesity," in order to see how many respondents thought these warranted selective abortion. We included obesity because of concerns that, if ever given the opportunity, some parents may make prenatal selections on cosmetic grounds, such as stature or the color of hair, eyes, or skin. In a nation obsessed with thinness, obesity would be one of the first characteristics selected against. In addition to the abortion questions, we included questions about child's health, future expectations for the child, knowledge about new genetic tests, reproductive plans, and the attitudes of spouses and members of the extended family toward abortion for CF.

Starting in January 1989, all 12 CF centers in New England distributed anonymous questionnaires to parents of children enrolled as patients. Parents returned their questionnaires directly to project staff. Of 395 parents asked to participate, 271 (68 percent, 228 families) responded. We spoke with all 120 families who volunteered for interviews and interviewed in depth 17 who were still fertile and at risk for having children with CF. For details of children's health status and sociodemographic background, see Wertz et al. 1991.

The majority of these mostly married, majority Catholic, middle-class white parents supported legal abortion in the first trimester for all of the 23 situations described and for 20 of the 23 in the second trimester (see Figure 1 in Wertz et al. 1991). Substantial minorities (41 to 49 percent) thought second trimester abortion should be legal in the remaining three situations.

Although in all situations fewer supported legal abortion in the second trimester than in the first, the differences were not great, averaging 11 percentage points. If these results are in any way indicative of views of the general population, they should give pause to efforts to ban abortions for specific purposes or for specific fetal conditions. A large percentage of Americans may favor leaving abortion decisions to the woman, even if they themselves would not abort in a particular situation. In our study most would support the right of others to abort, even for their own child's illness.

Parents' ratings of the *personal* acceptability of abortion for fetal characteristics suggest that most would themselves be reluctant to abort unless

Figure 11–1 Abortion for Fetal Characteristics
N=271 [a]

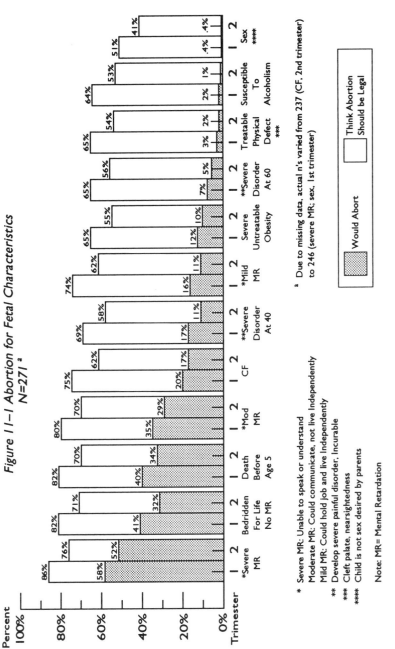

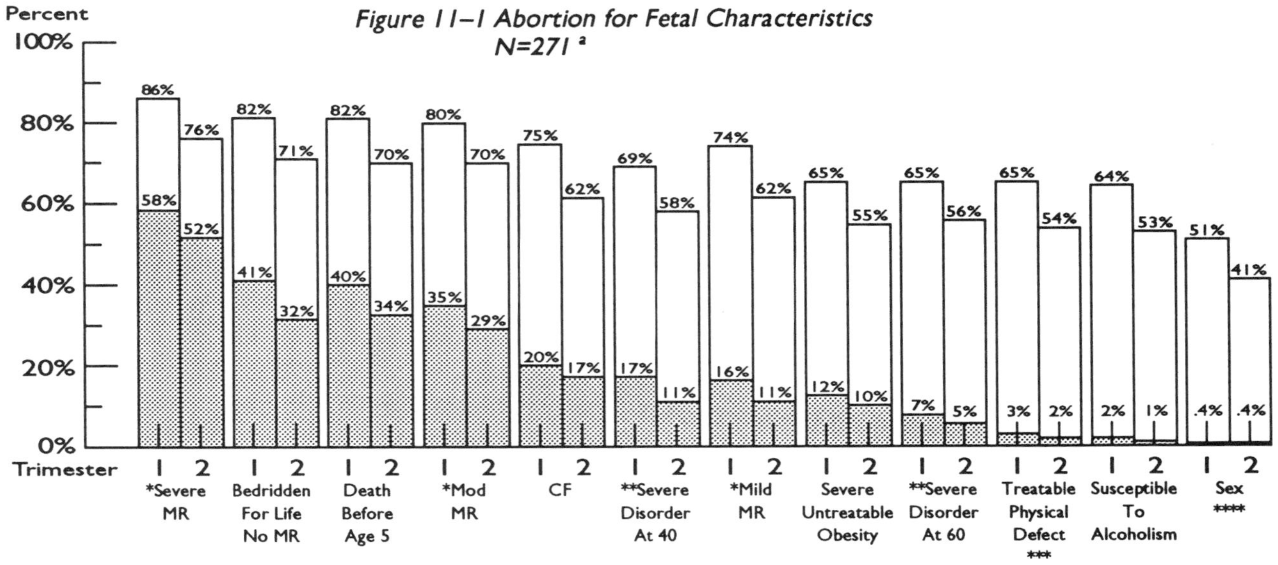

* Severe MR: Unable to speak or understand
Moderate MR: Could communicate, not live Independently
Mild MR: Could hold job and live Independently
** Develop severe painful disorder, Incurable
*** Cleft palate, nearsightedness
**** Child is not sex desired by parents

Note: MR= Mental Retardation

[a] Due to missing data, actual n's varied from 237 (CF, 2nd trimester) to 246 (severe MR; sex, 1st trimester)

Would Abort | Think Abortion Should be Legal

Adapted with permission from the *American Journal of Public Health* 81 No. 8 (1991).

extremely severe mental or physical disability or death in early childhood were involved. Our questions in these areas described the extreme limiting situations ("unable to speak or understand," "bedridden for life"). Figure 11–1 shows a steady gradient of perceived severity. The majority who would abort in a given situation are also included among those who would abort in the situation to the left. Severe mental retardation was the only fetal characteristic for which the majority (58 percent) would themselves abort.

For CF, the condition with which respondents had personal familiarity, 20 percent would abort in the first trimester and 17 percent in the second trimester. In the interviews, many said that after visiting pediatric clinics where they saw retarded children, they were thankful that their child "only had CF." Most were highly optimistic about their child's future and expected the child to live to at least age 40 (the highest age listed on the questionnaire) and to participate in most activities of "normal" life.

CF and thalassemia are comparable in severity and life expectancy. The 20 percent of New England parents who would abort for CF contrasts sharply with the nearly 100 percent of parents who actually do abort for thalassemia (Table 11–1). Perhaps community experience with thalassemia in close-knit southern European groups has led these cultures to condone abortion as an alternative to suffering. Most persons of northern European descent have no personal or cultural experience of CF prior to the birth of an affected child and thus have no community response. Mediterranean Catholicism and Greek Orthodoxy, although opposed to abortion, are perceived by the faithful as more forgiving of sinners than is the Irish Catholicism influential in New England.

Although their overall responses suggest that most parents would not use abortion frivolously, 12 percent would abort for severe obesity. Responses to the obesity question gave us pause. Apparently, there is a not insubstantial minority who would abort for cosmetic purposes if a prenatal assessment were possible.

The trimester of pregnancy had less relationship to personal willingness to abort than might be expected, given the public policy debates over second-trimester abortions. For most fetal conditions, only 5 percent fewer women would abort in the second trimester than in the first. This suggests that newer methods of prenatal diagnosis, such as chorionic villus sampling (CVS), that make first trimester abortions possible may have relatively little effect on deeply held attitudes.

For all maternal/family situations and all fetal characteristics except sex selection, attitudes toward abortion were associated with respondents' perception of the attitudes of spouse, mother, father, and sibs toward abortion of a fetus with CF. The majority thought that their spouses, mothers, fathers, and siblings would disapprove.

Parents' perceptions of the views of their CF doctors toward abortion for CF were among the factors most strongly related to their own attitudes toward abortion for CF. These perceptions may reflect in part the clinically necessary optimism conveyed by many pediatricians in their interactions with parents; we did not survey physicians' personal attitudes toward prenatal diagnosis or abortion for CF.

As we report elsewhere (Wertz et al. 1991), parents with higher education, income, and occupational status were more willing than others to abort. This finding reinforces concerns that differential use of selective abortion by different social groups could lead to discrimination against the disabled.

In all, the results of the study of CF families suggest a wide range of variability among families in terms of what they will accept. This points to the need to protect freedom of choice. The results also suggest that most families who have experienced life with a child made ill, but not retarded or severely disabled, by a genetic disorder are reluctant to abort a fetus with the same disorder. At the same time, as many told us in interviews, they are hesitant to risk conceiving another child with the same disorder. For these families, prenatal diagnosis is not the answer to their quest for a healthy child. They would prefer to wait—for a treatment, a cure, or a reproductive technique that avoids abortion.

The Social Context of Choice

Parents make their decisions, not on the basis of odds or medical information alone, but in a context of perceived social consequences. Our interviews with parents, the experience of genetic counselors, and some published reports have described the major factors affecting their decisions. These include (1) guilt at rejecting their own child with a disablity, (2) the quality of life: self, child, and marriage, (3) "wantedness" of the pregnancy, (4) optimism, (5) spouses and compromises, (6) finances, (7) risk, and (8) other children.

Guilt at Rejecting Their Own Child with a Disability

According to social workers, this is the major reason why parents of disabled children are reluctant to abort. They see abortion of an affected fetus as a rejection of their own, much loved child. "How could I throw away someone as lovable (read delightful, happy, loving, bright, talented, good-looking, depending on the disorder) as you?" Our own study does not support this line of reasoning. Not one parent of a child with cystic fibrosis gave this response, although we tried to elicit it in both questionnaires and interviews. Those who contemplated prenatal diagnosis would simply not tell their children about their plans. Concealing both pregnancy and abortion from the affected child, who is usually very young at the time parents attempt another pregnancy, would be fairly easy. With chorionic villus sampling (CVS) in the first trimester of pregnancy, the whole matter could be concealed even from the family's teenaged children.

Quality of Life: Self, Child, and Marriage

Parental guilt over rejection of their existing child does not seem to be the major factor in decision making. Instead, parents use a complex balance of social, psychological, and moral factors, which they sum up as "the kind of life the child would have" or "what our life would be like"—in other words, quality of life. Women speak of their own quality of life, the family's quality of life, and the child's quality of life as parts of an inseparable train of thought. Usually they mention their own quality of life first, closely followed by considerations about the potential child, the marriage, and the rest of the family. Women often use the word "selfish" to describe what they wish to avoid or to condemn. In women's ethical reasoning, "selfishness" (that is, acting without consideration of others) may well be the worst sin. Some women carry this to extremes; they believe that for a woman to have a space of her own or to do anything for herself is selfish. Many think that if they fail at being "superwomen" or "supermoms" who can cope with any disability, they will be regarded as selfish. Often they preface their decisions with "This may be selfish, but" and then go on to confess that they just could not cope with a child (or another child) who is sick or disabled. Conversely, some use the word "selfish" to condemn women who have made decisions to which they object. One woman, in speaking of an acquaintance who had carried a child with CF to term after prenatal diagnosis, said, "She did that for herself. She didn't think of the child at all. She just wanted another child, and she didn't think about what the child's life would be like." The speaker said that she herself would have prenatal diagnosis in her next pregnancy and would abort a fetus with CF because "it wouldn't be fair to the child to be born with that."

Married women always consider the possible effects of a disabled child on the marriage itself. Some think that they themselves could accept the child, but "this isn't the kind of child my husband wants." This line of reasoning appears most frequently with milder disorders, such as mild retardation, and especially with sex chromosome anomalies where the child will not mature sexually or will be infertile. Men find it more difficult than women to accept a boy who will not turn out to be a "man" according to accepted social definitions. They are somewhat more willing to accept the infertile girl, as long as she appears normal. Faced with this situation, the woman must weigh her belief that she could cope with the child against the fact that she will have to live with a man who may continue to reject the child. Under these circumstances, the child's chance for a normal life and the marriage's chance for survival are greatly diminished. In weighing the alternatives, many women decide to accede to the husband's view in order to protect the best interests of all concerned. These women's moral reasoning is based on a *network* of relationships rather than on the "rights" or interests of individuals (Gilligan 1982). They do not regard their own, the child's, and the family's quality of life as separate entities.

When parents speak of the child's quality of life, their perceptions tend to follow the logic presented in Figure 11–1. Although much disability is "socially constructed" (Asch 1989; Saxton 1984, 1988; Wexler 1989) and could be eliminated or greatly reduced by social changes such as laws guaranteeing fair employment, education, and access to buildings, some conditions are so severe that no amount of social change or social services could guarantee entry into the wider society. Even in the presence of outstanding social services, many parents will have to make considerable personal and financial sacrifices. A child that will die in infancy or early childhood or will be severely retarded is considered not to have had a real chance at life. A child that will be bedridden for life but not retarded gives mothers a peculiar horror. They dread having to care, perpetually, for a sound mind in a disabled body. Women we interviewed said, "I find this really difficult" or "I don't want to think about this." If a disorder is treatable, or occurs only after a period of 40 to 60 years of productive life, most would regard the individual's quality of life as good. Some "disorders" represent a failure to follow current fashion. Parents are reluctant to acknowledge the concept of socially constructed disability. They often describe socially constructed disabilities, such as obesity, in medical terms (higher risk of heart disease, shortened life expectancy) rather than in social terms.

In speaking of a fetus, parents almost never use ethical, legal, or religious terms such as "rights of the fetus," "right to life," "rights of the unborn child," or "personhood." Women feel that the fetus is a *potential* person, however, not merely "a collection of cells that made a mistake" (doctor quoted in Rapp 1988b, 103). Women think in terms of the child that the fetus could become, not only in terms of what it is now. Often they envisage the child over its entire life course. Few, however, seek out and talk with families who have raised such children to adulthood when counselors refer them to such families. Most women, faced with a decision about abortion, wish to make the decision as quickly as possible, even if they are still within the first trimester. They do not wish to delay their decisions by taking time to talk to other families.

As we learn more about the fetus and embryo, and as prenatal diagnosis assigns individual characteristics to fetuses earlier in pregnancy, more women have come to regard the fetus as a potential human being from the beginning of pregnancy (Imber 1990), regardless of their religious belief. Making selective abortion possible in the first trimester of pregnancy does not alter these fundamental beliefs, though it does make the abortion procedure physically easier.

Although religious beliefs play a large part in their decisions, women rarely give religious explanations. They say simply, "I couldn't go through with that [selective abortion]" or "I think God is forgiving." Catholic women who chose abortion may go to confession and may have the aborted fetus baptized (Rapp 1988b, 112–113).

"Wantedness" of the Pregnancy

Perhaps the most important factor after quality of life is the degree to which a pregnancy is "wanted" or "unwanted." Families with unwanted or semiwanted pregnancies usually do not hesitate to abort, even for fairly minor abnormalities. It is as if a positive diagnosis gives them a morally acceptable way out of an undesired situation. Families with wanted pregnancies, on the other hand, find the decision extremely difficult, even for severe abnormalities. Sometimes they have tried for years to achieve this pregnancy or have a history of miscarriages. Even if they have become pregnant without difficulty, abortion means abandoning hopes and dreams for a much-wanted child.

Optimism

Most parents who consider having more children after the birth of a disabled child are coping rather well, simply because the affected child is still quite young and has not yet exhibited major symptoms of the disorder. Even with severe disorders, an infant or small child may appear close to normal. The differences show up later, when the child's age-mates start to mature. Parents of small children, finding that the child seems healthier and more normal appearing than they had expected, and themselves feeling a sense of achievement because they have been able to cope, are frequently optimistic about the child's future. In our CF study the majority of parents thought that their children would reach age 40 (the oldest age listed in the questionnaires), even though few people with CF have lived this long. Most expected their children to live independently, hold full-time jobs, marry, become parents (if boys, through artificial insemination because men with CF are infertile), travel, engage in sports, and do whatever else is associated with "normal" life. In the interviews many said that they expected science to find a cure before their children started to experience severe symptoms. "It would be really hard for me to think about that [abortion] right now. She's doing so well. I know I'll think about it when she's a teenager and maybe starts getting real sick, if they still haven't found a cure" (mother of a four–year-old with CF).

Optimism is pervasive among parents of disabled children. Optimism is part of the "denial" that goes with normal psychological coping mechanisms; parents find it easier to get by from day to day if they believe that the worst symptoms will never appear or that science will find a cure in time. Optimism, much of it unrealistic, accompanies many disorders. For example, one-quarter of adults at risk for Huntington disease think that science will find a cure before they develop symptoms (Kessler et al. 1987), even though no cure is in sight. "Can't you fix it?" is a constant refrain from patients who receive a diagnosis of an affected fetus. Even if every cell in the child's body has an extra chromosome (a situation that most geneticists despair of ever rectifying), parents expect science to find a remedy.

In some cases, however, expectations of cure, or at least treatment, may be realistic. For example, 25 years ago children with CF lived to the age of about 7; now the median life expectancy is 27 and rising. Children with CF often live for long periods—10 years or more—with no symptoms.

Spouses and Compromises

Most people choose spouses with similar underlying values about abortion. Nevertheless, some studies have shown that in a substantial minority of marriages—up to two-fifths—spouses hold somewhat different views about aborting abnormal fetuses (Beeson & Golbus 1985; Sjögren & Uddenborg 1988) or about the burdens of raising an affected child (Sorenson & Wertz 1986). Since men have a certain emotional distance from the pregnancy and do not take primary responsibility for children's daily care, they may find it considerably easier than their wives to decide what should be done. In our study of CF, men tended toward the extremes, either "I would have an abortion" or "abortion should be prohibited by law," while more women preferred the middle ground.

Who compromises when spouses differ? Counselors report that often the woman's views prevail because she is carrying the pregnancy and will later care for the child. On the other hand, sometimes the woman, after considering the effects on the marriage, accedes to the man's view. According to a woman who carried a fetus with CF to term after receiving the diagnosis only a week before the time limit on abortion ran out,

> I wanted to have an abortion. I didn't want to bring a child into the would to see it suffer. But my husband, he was brought up Catholic, though he isn't religious anymore. But he was bothered by the idea of abortion. He said to me, 'How many more times are you going to go through this? ' That really got me thinking, because I knew if I had an abortion I would have to do this again. So I went ahead and had _______, and then I had my tubes tied. If I'd really insisted on it he would have let me have an abortion. I know if I'd had more time [to decide], I would have had an abortion.

This woman, after considering the quality of life with a potentially disgruntled husband, the certainty that she would have to go through prenatal diagnosis on the next pregnancy, the possibility that the next pregnancy might also be affected, and the fact that her previous child with CF was doing well, opted to have a second child with CF. For her, this was the "least-lose" option, there being no real "most-win" options in her situation.

Finances

Financial considerations play a role in most decisions, and are really part of "quality of life." Upper-income as well as lower-income families use cost as a rationale.

> One genetic counselor encountered two patients, each of whom chose to abort a fetus after learning that its status included XXY sex chromosome (Klinefelter's syndrome). One professional couple [said,] "If he can't grow up to have a shot at becoming the President, we don't want him." A low-income family said of the same condition, "A baby will have to face so many problems in this world; it isn't fair to add this one to the burdens he'll have" (Rapp 1992).

On the other hand,

> A Puerto Rican single mother who chose to continue a pregnancy after getting a prenatal diagnosis of Klinefelter's said, "He's normal, he's growing up normal. As long as there's nothing wrong that shows, as long as he's not blind or deaf or crippled, he's normal as far as I'm concerned" (Rapp 1992).

Lower-income women sometimes point out that parent support groups and social activists for disabled children are usually upper middle class. They cannot count on the same level of support for their own disabled children.

> All those groups, those films and stuff, I don't know if that really helps Malik. In fact, it *don't* help Malik. What good does it do to put all those

> fancy white kids on television?... I bet the Reagans, they sit home nights watchin' it. Gives them a good excuse not to worry when they cut the social services back. Those films don't say that the kids got parents who can pay for speech therapists, foot doctors, special computer tapes in their homes. Not my son, why don't they put my son on the television? Then people would see what it's really like (Leila Robertson, mother of a seven–year-old with Down syndrome, quoted in Rapp 1992).

Risk

Risk itself is less important than *what* is risked. For example, many parents find even a small risk of retardation unacceptable.

> We were told of a possible 10% risk of mental retardation in our child; the degree of impairment could not be predicted. We clutched at straws. The baby was moving and growing normally; two ultrasound scans had been normal. Were not these important signs? But then the baby would be physically normal even if mentally retarded. No comfort there....
>
> It seemed crazy that although we had not been prepared to risk a chance of one in 200 of having a child with Down's syndrome we were now in an agony of indecision over a one in 10 risk of mental retardation (When ... risk 1989, 1600).

This family decided upon abortion. On the other hand, a similar risk for a sex chromosome abnormality would have led many families to a different decision (Robinson et al. 1989; Verp et al. 1988).

Other Children

According to some, simply being a *parent* of a normal child makes women less willing to abort, especially a wanted pregnancy (Black & Furlong 1984; Rothman 1986). On the other hand, some women choose to abort an abnormal fetus largely on behalf of their normal children.

> Our first child and her welfare became a major factor in the equation. Not only were we aware of the possible effects on her of having a mentally retarded sibling but also we were continually thankful for her existence. It would have been much worse if it had been our first pregnancy (When risk ... 1989, 1600).

Adult and teenage siblings of affected children are usually quite accepting of prenatal diagnosis and often plan to have it themselves (Miller et al. 1987). Affected children themselves may accept the idea, even though in principle it negates their own existence. In one study, the majority of teenagers and young adults with thalassemia said that they wished their parents had had prenatal diagnosis and selective abortion before their own births, even though they themselves would not have been born (Schiliro et al. 1988).

Reproductive Alternatives

Some families could avoid the abortion decision by adopting or using artificial insemination with a donor. Few do. Adoption has become both difficult and expensive, with an average payment of about $14,000 to agencies, lawyers, and hospitals, that is, if a healthy infant can be found (Caplan 1990). If at all possible, most families prefer to have their own children. As one couple in our cystic fibrosis study put it, "An adopted child wouldn't really be our own."

Many people might favor donor insemination (McCormack et al. 1983) if a "risk-free" donor could be found. Several families in the CF study said that they had considered and rejected donor insemination because at the time it was impossible to be certain that the donor did not carry the gene for CF. Discovery of the gene for CF and development of carrier tests have since made donor insemination a stronger possibility, though current tests leave a small, but real, possibility (perhaps 1 in 650) that the woman could still have a child with CF after insemination.

Another possibility, spontaneously mentioned by several families we interviewed, was IVF and selection of a healthy embryo for implantation. Although we did not ask about reproductive alternatives, a number of couples had read about embryo selection and were enthusiastic. "I'd be willing to go from door to door and take up a collection for [research on] this," said one man whose wife opposed abortion and who had been unable to adopt. No one regarded embryo selection as abortion because there was no pregnancy. They did not see the embryo as a human being and were not concerned about destroying defective embryos. Women clearly regarded pregnancy as a process taking place inside their bodies and abortion as removal of something from *them*. What happened in a petri dish, before implantation in the womb, was another matter entirely. If and when it becomes possible to select embryos free of cystic fibrosis or other disorders, many families at risk will see this as the best alternative, in spite of the high costs and low chances of success of IVF.

Conclusion

Will selective abortion lead to eugenics? Public policy makers, in arguing that prenatal diagnosis be made available to everybody at low cost, expect "terminations of affected pregnancies" and "control" of genetic disorders. Women, on their part, usually expect "good" babies, who are as perfect as possible.

The days of coercive eugenics through public policy are probably over; geneticists fear comparisons with Nazi campaigns to exterminate the retarded. Instead, most say that patients should make whatever decisions are best for them, in the light of their own reproductive goals. Genetic counselors aim to provide information and to be willing to support whatever decisions patients make (Sorenson et al. 1981; Wertz & Fletcher 1988, 1989a, 1989b, 34–35). Since *individuals* rather than governments are making these decisions, they are not considered eugenic. Yet individuals can practice eugenics, perhaps more effectively than governments. Informal social pressure is a very effective measure of coercion. Once tests are offered, to reject them is a rejection of modern faith in science and also a rejection of our belief that we should do everything possible for the health of the future child (Lippman 1991, 27). To bear, knowingly, a less than perfect child affronts the mores of many social circles. The sharp reduction in incidence of certain birth defects, such as Tay-Sachs in the United States and spina bifida in Britain, suggests that families are making what amount to eugenic decisions.

Nevertheless, we are a pluralistic society. Individuals, families, and cultural groups have different thresholds of acceptance for different kinds of disability. Our study of families of children with cystic fibrosis shows wide variation in acceptance of various conditions. What one person could accept, another could not. It is appropriate that the person who will raise the child make the decision, whatever that decision may be. Usually this is the mother. Social workers, doctors, and ethicists should not interfere with parents' decisions, unless they themselves intend to raise the child. (Although carrying the child to term and placing it for adoption is usually a possibility, few women are willing to turn over a "wanted" baby to someone else.) It is probably better to allow some parents to make what some would consider "frivolous" decisions (e.g., aborting a fetus with a treatable defect) than to interfere legally and thereby jeopardize the entire structure of patient autonomy.

In reality, most parents find decisions about selective abortion of a wanted fetus very painful. Their decisions are made in a social context and on the basis of how an affected child would affect their own and their family's quality of life. Practically speaking, it is impossible to separate their own quality of life from the child's quality of life in trying to assess the consequences of having such a child. Most use a "least-lose" pattern of reasoning. Women stand to lose, whatever decision they make. A woman who chooses abortion has to give up the Madonna image of the long-suffering mother who nurtures without conditions; she may instead feel like an "agent of quality control in the reproduction production line" (Rapp 1988b, 115).

On the other hand, a woman who chooses to carry an affected child to term may be "a mother forever," losing out on the new job or career opportunities available to other women and often raising the child without adequate social and financial support. She may also be accused of "selfishness" for bringing the child into the world without thinking of its quality of life.

One answer to this dilemma would be to make more social and financial support available for people with disabilities. Educational programs for children with Down syndrome, for example, have brought out the children's potential and greatly eased the lives of parents. These programs may lead more parents to carry fetuses with Down syndrome to term.

Disability rights activists argue that disability is a social construct and that most disability can be overcome through social change. To an extent this is true; we create problems for people who are far from the "average" by declaring them deviant. Society needs to be more accepting of human diversity. On the other hand, it is parents, not society, who raise the children. Parents should not be expected to bear the burden while waiting for social changes that may never come. And for some disabilities, no amount of social change will be sufficient.

The availability of selective abortion should not divert our attention from care and treatment of persons with disabilities. At the same time, we should not allow disability to became a mark of social class. Tests (and treatments) should be accessible to women of all social groups.

Notes

1. Prenatal diagnosis is mandatory in some cases in the People's Republic of China. Under the "one-child policy," a woman who has given birth to a "defective" child must agree to have prenatal diagnosis in order to obtain an official certificate allowing her to have a second child. Although abortion is not legally mandatory if the prenatal diagnostic results are positive, social pressures will force a woman to terminate the pregnancy. A woman will be "laughed at for her silliness" if she carries an affected fetus to term (Sun 1990).
2. When infertility accompanies a disorder that does not affect the sex chromosomes, it appears to have little effect on parental decisions. For example, boys with cystic fibrosis are always infertile, though otherwise sexually normal. Parents in our CF study did not consider male infertility important.
3. Sickle cell anemia and cystic fibrosis are both Mendelian recessive disorders. This means that in order for the child to be affected, both parents must carry a gene for

the disorder. If both parents carry the gene, each child has a 25 percent chance of being affected. If only one parent carries the gene, none of their children will be affected.

Acknowledgments

The cystic fibrosis study was supported by the New England Regional Genetics Group (NERGG) with funds from the Bureau of Maternal and Child Health Resources Development, D.H.H.S. Janet M. Rosenfield of the Shriver Center for Mental Retardation, Waltham, Mass., and Barbara Thayer of the Prenatal Diagnostic Center, Lexington, Mass., provided valuable insights on families' decision making.

References

Al-Jader, L.N., M.C. Goodchild, and Peter S. Harper. 1990. Attitudes of parents of cystic fibrosis children towards neonatal screening and prenatal diagnosis. *Clinical Genetics* 38:460–465.

Asch, Adrienne. 1989. Reproductive technology and disability. In *Reproductive laws for the 1990s*, ed. Sherrill Cohen and Nadine Taub, 69–128. Clifton, N.J.: Humana Press.

Beeson, Diane, and Mitchell S. Golbus. 1985. Decision making: Whether or not to have prenatal diagnosis and abortion for X-linked conditions. *American Journal of Medical Genetics* 20:107–114.

Benn, Peter A., Lillian Y.F. Hsu, Ann Carlson, and Hody L. Tannenbaum. 1985. The centralized prenatal genetics screening program of New York City III: The first 7,000 cases. *American Journal of Medical Genetics* 20:369–384.

Black, Roberta Beck, and R. Furlong. 1984. Prenatal diagnosis: The experience in families who have children. *American Journal of Medical Genetics* 19:729–739.

Blumberg, B.D., M.S. Golbus, and K.H. Hanson. 1975. The psychological sequelae of abortion performed for a genetic indication. *American Journal of Obstetrics and Gynecology* 122:799–808.

Boat, T.F., M.J. Welsh, and A.L. Beaudet. 1989. Cystic fibrosis. In *The metabolic basis of inherited disease*, 6th ed., Vol. II, ed. Charles F. Scriver, A.L. Beaudet, W.S. Sly, and D. Valle, 2649–2680. New York: McGraw-Hill.

Boue, A., Françoise Muller, C. Nezelof, et al. 1986. Prenatal diagnosis in 200 pregnancies with a 1-in-4 risk of cystic fibrosis. *Human Genetics* 74:288–297.

Cao, Antonio, P. Cossu, G. Monni, and M.C. Rosatelli. 1987. Chorionic villus sampling and acceptance rate of prenatal diagnosis. *Prenatal Diagnosis* 7:531–533.

Caplan, Lincoln. 1990. An open adoption. *New Yorker* 28 May: 73–94.

Carstairs, V., and S. Cole. 1984. Spina bifida and anencephaly in Scotland. *British Medical Journal* 289:1182–1184.

Chemke, Juan, and Avraham Steinberg. 1989. Ethics and medical genetics in Israel. In *Ethics and human genetics: A cross-cultural perspective*, ed. Dorothy C. Wertz and John C. Fletcher, 271–284. Berlin and New York: Springer-Verlag.

Craufurd, David, and Rodney Harris. 1988. Predictive testing for Huntington's disease. *British Medical Journal* 298 (6677):892.

Cuckle, H.S., and Nicholas J. Wald. 1987. Impact of screening for open neural tube defects in England and Wales. *Prenatal Diagnosis* 7:91–99.

Cuckle, H.S., Nicholas J. Wald, and P.M. Cuckle. 1989. Prenatal screening and diagnosis of neural tube defects in England and Wales in 1985. *Prenatal Diagnosis* 9:393–400.

Czeizel, Andrew. 1988. *The right to be born healthy: The ethical problems of human genetics in Hungary*, trans. Catherine Koltoi Bokor and Gabe Bokor. New York: Liss.

Denayer, Lieve, Gerry Evers-Kiebooms, and Herman van den Berghe. 1990. A child with cystic fibrosis: I. Parental knowledge about the genetic transmission of CF and about DNA-diagnostic procedures. *Clinical Genetics* 37:198–206.

Donnai, P., N. Charles, and Rodney Harris. 1981. Attitudes of patients after "genetic" termination of pregnancy. *British Medical Journal* 282:621–622.

Driscoll, M. Catherine, Norma Lerner, Kwame Anyane-Yeboa, et al. 1987. Prenatal diagnosis of sickle hemoglobinopathies: The experience of Columbia University Comprehensive Center for Sickle Cell Disease. *American Journal of Human Genetics* 40:548–558.

Duster, Troy. 1990. *Backdoor to eugenics*. New York and London: Routledge.

Elkins, T.E., T.G. Stovall, S. Wilroy, and J. Dacus. 1986. Attitudes of mothers of children with Down syndrome concerning amniocentesis, abortion, and prenatal genetic counseling techniques. *Obstetrics and Gynecology* 68:181–189.

Engel, Eric, and Celia Dawn DeLozier-Blanchet. 1989. Ethics and medical genetics in Switzerland. In *Ethics and human genetics: A cross-cultural perspective*, ed. Dorothy C. Wertz and John C. Fletcher, 353–379. Berlin and New York: Springer-Verlag.

Evans, D.I.K., and A. Shaw. 1979. Attitudes of hemophilia carriers to fetoscopy and amniocentesis. *Lancet* 2:1371.

Evers-Kiebooms, Gerry. 1987. Decision making in Huntington's disease and cystic fibrosis. *Birth Defects: Original Article Series* 23(2):115–149.

Faden, Ruth R., A. Judith Chwalow, Kimberly Quaid, et al. 1987. Prenatal screening and pregnant women's attitudes toward the abortion of defective fetuses. *American Journal of Public Health* 77(3):288–290.

Ferguson-Smith, Malcolm A. 1983. The reduction of anencephalic and spina bifida births by maternal serum alpha-fetoprotein screening. *British Medical Bulletin* 39(4):365–372.

Frets, Petra G., and Martinus F. Niermeijer. 1990. Reproductive planning after genetic counselling: A perspective from the last decade. *Clinical Genetics* 38:295–306.

Gilligan, Carol. 1982. *In a different voice: Psychological theory and women's development*. Cambridge: Harvard University Press.

Golbus, Mitchell S., W.D. Loughman, C.J. Epstein, et al. 1979. Prenatal diagnosis in 3,000 amniocenteses. *New England Journal of Medicine* 300 (3):157–163.

Great Britain, Northern Regional Health Authority. 1988. *A regional fetal anomaly survey: First progress report*. London: Her Majesty's Stationery Office.

Harris, Rodney, and Dorothy C. Wertz. 1989. Ethics and medical genetics in the United Kingdom. In *Ethics and human genetics: A cross-cultural perspective*, ed. Dorothy C. Wertz and John C. Fletcher, 388–418. Berlin and New York: Springer-Verlag.

Holmes-Siedle, M., M. Ryyanen, and R.H. Lindenbaum. 1987. Parental decisions regarding termination of pregnancy following prenatal detection of sex chromosome abnormality. *Prenatal Diagnosis* 7:239–244.

Holtzman, Neil A. 1989. *Proceed with caution: Predicting genetic risks in the recombinant DNA era*. Baltimore: Johns Hopkins University Press.

Imber, Jonathan B. 1990. Abortion policy and medical practice. *Society* 27(5):27–35.

Kessler, Seymour, Tracy Field, Laura Worth, and Heidi Mosbarger. 1987. Attitudes of persons at risk for Huntington disease toward predictive testing. *American Journal of Medical Genetics* 26:259–270.

Lalatta, Faustina, and Gianni Tognoni. 1989. Ethics and medical genetics in Italy. In *Ethics and human genetics: A cross-cultural perspective*, ed. Dorothy C. Wertz and John C. Fletcher, 285–293. Berlin and New York: Springer-Verlag.

Laurence, K.M. 1985. The apparently declining prevalence of neural tube defect in two counties in South Wales over three decades illustrating the need for continuing action and surveillance. *Zeitschrift für Kinderchirurgie* 40:58–60.

Lippman, Abby. 1991. Prenatal genetic testing and screening: Constructing needs and reinforcing inequities. *American Journal of Law and Medicine* 17:15–50.

Luker, Kristin. 1984. *Abortion and the politics of motherhood*. Berkeley: University of California Press.

McCormack, M.K., S. Leiblum, and A. Lazzarini. 1983. Attitudes regarding utilization of artificial insemination by donor in Huntington disease. *American Journal of Medical Genetics* 14:5–13.

Markel, Dorene S., Anne B. Young, and John B. Penney. 1987. At-risk persons' attitudes toward presymptomatic and prenatal testing of Huntington disease in Michigan. *American Journal of Medical Genetics* 26:295–305.

Markova, Ivana, C.D. Forbes, and M. Inwood. 1984. The consumers' views of genetic counseling for hemophilia. *American Journal of Medical Genetics* 17:741–752.

Meissen, Gregory J., and Roxanna L. Berchek. 1987. Intended use of predictive testing by those at risk for Huntington disease. *American Journal of Medical Genetics* 26:283–293.

Meryash, David L. 1989. Perception of burden among at-risk women of raising a child with the fragile-X syndrome. *Clinical Genetics* 36(1):15–24.

Meryash, David L., and Dianne Abuelo. 1988. Counseling needs and attitudes toward prenatal diagnosis and abortion in fragile-X families. *Clinical Genetics* 33:349–355.

Miller, Connie H., Margaret W. Hilgartner, and Louis M. Aledort. 1987. Reproductive choices in hemophiliac men and carriers. *American Journal of Medical Genetics* 26:591–598.

Modell, Bernadette D., and M. Mouzouras. 1982. Social consequences of introducing antenatal diagnosis for thalassemia. In *Thalassemia: Recent advances in detection and treatment*, ed. Antonio Cao, U. Carcassi, and Peter T. Rowley. *Birth Defects* 19 (7):285–291.

Modell, Bernadette D., and M. Petrou. 1988. Review of control programs and future trends in the United Kingdom. In *Thalassemia: Pathophysiology and management*, Part B, ed. S. Fucharoen, Peter T. Rowley, and N.W. Paul, 422–433. New York: Liss.

National Center for Health Statistics. 1990. *Health: United States, 1989*. Hyattsville, Md.: U.S. Public Health Service.

Pearson, H.A., D.K. Guiliotis, L. Rink, and J.A. Wells. 1987. Patient age distribution in thalassemia major: Changes from 1973 to 1985. *Pediatrics* 80:53–57.

President's Commission for the Study of Ethical Problems in Medicine and Biomedical and Behavioral Research. 1983. *Screening and counseling for genetic conditions*. Washington: U.S. Government Printing Office.

Priest, J.H., P.M. Fernhoff, and L.J. Elsas. 1988. Prenatal diagnosis in metropolitan Atlanta and the impact on autosomal trisomies. *American Journal of Obstetrics and Gynecology* 159(5):1306–1307.

Rapp, Rayna. 1988a. Chromosomes and communication: The discourse of genetic counseling. *Medical Anthropology Quarterly* 2(2):143–157.

Rapp, Rayna. 1988b. The power of "positive" diagnosis: Medical and maternal discourses on amniocentesis. In *Childbirth in America: Anthropological perspectives*, ed. Karen L. Michaelson, 103–116. South Hadley, Mass.: Bergin & Garvey.

Rapp, Rayna. 1991. Constructing amniocentesis: Maternal and medical discourses. In *Negotiating gender in American culture*, ed. Faye Ginsburg and Anna Tsing, 28–42. Boston: Beacon Press.

Rapp, Rayna. 1992. Accounting for amniocentesis. In *Analysis in medical anthropology*, ed. Shirley Lindenbaum and Margaret Lock. Berkeley: University of California Press.

Richwald, Gary A., Robin D. Clark, Barbara F. Crandall, et al. 1990. Cost and acceptance of maternal serum alpha fetoprotein (MSAFP) screening in public prenatal clinics. *American Journal of Human Genetics* 47(3) Suppl: A291.

Robinson, Arthur, Bruce G. Bender, and Mary C. Linden. 1989. Decisions following the intrauterine diagnosis of sex chromosome aneuploidy. *American Journal of Medical Genetics* 34:552–554.

Rogers, John, and Anna Marie Taylor. 1989. Ethics and medical genetics in Australia. In *Ethics and human genetics: A cross-cultural perspective*, ed. Dorothy C. Wertz and John C. Fletcher, 28–42. Berlin and New York: Springer-Verlag.

Rothman, Barbara Katz. 1986. *The tentative pregnancy: Prenatal diagnosis and the future of motherhood*. New York: Viking.

Rowley, Peter T. 1989. Prenatal diagnosis for sickle cell disease: A survey of the United States and Canada. *Annals of the New York Academy of Sciences* 565:48–52.

Rowley, Peter T., Starlene Loader, Carol J. Sutera, Margaret Walden, et al. 1991. Prenatal screening for hemoglobinopathies. I. A prospective regional trial. *American Journal of Human Genetics* 48:439–446.

Saxton, Marsha. 1984. Born and unborn: The implications of reproductive technologies for people with disabilities. In *Test-tube women: What future for motherhood?* ed. Rita Arditti, Renate Duelli Klein, and Shelley Minden, 298–312. Boston: Pandora Press.

Saxton, Marsha. 1988. Prenatal screening and discriminatory attitudes about disability. In *Embryos, ethics, and women's rights: Exploring the new reproductive technologies*, ed. Elaine Hoffman Baruch, Amadeo F. D'Adamo, and Joni Seager, 217–224. New York: Harrington Park Press.

Schiliro, Gino, Maria Antonietta Romeo, and Florindo Mollica. 1988. Prenatal diagnosis of thalassemia: The viewpoint of patients. *Prenatal Diagnosis* 8:231–233.

Schoenfeld, Miriam, Richard H. Myers, Barbara Berkman, and Eleanor Clark. 1984. Potential impact of a predictive test on the gene frequency of Huntington disease. *American Journal of Medical Genetics* 18:423–439.

Sjögren, Berit, and Nils Uddenborg. 1988. Decision making during the prenatal diagnostic procedure. A questionnaire and interview study of 211 women participating in prenatal diagnosis. *Prenatal Diagnosis* 8(4):263–273.

Sorenson, James R., Judith P. Swazey, and Norman A. Scotch. 1981. *Reproductive pasts, reproductive futures: Genetic counselling and its effectiveness*. New York: Liss.

Sorenson, James R., and Dorothy C. Wertz. 1986. Couple agreement before and after genetic counselling. *American Journal of Medical Genetics* 25(3): 549–555.

Sun, Nianhu. 1990. Bioethics in medical genetics in China. Japan Society of Human Genetics, Fukui, 3 August.

Swerts, A. 1987. Impacts of genetic counseling and prenatal diagnosis for Down syndrome and neural tube defects. In *Genetic risk, risk perception and decision making*, ed. G. Evers-Kiebooms, J.J. Cassiman, H. van den Berghe, and G. D'Ydewelle. *Birth Defects* 22 (2):61–83.

Therkelsen, Aage J., Lars Bolund, and Viggo Mortensen. 1989. Ethics and medical genetics in Denmark. In *Ethics and human genetics: A cross-cultural perspective*, ed. Dorothy C. Wertz and John C. Fletcher, 141–155. Berlin and New York: Springer-Verlag.

University of Chicago, National Opinion Research Center. 1990. *General social surveys, 1972–1989 cumulative codebook*. Chicago: The Center.

Verp, M.S., A.T. Bombard, J.L. Simpson, and S. Elias. 1988. Parental decision following prenatal diagnosis of fetal chromosome abnormality. *American Journal of Medical Genetics* 29:613–622.

Wertz, Dorothy C., and John C. Fletcher. 1988. Attitudes of genetic counselors: A multinational survey. *American Journal of Human Genetics* 42(4):592–600.

Wertz, Dorothy C., and John C. Fletcher. 1989a. Ethical problems in prenatal diagnosis: A cross-cultural survey of medical geneticists in 18 nations. *Prenatal Diagnosis* 9:145–157.

Wertz, Dorothy C., and John C. Fletcher, eds. 1989b. *Ethics and human genetics: A cross-cultural perspective*. Berlin and New York: Springer-Verlag.

PART III

CRYOPRESERVATION OF HUMAN EMBRYOS

Chapter 12

TO FREEZE OR NOT TO FREEZE: IS THAT AN OPTION?

Helen Bequaert Holmes

"If I could save time in a bottle. . . "

Jim Croce

Over the centuries humans have yearned to extend their life spans to reach toward immortality. The tale of Rip van Winkle's 100-year sleep illustrates this longing. Recently, science's skill with deep freezing has encouraged research on whole-body freezing. Should this method work, adults could choose to be frozen to be "thawed alive" later, presumably under more congenial social circumstances or when cures for their diseases had been discovered (Ben-Abraham 1989; Vogel 1988). It is, therefore, a bit ironic that cryopreservation of *Homo sapiens* has so far worked only with tiny embryos, with entities that the authors in this section consider not really persons (albeit not really property, either).

The first author in this section, Mina Alikani, senior embryologist at Cornell Medical Center, describes the technical problems that have been partially solved for freezing and then thawing early embryos. Next, Howard W. Jones, Jr., the United States' pioneer of in vitro fertilization, presents explicit policy recommendations to cope with nonmedical problems that have arisen—or are likely to arise—with cryopreservation. Andrea L. Bonnicksen, political scientist, looks with care at the clinical stage on which the freezing drama is played. Thomas C. Shevory, also a political scientist, by focusing on one specific drama (the Davis case in Tennessee) demonstrates that having an already established policy might have alleviated—yet not wholly prevented—courtroom trauma.

The ethical questions that Jones, Bonnicksen, and Shevory raise would also occur should mature adults, not just tiny nonpersons, be cryopreserved. There would still have to be a carefully thought-out prefreeze agreement; the designated next of kin would still be required to make the awesome decision on the appropriate moment to thaw; older siblings might still have fewer candles on their birthday cakes than their younger siblings. As for capacity for informed consent in choosing the moment for thawing, the frozen mature adult would have the same number of functioning brain cells as the frozen four-cell embryo, to wit, zero. Most worrisome in either situation would be the tremendous powers of third parties. Members of the Cryonics Society should be grateful to concerned clinicians like Jones for their ethical groundwork.

An Embryo by Any Other Name . . .

Does it really matter, therefore, what we call the entity that now (if lucky) we can preserve by freezing? Those of us who studied embryology in the 1940s and 1950s learned that once the sperm merged with the egg, the entity was called a zygote: the one-cell stage, the very earliest embryonic stage. Yet may we use the term "zygote" with humans? After entering an egg, a sperm nucleus swells into a sphere, the "pronucleus" next to the egg's pronucleus—fun to see in frog eggs under student microscopes. But, as Jones points out, in humans there is no zygote because the chromosomes in those two pronuclei do not join together but arrange themselves for cell division, and lo! you have a two-cell stage without ever having had a one-cell stage. In some of the laboratories where they freeze that human pronuclear stage, they called it "prezygote," which is rather euphemistic if there never can be a zygote. Though both Jones and Bonnicksen use this term, few experts (like Alikani) who freeze this stage use "prezygote."

As we see from Alikani's essay, cryopreservation is usually done in the two- to eight-cell stages. What is the entity then? An outstanding embryologist in the first half of the twentieth century, Leslie B. Arey (1930), divided development into periods: the ovum (which included many cell divisions), the embryo, and the fetus. But the two dividing points between ovum period and embryo, between embryo period and fetus, have always been rather arbitrary.[1] Development is a continuous process—any terminology applied to it is a human artifact. The term "preembryo" used by Jones and by some practitioners of in vitro fertilization might be simply considered Arey's "period of the ovum" (Biggers 1990). Grobstein (1988) and Jones (1989), however, justify it on different biological grounds. Its first very explicit, logically reasoned use seems to be that by a regulatory group, the Voluntary Licensing Authority (VLA) in Great Britain (Voluntary 1986, 8).

According to Biggers (1990), Shevory (this volume), Spallone (1989), and others, the VLA's coining of the term "preembryo" was a political, not a biological, move. When the Warnock report (1985) to the British government produced no immediate action, the VLA set itself up, essentially as recommended by that report.[2] To facilitate the public's acceptance of experiments with and manipulations of the early embryo, and to avoid concern about moral status (according to the above critics), the VLA started speaking of "preembryo."

Biggers's (1990) greatest objection seems to be that use of "preembryo" is not wise for accurate communication. Since development is a continuum, the moral status of the embryo should also be. However, Jones—this book's strong advocate for that term—explicitly argues that the preembryo should have its own special status, neither that of person nor that of property. Most people would also accept a distinctive status for later embryos, and many, for fetuses. My view is that concern about the term (unless deliberately used to obfuscate) is not nearly as important as concern about the best interests of those tiny *Homo sapiens* creatures who are not persons and yet not property. I believe that the term preembryo has *not* softened the political, social, and moral objections to research on early embryos: those who consider that embryos have the moral status of humans also believe it for preembryos and (pre)zygotes. Indeed, most authors and researchers (viz. Alikani) have not used "preembryo."

Is there any validity to a property analogy? Let us compare a frozen embryo with a summer cottage that a couple has built together, using money and labor from both. If they divorce, who will get custody of the cottage? In making this decision, lawyers are not apt to consider the question of who put in the most effort hammering and sawing. Also, they are not likely to consider what will be in the cottage's best interests, e.g., who will best keep the roof repaired, who will vacuum it most faithfully. Should we pull out one appropriate similarity between property and persons by advocating that both invested effort and an entity's best interests be used in deciding a custody case?

We might also utilize the property analogy by imagining that the cottage once existed but now has only a 50 percent chance of continuing to exist, as

Alikani reports the roughly 50-50 chance of successful embryo thaw at the better centers. Such a cottage or embryo is like a junk bond—perhaps very valuable, perhaps of no value. Only after the custody decision is made can we learn whether the cottage/embryo actually exists; this means someone must guess what value to assign if we wish to make a 50-50 property settlement.

Why Freeze?

Let us backtrack and consider why a couple would have their embryos frozen. The medical reasons are excellent: less physical stress on a woman if she can avoid repeated hormonal stimulations and egg retrievals; better chance for embryo implantation (in general) if it occurs in a natural, not a stimulated, cycle. If preimplantation genetic diagnosis is done on a cell biopsied from the embryo, more time can be allowed for test results to be returned, for accuracy to be checked, and for a decision to be made whether to toss that particular embryo in the landfill.[3] Freezing may seem to let someone put time in a bottle to make a later decision (how large a family, whether one can raise a disabled child, etc.).

Yet, precisely because these reasons are so good, cryopreservation has become (as Bonnicksen quotes) "firmly established and routine" (Trounson 1990, 695) and "a necessity" (Alikani & Cohen 1990, 714). Precisely because these reasons are so good, a couple may not really be asked *whether* they elect freezing. The question will probably be raised on presentation of the prefreeze agreement, but in such a way that vast amounts of assertiveness would be needed to say, "No, I don't want any surplus embryos frozen." Or with fresh embryos, the alternatives may be unpalatable (destroy, give to another couple, use for research). Those three alternatives may arise with frozen embryos, too, but procrastination (time in a bottle) may seem like a boon.

Think about the psychic burden on a couple. Under storage for them is an entity with more moral status than a summer cottage, but with only a 50 percent likelihood of existence. They must decide when to try to turn this entity into a human being, an awesome "choice." Yet choice here is only an illusion because not only Mother Nature but also some half dozen third parties must cooperate. Required are no power failures, the right chemicals along with an effective protocol for slow-freeze or fast-freeze, proper thawing protocol, correct timing for the moment of insertion, no mislabeling of straws or loss of labels, no change in deep-freeze policy when laboratory personnel change, no decision to throw out all "outdated" embryos, and you name it. Those agonizing decisions to try to make a person exist—or perhaps more painful, not to try—have to be made even if the embryos later turn out to have been nonviable.

Psychic pain derives from the knowledge that the tiny frozen nonperson has 23 chromosomes from its mother, 23 from its father, in an unique combination like no existing person. It has chromosomes from grandparents and great-grandparents, and yet its potential of passing its chromosomes to another generation hangs on the decisions of its parents and the skill of technicians.

Would the freezing of *eggs* cause less psychic pain and "solve all ethical questions"? So far, as Alikani reports, this process has rarely worked. Reported successes have not been repeated. One theory is that in the egg stage the spindle proteins, those very proteins standing ready to help the chromosomes of two pronuclei to line up and turn the prezygote into a two-cell stage, are damaged by freezing.

Yet, suppose egg freezing does become successful—as it may if the avid research interest pays off. Would all ethical dilemmas vanish? After all, such frozen entities would have only 23 chromosomes. They thus would be nonpersons and thus would "belong" to only one parent, not to two. And belonging to two is the situation that can lead to custody conflicts.

I believe that success in freezing eggs would be disastrous for women. It would be another tooth in the saw that dismembers women into body parts, another spoke in the wheel that requires reproduction as validation of true womanhood.

The ideas and experiments are already in the literature. There are suggestions that women freeze their eggs while they are young so that those eggs will be of prime quality, plus several experiments to show that embryos from young donated eggs do well in middle-aged uteruses (Bergh et al. 1991; Sauer et al. 1990). In New York women with cancer have stored embryos before chemotherapy (Applegarth et al. 1991). In IVF programs worldwide women are urged to donate eggs in altruism for their unfortunate sisters without ovaries.[4] This last is most worrisome, for it is quite true that women produce many more eggs than they can ever use, as most healthy humans produce more blood than they need. Now that freezing blood—hence storing and shipping it—is perfected, all decent folk are expected to donate their surplus blood; similarly, all decent women might be expected to donate their surplus eggs.

Although I am disturbed by the "guilty unless you donate" propaganda of blood collection campaigns, and by the extreme pressure put on middle-aged people to sign living wills to donate their organs (for instant removal after death) to prolong other people's lives, the pressure to donate eggs I find even more disturbing—indeed, unconscionable. Part of my worry for women is, of course, about the physical stress of fertility drug treatments and egg retrieval procedures, none of which are simple. But my deep uneasiness arises from the fact that an egg carries half one's genes. Any successful use of that egg means that one has a(nother) child on this planet. Unconscionable acts include producing a child whom one cannot love, producing a child who can never know its grandparents (i.e., one that must live with a false genealogy), producing a child whose grandparents never know of its existence, producing a child who may inadvertently marry its own siblings or cousins.[5] All these outcomes occur now because the pressure to donate eggs is already intense[6]—but synchronizing two women's menstrual cycles involves tricky medical manipulations. How much easier will the manipulations be once eggs can be frozen. And how much greater will the temptation be for clinicians to store eggs without informed consent.

In their chapters all four authors raise yet other issues and provide more food for thought. Alikani describes technical difficulties but seems confident that they will be surmounted. But even if they are not quickly solved, we must remember that many technologies at the forefront of medicine continue to be applied for years, despite continuing poor success rates. To Alikani, more effective cryopreservation will be valuable in other extensions of assisted reproduction. Also strongly convinced of the value of this technology, Jones advocates the immediate formulation of sensible policies. Bonnicksen, I believe, thinks that sound policies are better than the current vacuum but that, regardless, some social, psychological, political, and legal problems will still remain. Shevory gives a case study analysis of the fate of the seven Junior and Mary Davis embryos in a Tennessee freezer—showing that absence of policy in an option 2 situation (from Jones's classification) has been disastrous.[7] Yet, could the courtroom trauma really have been avoided by having a policy in place? Shevory's analysis synchronizes with Dietrich's discussion of utilitarian, libertarian ethics and with Oliver's and Lucier et al.'s analyses of custody issues, all three of which appear in this book's section on contract pregnancy.

What to do? Nowadays when a couple enters an IVF program and treatment actually succeeds in producing embryos, some of those embryos (almost inevitably) get frozen. And most couples will not object, if asked, for it seems to be a tidy technical solution to a formidable and complex problem. And we do not all have an inner longing to save time in a bottle?

Notes

1 For a strong criticism of the term "preembryo," especially of the different arguments from biology given by Grobstein (1988) and Jones (1989), see Biggers 1990.

2. As of 1990, the Voluntary Licensing Authority became official.

3. For information on methods of preimplantation biopsy, advocacy of it, and its proposed uses, see the references cited in Note 4 in Bonnicksen's chapter.
4. At the Seventh World Congress on IVF and Assisted Procreations in Paris, July 1991, the 4 presentations and 23 posters on egg donation came from Argentina, Belgium, Brazil, France, Great Britain, Greece, Israel, Italy, Mexico, Singapore, Taiwan, and the United States. Not all the human eggs used in these clinical ventures are donated: some are sold (usually anonymously) to the recipients, at an average of $2000 per egg in the United States (Kolata 1991). Sale of any human body product raises yet more ethical questions.
5. Of course, comparing and contrasting sperm donation/cryopreservation with blood and egg donation would also be pertinent. Obviously, men produce vastly more sperm than they need, and freezing sperm has long been successful. Moreover, like egg donors, sperm donors produce children they cannot love, with false genealogies. On the other hand, giving semen = no risk or pain to donor; giving blood = slight risk or pain to donor; giving eggs = much risk and pain to donor. When these body products are sold, the prices do reflect the risks.
6. For example, what were the pressures on the woman who first had two ectopic pregnancies, then five unsuccessful IVF attempts, and then, when 15 eggs were retrieved in her sixth try at IVF, "donated" four of them to other infertile couples (Rizk et al. 1991)?
7. Since most judges yearn to be considered as wise as their eminent forebear Solomon, I am disappointed that Judge Young in Blount County, Tennessee, failed to take advantage of this excellent opportunity. Since embryo splitting leads to viable twins (in sheep anyway), why did he not order that the seven embryos be thawed and then each one split in order to give one half of each to each partner?

References

Alikani, Mina, and Jacques Cohen. 1990. Human oocyte and embryo cryopreservation. *Current Opinion in Obstetrics and Gynecology* 2:714–717.

Applegarth, L., A. Berkeley, M. Graf, et al. 1991. Embryo cryopreservation prior to cancer therapy: Medical, psychosocial, and ethical issues. Poster presentation. Poster presented at the Seventh World Congress on IVF and Assisted Procreations, Paris, 30 June–3 July. *Abstract Book*:161.

Arey, Leslie B. 1930. *Developmental anatomy*, 2nd ed. Philadelphia: Saunders.

Ben-Abraham, Avi. 1989. Putting death on ice. *Saturday Evening Post* April:60–62.

Bergh, P., M. Williams, I. Guzman, et al. 1991. Infertility at older age is due to declining oocyte quality and may successfully be treated by ovum donation. Paper presented at the Seventh World Congress on IVF and Assisted Procreations, Paris, 30 June–3 July. *Abstract Book*:115.

Biggers, John D. 1990. Arbitrary partitions of prenatal life. *Human Reproduction* 5(1):1–6.

Grobstein, Clifford. 1988. Biological characteristics of the preembryo. *Annals of the New York Academy of Science* 541:346–348.

Jones, Howard W., Jr. 1989. And just what is a pre-embryo? *Fertility and Sterility* 52:189–191.

Kolata, Gina. 1991. Young women offer to sell their eggs to infertile couples. *New York Times National* 10 Nov.:1, 30.

Rizk, Botros, Robert G. Edwards, Umberto Nicolini, et al. 1991. Edwards' syndrome after the replacement of cryopreserved-thawed embryos. *Fertility and Sterility* 55(1):208–210.

Sauer, Mark V., Richard J. Paulson, and Rogerio A. Lobo. 1990. A preliminary report on oocyte donation extending reproductive potential to women over 40. *New England Journal of Medicine* 323:1157–1160.

Spallone, Patricia. 1989. *Beyond conception: The new politics of reproduction*. Granby, Mass.: Bergin & Garvey.

Trounson, Alan O. 1990. Cryopreservation. *British Medical Bulletin* 46(3):695–708.

Vogel, Shawna. 1988. Cold storage. *Discover* Feb.:52–54.

Voluntary Licensing Authority for Human In Vitro Fertilization and Embryology. 1986. *First Report*. London.

Warnock, Mary. 1985. *A question of life: The Warnock report on human fertilisation and embryology*. Oxford: Basil Blackwell.

Chapter 13

PRESERVATION OF HUMAN EGGS AND EMBRYOS THROUGH FREEZING

Mina Alikani

Methodology: A General Description

Successful mammalian embryo freezing was first established in 1971 when pregnancies were achieved in mice after transfer of frozen-thawed embryos (Whittingham 1971). The first human pregnancies resulting from cryopreserved embryos were attained in 1983 (Trounson & Mohr 1983; Zeilmaker et al. 1984). Since then, cryobiologists have focused on improving the efficiency of human embryo freezing by answering key questions regarding methodology.

Early embryonic development in vitro is marked by successive cell divisions. An early embryo can withstand the freeze/thaw process at various stages, from shortly after fertilization, two days after fertilization when it is four-celled, or five to six days post fertilization as a blastocyst (a hollow ball of approximately 100 cells). However, embryos are dynamic structures with different sensitivities and requirements during each phase of development. Thus a single method for cryopreservation cannot be universally applied.

During the early attempts at human embryo freezing, one of two cryoprotective agents, dimethylsulfoxide (DMSO) and glycerol, were mainly used. Such compounds are added to embryos before freezing in order to prevent the formation of ice crystals within cells that would incur irreversible damage as cooling occurs. Since it had already been established that fresh four- to eight-cell embryos can produce pregnancies, these stages were chosen for cryopreservation. The freezing regimen consisted of stepwide addition of cryoprotectant, slow cooling in a programmable cell freezer to low subzero temperatures (–80°C), transfer of embryos into plastic straws or vials (and occasionally glass ampules), and then submersion in liquid nitrogen (–196°C) (Trounson 1986). Embryos were thawed by gradually increasing the temperature. All traces of cryoprotectant were removed stepwise.

Alternatively, blastocysts were successfully frozen using a glycerol-based cryoprotectant and slow cooling to higher subzero temperatures (–40°C) prior to the plunge into liquid nitrogen (Cohen et al. 1985). Thawing was done rapidly by immersing the glass ampule containing the embryo in a water bath at 30°C, followed by gradual dilution of glycerol.

As the cryopreservation data accumulated, however, it became increasingly apparent that overall results were not optimal. Cleaved embryo (four- to eight-cell) survival rates were 60 percent at best, and the incidence of pregnancy in patients who had frozen/thawed embryos replaced usually did not exceed 15 percent. The introduction of an alternative cryoprotectant, propanediol combined with sucrose (PROH-S), for freezing early embryos, excluding the eight-cell embryos, helped improve embryo survival as well as pregnancy rates (Lassalle et al. 1985). Again, a cell freezer was used to slowly lower the temperature to –30°C to –36°C, prior to rapid cooling to –196°C in liquid nitrogen.

Two large-scale retrospective studies from two European centers demonstrate the improving results rather clearly. Camus and his co-workers (1989) evaluated the survival and implantation potential of 319 DMSO-frozen three- to eight-cell embryos and reported an average survival incidence of 52 percent for all embryos thawed. Of the replaced embryos, 6 percent produced a pregnancy. The second study involved 310 embryos (of one to six cells) for which the PROH-S protocol was used. Of these embryos, 64 percent survived the freezing procedure and 14 percent implanted after replacement (Testart et al. 1988). The dilemma in using cryoprotectants is the toxicity they impose on the cells they are meant to protect. There is sufficient evidence to support that PROH is less toxic to embryos than DMSO, which in part explains the improved results.

Several other key observations have simultaneously contributed to the improvement trend. As attempts have been made to cryopreserve various embryonic stages, a correlation has been established between embryonic age and structural integrity at the time of freezing and subsequent survival and implantation rates (Cohen et al. 1988). Although the incidence of postthaw survival seems to be similar for one- to five-cell embryos frozen in PROH-S, thawed two-cell embryos do not tend to implant once replaced in the uterus. Therefore, freezing of two-cell embryos is generally not practiced. Moreover, the one-cell human embryo (the zygote or the fertilized egg) with postthaw survival rate of around 70 percent, may be a more ideal stage for freezing (Fugger et al. 1988; Wright et al. 1990). The methods used for cryopreservation and thawing of zygotes are identical to those for cleaved embryos.

Can the Human Egg Survive Freeze/Thaw Procedures?

The feasibility of oocyte (here synonymous to egg) cryopreservation has been established in many mammalian species. Mouse oocytes, for instance, that were stored at –196°C were successfully fertilized upon thawing (Whittingham 1977). These experiments have been repeated in the hamster, rat, rabbit, and monkey. Despite experience in animal models, human oocyte freezing remains largely experimental. In the first report of a successful birth after oocyte freezing, Chen (1986) announced a singleton (one fetus) pregnancy after replacement of embryos generated from frozen, thawed, and in vitro fertilized oocytes. He later reported a twin pregnancy (1988). In the two years following the first pregnancy, two other births were reported by van Uem et al. (1987) and Diedrich et al. (1988), although the latter case was not fully described.

The conservative approach to human oocyte freezing is justifiably based on a series of experimental data that has demonstrated the technique's profound adverse consequences. Electron microscopic studies of oocytes after exposure to DMSO and cooling to 0°C have revealed substantial structural discrepancies, believed to have been caused by the drop in the temperature (Sathananthan et al. 1988). As seen in animal models, these abnormalities potentially can generate chromosomally abnormal embryos that may lead to birth defects (Kola et al. 1988).

Another problem associated with oocyte freezing is that exposure to cryoprotectant may alter the fertilizing capacity of oocytes (Johnson 1989). Whereas PROH is considered a better choice than DMSO for freezing embryos, its use is not advocated for eggs since it may bring about a condition referred to as "parthenogenetic activation." In this condition eggs start to divide spontaneously, without fertilization by a sperm, and behave as embryos despite gross deficiencies in genetic information that is required for further development.

The preservation of human eggs is still a technical challenge. It appears, however, that an "ultrarapid" freezing procedure in which eggs are immersed in liquid nitrogen immediately following exposure to cryoprotectant (as opposed to slow cooling to low temperatures) may in fact be the method of choice (Pensis et al. 1989). This technique has been used successfully to cryopreserve mouse embryos (Trounson et al. 1988). A very limited number of human embryos have also been subjected to ultrarapid freezing, but the viability of such embryos must be investigated.

The Current Efficiency of Cryopreservation

The first pregnancy and birth from a cryopreserved human embryo in the United States occurred in 1986 (Marrs et al.).

The Society for Assisted Reproductive Technology conducted a survey among its member institutions on their experience with human egg and embryo cryopreservation prior to 1989. The results of 25 centers with active cryopreservation programs were included in the final report (Fugger 1989). Five centers reported oocyte cryopreservation with a total of 463 oocytes frozen. Of these oocytes, 127 were thawed, of which only 8 (6.3 percent) generated embryos suitable for replacement. None of these led to a pregnancy. These data reflect the primitive nature of our experience with oocyte freezing and a lack of efficiency of the current techniques.

The centers reported that 2085 patients had a total of 6934 zygotes, cleaved embryos, and blastocysts frozen, of which 2531 were thawed and 1767 were replaced, resulting in 118 clinical pregnancies (fetal heart activity seen on ultrasound examination) in 884 patients (approximately 13 percent).

An equivalent European survey of 24 groups that reported replacements of cryopreserved embryos up to the end of 1986 indicated 163 pregnancies: 63 babies born, 43 abortions, and 60 ongoing pregnancies (van Steirteghem & van den Abbeel 1988). Approximately 50 percent of 3577 frozen/thawed embryos were found suitable for replacement in 1219 patients.

Cryopreservation had indeed improved the efficiency of IVF by providing an additional opportunity for a pregnancy after a single treatment cycle. Patients who fail to become pregnant from their "fresh" embryos may subsequently return for the thaw and replacement of their frozen embryos. Successful freezing, however, is still more an art than a science. Results may vary greatly from one center to another and sometimes among different individuals performing the procedures. These variations eventually may be resolved when the methodology becomes more standardized.

Future Applications of Cryopreservation in Assisted Reproduction

A fascinating new area associated with IVF is genetic diagnosis of embryos that may be at risk for genetic disease. This procedure involves creating a large hole in the protective outer coating of the embryo, the zona pellucida, in order to remove a single cell for genetic analysis. Though most of the analysis can be performed within one day, some time-consuming assays may require cryopreservation of the biopsied embryo. In addition, assisted fertilization techniques also require introduction of gaps in the zona, a situation that will generate embryos physically different from nonmanipulated ones. Experience in freezing manipulated embryos is very limited, although it has been successful in the animal model (Wilton et al. 1989). Further investigations in this area will be necessary as procedures such as the above are applied more commonly.

Although ethically complex, human egg and embryo banking is certainly a viable possibility. One group to whom the idea may be of great practical value would be those patients who are in need of certain treatments for life-threatening diseases, such as cancer, that would undoubtedly jeopardize their reproductive potential. Such patients would have the option of undergoing IVF in order to cryopreserve embryos before they begin invasive chemotherapy or radiation treatment.

Patients whose infertility is due to premature ovarian failure and are thus unable to produce eggs, would certainly benefit from eggs that may be available through a bank. Just as it has been practiced with sperm for many years, donated oocytes could be cryopreserved for later matching to a recipient. Moreover, menopause naturally renders the ovaries inactive, though the uterus can be hormonally conditioned to support a pregnancy. Although in most Western societies postponing childbirth is not an accepted and common practice among women, increased maternal age does reduce the likelihood of a successful pregnancy, partly because of the increased incidence of chromosomal abnormalities in eggs. If oocyte freezing becomes safe and reliable, it could dramatically add to the reproductive options of women. In the future, many women might contemplate oocyte freezing at a young age and cryobanking until a pregnancy is desired.

References

Camus, M., E. van den Abbeel, L. van Waesberghe, et al. 1989. Human embryo viability after freezing with dimethylsulfoxide as a cryoprotectant. *Fertility and Sterility* 51:460–465.

Chen, C. 1986. Pregnancy after human oocyte cryopreservation. *Lancet* i:884–886.

Chen, C. 1988. Pregnancies after human oocyte cryopreservation. *Annals of the New York Academy of Sciences* 541:541–561.

Cohen, J., G.W. DeVane, C.W. Elsner, et al. 1988. Cryopreservation of zygotes and early cleaved human embryos. *Fertility and Sterility* 49(2):283–289.

Cohen, J., R.F. Simons, R.G. Edwards, et al. 1985. Pregnancies following the frozen storage of expanding human blastocysts. *Journal of in Vitro Fertilization and Embryo Transfer* 2(2):59–64.

Cohen, J., K.E. Wiemer, and G. Wright. 1988. Prognostic value of morphologic characteristics of cryopreserved embryos: A study using videocinematography. *Fertility and Sterility* 49(5):827–833.

Diedrich, K., H. Al-Hasani, H. van der Ven, et al. 1988. Successful in vitro fertilization of frozen thawed rabbit and human oocytes. *Annals of the New York Academy of Sciences* 541:562–570.

Fugger, E.F., M. Bustillo, L.P. Katz, et al. 1988. Embryonic development and pregnancy from fresh and cryopreserved sibling pronucleate human zygotes. *Fertility and Sterility* 50(2):273–278.

Fugger, E. 1989. Clinical status of human embryo cryopreservation in the United States of America. *Fertility and Sterility* 52(6):986–990.

Johnson, M.H. 1989. The effect on fertilization of exposure of mouse embryos to dimethylsulfoxide: An optimal protocol. *Journal of in Vitro Fertilization and Embryo Transfer* 6:168–175.

Kola, I., C. Kirby, J.Shaw, et al. 1988. Vitrification of mouse oocytes results in aneuploid zygotes and malformed fetuses. *Teratology* 38:467.

Lassalle, B., J. Testart, and J.P. Renard, 1985. Human embryo features that influence the success of cryopreservation with the use of 1,2-propanediol. *Fertility and Sterility* 50:273–278.

Marrs, R.P., J. Brown, F. Sato, et al. 1986. Successful pregnancies from cryopreserved human embryos produced by in vitro fertilization. *American Journal of Obstetrics and Gynecology* 156:1503.

Pensis, M., E. Loumaye, and I. Psalti. 1989. Screening of conditions for rapid freezing of human oocytes: Preliminary study toward their cryopreservation. *Fertility and Sterility* 52(5):787–794.

Sathananthan, A.H., A. Trounson, L. Freeman, et al. 1988. The effects of cooling human oocytes. *Human Reproduction* 3(8):968–977.

Testart, J., B. Lassalle, J. Belaisch-Allart, et al. 1988. Human embryo freezing. *Annals of the New York Academy of Sciences* 541:532–540.

Trounson, A. 1986. Preservation of human eggs and embryos. *Fertility and Sterility* 46(1):1–2.

Trounson, A.O., and L. Mohr. 1983. Human pregnancy following cryopreservation, thawing and transfer of an eight-cell embryo. *Nature* 305:707.

Trounson, A., A. Perura, L. Freemann, et al. 1988. Ultrarapid freezing of early cleavage stage human embryos and eight-cell mouse embryos. *Fertility and Sterility* 49(5):822–826.

van Steirteghem, A.C., and E. van den Abbeel, 1988. Survey on cryopreservation. *Annals of the New York Academy of Science* 541:571–574.

van Uem, J., E.R. Siebzehnrubl, and B. Schuh, 1987. Birth after cryopreservation of unfertilized oocytes. *Lancet* i:752–753.

Whittingham, D.G. 1971. Survival of mouse embryos after freezing and thawing. *Nature* 233:125.

Whittingham, D.G. 1977. Fertilization *in vitro* and development to term of unfertilized mouse oocytes previously stored at –196C. *Journal of Reproduction and Fertility* 49:89.

Wilton, L.J., J.M. Shaw, and A.O. Trounson. 1989. Successful single-cell biopsy and cryopreservation of preimplantation mouse embryos. *Fertility and Sterility* 51(3):513–517,

Wright, G., S. Wiker, C. Elsner, et al. 1980. Observations on the morphology of pronuclei and nucleoli in human zygotes and implications for cryopreservation. *Human Reproduction*. 5:109–115.

Zeilmaker, G.H., A.Th. Alberda, I. van Gent, et al. 1984. Two pregnancies following transfer of intact frozen-thawed embryos. *Fertility and Sterility* 42(2):293–296.

Chapter 14

POLICY CONSIDERATIONS FOR CRYOPRESERVATION IN IN VITRO FERTILIZATION PROGRAMS

Howard W. Jones, Jr.

Introduction

The option of cryopreservation has proven to be an extraordinarily useful procedure for reducing the risk of multiple pregnancies by reducing the number of prezygotes/preembryos in the initial transfer procedure. At present, the best programs report about a 70 percent survival rate of cryopreserved material. Furthermore, the pregnancy expectation per thawed prezygote/preembryo approximates the pregnancy rate for the transfer of fresh prezygotes/preembryos. With improved methods of stimulation in responsive patients, the expectancy of pregnancy from a single egg harvest, including cryopreservation, approaches and, in specific circumstances, exceeds 50 percent. It is obviously of the utmost importance that these excellent results not be negated by neglect of the problems of cryopreservation. The ultimate fate of cryopreserved prezygotes and preembryos that, for whatever reason, cannot be transferred into the uterus of the prospective, willing mother under optimum conditions will become more and more a dilemma as more and more prezygotes and preembryos are cryopreserved.

This essay is modified from Howard W. Jones, Jr., Cryopreservation and its problems, *Fertility and Sterility* 53(1990):780–784. It is reproduced with permission of the publisher, the American Fertility Society.

The Prezygote and Preembryo: Definitions and Status

Because ultimate disposition involves an evaluation of moral status and because moral status has traditionally been related to biology, understanding the biology of the prezygote and the preembryo is necessary. A prezygote may be defined simply as a fertilizing egg up to the time of syngamy, which is when the egg and sperm chromosomes assemble just before the first cell division.

Fertilization is not an event. It is a process that takes place over a minimum of 24 hours. This process may be considered to begin with the first contact of the sperm with the dense, firm layer (the zona pellucida) surrounding the egg. The end of the process of fertilization remains a debatable point, but for the purposes of this discussion, fertilization will be considered to end some 24 hours later with the first commingling of the genetic material of the two progenitors within a nuclear envelope, i.e., at the formation of the two nuclear envelopes at the two-cell stage. Thus, there is no such thing as a "moment of fertilization" (see Jones & Schrader 1987, 1989).

The prezygote with no commingling of the chromosomes is considered by some to have a different moral status from the preembryo, where the genetic material is commingled.

The short definition of a preembryo is that structure that exists from the end of the process of fertilization until the appearance of a single primitive streak.

During the embryonic period developmental events are quite special. Often, abnormalities occur, so often, in fact, that it is the exception rather than the rule that a single biological individual will result.

It is only the appearance of a single primitive streak in the embryoblast that guarantees that a biological individual is in the process of formation from the preembryo. The development of the primitive streak has been described as varying from perhaps day 12 to as late as day 16, but, on average, 14 days is not far off the mark.

Moral theologians, philosophers, and others have turned to biologists to ask for some event that would help them identify important periods of development that could be associated with moral status. Moral status in this sense is meant to designate the worth, rights, and responsibilities, if any, that could be assigned to an individual in the developing phase. There cannot be the slightest doubt that the preembryo is human in a genetic sense. However, it is equally clear that during the preembryonic stage it has not yet been determined with certainty that a biological individual will result. In the absence of such a single individual, the assignment of full rights of a human person is inconsistent with biological reality.

Can the frozen prezygote/preembryo be regarded as property? To be sure, it cannot be sold. Selling sperm, eggs, or preembryos is considered unethical by the Ethics Committee of the American Fertility Society (1990) and was specifically prohibited by the Warnock report (United Kingdom 1984) and, indeed, by other ethics committees. Furthermore, there are laws in some jurisdictions that prohibit the sale of body parts such as kidneys and hearts. These considerations would surely indicate that a prezygote/preembryo cannot be dealt with as property.

Thus, if the prezygote/preembryo is not property and does not have the status of a human person, what is it? The preembryo represents a special era in biological development. This requires the establishment of special rules for its place in society. This niche is different from that of the egg, sperm, and the fertilizing egg (prezygote), on the one hand, and from the niches of the embryo, fetus, and infant, on the other. For the purposes of this discussion of cryopreservation, however, the status of the fertilizing egg (prezygote) and the preembryo can be considered equivalent except for one situation, which will be discussed below.

Problems of Disposition

In 1989, attention was centered on the ultimate disposition of the preembryos in a divorce case, but divorce is only one of the many situations that could alter the original intent of all concerned. For example:

1. Death or disability of one or both of the prospective parents.
2. Legal separation or divorce of the prospective parents.
3. The cryopreserved material may remain in storage beyond the reproductive limit of the prospective mother or beyond some other agreed-on time limit.
4. Loss of contact with the prospective parents may occur, including their failure to pay current or delinquent cryopreservation fees and charges, if any.
5. There may be loss of interest by the prospective parents in attempting a pregnancy.
6. One or both prospective parents may wish to remove the cryopreserved prezygote/preembryo from the original program.
7. There may be voluntary or involuntary discontinuation of a cryopreservation program by an in vitro fertilization (IVF) program.

To maintain credibility before the public and to place responsibility on the source of the dilemmas, IVF programs must call attention to the troublesome possibilities and provide specific alternatives by prefreeze agreements that give consideration to the best interests of those immediately involved, as well as to the public interest. Individual autonomy must be modulated by good medicine, and good ethics should be paramount.

Of course, legal considerations are likewise important. However, laws are made by citizens, and if existing laws made at other times to fit other situations do not apply to the fruits of contemporary biology, such laws must not be convoluted to fit an entirely new situation. The pitfalls of convolution may be illustrated by two 1989 legal proceedings. In Tennessee, where the court had to decide the disposition of cryopreserved preembryos, it was held that the preembryos had the full moral status of children (*Davis v. Davis* 1989). On the contrary, in Virginia, where the court had to rule on an injunction regarding the disposition of a prezygote, it ruled that the prezygote was property, i.e., it had no moral status (*Jones v. York* 1989). The same biological process is judged to have different statuses in different courts.

Clearly, the legal system is uncertain, and, to a great extent, it ought to be spared the decision-making responsibility on issues that would benefit from a continuing discussion, which should involve the views of reproductive biologists, patients, theologians, ethicists, lawyers, and public representatives, especially those with practical experience in the field.

Necessity for and Nature of a Prefreeze Agreement

Because of the possibility of an unexpected catastrophe to one or both of the prospective parents after cryopreservation or of other events listed above, a prefreeze agreement to provide for the disposition of the prezygote/preembryo is essential to carry out the intent of the prospective parents. It would seem reasonable to be able to amend this agreement from time to time before it becomes operational, with the approval of all parties. This agreement is to be distinguished from a document of informed consent, which deals with the willing acceptance of medical intervention after adequate disclosure.

The prospective parents should be expected to provide the principal input for the ultimate disposition of the cryopreserved prezygote/preembryo. This input, however, cannot be an absolute right but must be consistent with the interests of good medicine, good public policy, and good ethics. A simple example can illustrate the importance of these latter points. It would be dehumanizing and prone to abuse, therefore undesirable and against good public policy, to allow the prospective parents the option of offering their cryopreserved prezygotes/preembryos for sale.

If the concept can be accepted by the agreeing parties that the prezygote/preembryo is neither property nor a human individual, one can then propose a prefreeze agreement based on a social theory unencumbered by a backward look at precedents based on property or custodial theory. The opportunity would then exist to look forward freely, with a view to balancing the interest of the prospective parents, the prezygote/preembryo, and society.

If, at cryopreservation, the intent of the prospective parents was to fulfill their joint reproductive goal by bearing a child by joining their genetic material, it follows that if both cannot participate in the use of the cryopreserved prezygotes/preembryos as originally planned, the original intent can no longer be fulfilled. The proposed theory holds that if the original intent can no longer be fulfilled, then one of four standard options should be selected by the prospective parents before cryopreservation becomes operational. These four standard options specify that cryopreserved prezygotes/preembryos should be:

1. Made available to other couples for adoption on an anonymous basis.
2. Made available for pathological examination, as with any other discarded human tissue.
3. Discarded without further development or examination.
4. Made available for research approved by a properly constituted institutional review board and other boards with jurisdiction.

It should be emphasized that these options are now included in many documents of informed consent, but the circumstances that trigger the use of these options are often vaguely stated or only implied in the most general terms.

In selecting these options, some patients may distinguish between the moral status of a prezygote and a preembryo. As is evident from the description above, a prezygote is a fertilizing egg; fertilization is not complete. It is possible that under this circumstance many will consider the prezygote in the same category as an egg and therefore will have no moral problem with any type of disposition. On the other hand, these same individuals may consider a preembryo as morally distinct and would therefore be influenced by their moral consideration in the option that they select. This point is the exception to the previous statement that, for the purposes of this discussion, the prezygote and the preembryo could be considered together. Thus, the method of cryopreservation, i.e., the stage during development, may be of relevance in selecting a standard option.

The four standard options can apply to situations 1 through 5 listed above and can eliminate possibilities that might apply to property or custodial concepts.

Interprogram Transfer

Special comment is needed for situations 6 and 7, which concern the possibility of transferring a cryopreserved prezygote/preembryo from one program to another at the request of one or both prospective parents or considerations revolving around the discontinuation of a cryopreservation program by a medical facility.

The request of both prospective parents for the transfer of a cryopreserved prezygote/preembryo to another program presents several problems. In view of the diversity in the techniques of freezing and thawing, two-program entanglement could impose a substantial risk to the prezygote/preembryo. Furthermore, the necessity for synchronization of preembryo development with endometrial receptivity could present a major problem in interprogram transfer.

A further vexing problem could arise concerning the competence of one or another of the programs. There has been public consideration and concern about the competence of IVF programs. The often quoted study of the Office of Technology Assessment (OTA) (U.S. Congress 1988) indicated that about half of the IVF programs in the United States had not had a single birth. This situation led to congressional hearings on this matter by Representative Ron Wyden (U.S. House of Representatives 1989). Although the OTA data are probably now outdated, the fact remains that any given IVF program is not likely to have current information about the competence of other programs, especially about their results with cryopreservation. Thus, the involvement of two programs can expose the cryopreserved prezygote/preembryo to an avoidable hazard. Therefore, the assignment of legal responsibility in the event of a medical mishap either in the freezing or in the thawing program could become extraordinarily complex with two-program involvement.

In addition to these purely medical considerations, there are public policy issues involving the experimental use of human material. A number of years ago, the federal government issued regulations providing for the establishment of an Institutional Review Board (IRB) to review and supervise prospectively any experimental program using human tissue. Whereas the regulations apply only to programs supported by federal funds, most universities and hospitals—especially teaching hospitals—have required IRB approval of experiments using human tissue regardless of the source of financial support. According to the report of the Ethics Committee of the American Fertility Society (1990), a clinical experiment is considered to be an innovative procedure with very limited, if any, record of whether any success can be achieved through its application. Because, as of this writing, there are no published data on the effect of interprogram transfer, such transfer must be considered an experimental procedure with human tissue and therefore subject to IRB approval.

Interprogram transfer therefore needs to be distinguished from what might be referred to as basic cryopreservation, which is fast becoming a standard clinical procedure. Additionally, because experimental procedures involving preembryos in particular are so sensitive, due to the special nature of the preembryo that sets it apart from other human tissue, the Ethics Committee of the American Fertility Society (1990) recommended that IRBs should not rely on local opinion alone in the matter of interprogram transfer but should seek verification of their decision by reference to a more representative national body. Thus, to comply with a request to transfer a cryopreserved prezygote/preembryo is to participate in an action contrary to established public policy.

The ultimate disposition of cryopreserved prezygotes/preembryos becomes very troublesome in the event that a program of assisted reproduction ceases to operate, with cryopreserved prezygotes/preembryos on hand. There seems to be no option that can satisfactorily accommodate to the interests of all concerned. Nevertheless, the agreement must consider this possibility. At the very least, the program should be required to notify the prospective parents of the discontinuation of the cryopreservation program with a minimum lead time of two years, in the hope that during this interval the majority of the cryopreserved prezygotes/preembryos would be transferred into the prospective mothers. At the end of that time, it would seem necessary to accept the additional medical risks involved in interprogram transfer. The public policy issue is equally troubling, and special approval of IRBs would certainly seem to be required under present regulations.

Conclusion

The integrity of cryopreservation could be preserved by the use of a prefreeze agreement that would provide for the several contingencies. The above suggestions can only be a beginning, for there are likely to be other views. If IVF programs do not take the lead in suggesting specific plans for the ultimate disposition of prezygotes/preembryos, there is a danger that the advantages of cryopreservation will be lost.

References

Davis v. Davis. 1989. No. E-14496. Blount Co. Cir. Ct., Tenn.

Ethics Committee of the American Fertility Society. 1990. Ethical considerations of the new reproductive technologies. *Fertility and Sterility* 53(6)(Suppl. 2): 1S-109S.

Jones, Howard W., Jr., and Charlotte Schrader. 1987. The process of human fertilization: Implications for moral status. *Fertility and Sterility* 48:189–192.

Jones, Howard W., Jr., and Charlotte Schrader. 1989. And just what is a pre-embryo? *Fertility and Sterility* 52:189–191.

Jones v. York. 1989. No. 33455, E.D. Va.

United Kingdom, Department of Health and Social Security. 1984. *Report of the Committee of Inquiry into Human Fertilisation and Embryology*. London: Her Majesty's Stationery Office.

U.S. Congress, Office of Technology Assessment. 1988. *Infertility: Medical and social choices*. OTA-BA-358. Washington, D.C.: U.S. Government Printing Office.

U.S. House of Representatives. 1989. *Consumer protection issues involving in vitro fertilization clinics*. Serial No. 101–5. Washington, D.C.: U. S. Government Printing Office.

Chapter 15

ETHICAL ISSUES IN THE CLINICAL APPLICATION OF EMBRYO FREEZING

Andrea L. Bonnicksen

Introduction

Only seven years ago, embryo freezing (cryopreservation) was considered a technique raising "disturbing," "extremely difficult," "incredibly complex," and even "nightmarish" ethical issues. Today, however, embryo freezing is offered in many in vitro fertilization (IVF) clinics and is said to be "firmly established as a routine component" of IVF (Trounson 1990, 695) and "no longer considered a novelty but a necessity" (Alikani & Cohen 1990, 714). Of 163 IVF centers recording data for 1989, for example, 110 reported freezing programs. Physicians in these 110 clinics reported initiating 2124 IVF cycles involving frozen/thawed embryos (Medical Research International 1991, 20). The number of frozen embryos in this country has grown rapidly from 289 in 1985 to 23,468 in 1989 (Medical Research International 1988, 212–215; Medical Research International 1991, 20). Only an estimated 10 infants in the United States and 60 in the world were born as of 1988 after having been frozen as embryos (U.S. Congress 1988, 298), but in 1989, U.S. clinics alone reported 172 deliveries (Medical Research International 1991, 20).

An earlier version of this paper appeared in the December 1988 issue of *The Hastings Center Report*. It is reprinted with permission.

Some physicians have concluded that freezing reduces ethical dilemmas by allowing embryos to be stored rather than discarded, and researchers have contended that freezing poses few unique dilemmas (Trounson 1986).[1] It is true that if we look for evidence of public controversy, predictions of perplexing ethical quandaries have not been realized. Instead, public attention has been drawn to conflicts over who has jurisdiction over frozen embryos.[2] Unanswered questions do remain, however, about the daily practice of embryo freezing in the clinical setting. These questions suggest the need to keep alive the ethical debate about the benefits to patients and society of embryo freezing.

Questionable Benefits

During a woman's initial IVF cycle, three or four of the embryos created are transferred to her uterus, while the rest are frozen and stored for thawing and transfer to the uterus at a later date. Practitioners of IVF justify freezing as enhancing their ability to act in the patient's best interest.[3] In general, they presume freezing will benefit the patient physically, emotionally, and financially.

In theory, because a small number of embryos can be transferred in the first IVF cycle (with the remainder frozen for later use), freezing physically benefits a woman undergoing IVF by reducing the odds that a multiple pregnancy will occur. It also lets the woman recover from the emotional and physical stress (including hormonal stimulation) of the initial IVF cycle before a second transfer of embryos (Trounson 1990, 702), and it spares her from repeated ovarian hyperstimulation and egg retrievals (Ethics Committee 1990, 59S). It furthers her emotional needs by reducing anxiety when she knows she has succeeded in one part of IVF and has tangible evidence, in the form of stored embyros, of that success. Finally, the patient benefits financially in that freezing avoids repeated start-up IVF expenses of hormonal monitoring and time lost from work during the two-week IVF cycle.

There is a real, although diminishing, distance between theory and practice, however. Directors interviewed by this author in the early years of embryo freezing reported freezing an average of fewer than three embryos per patient, with one-quarter to one-half not surviving the freeze/thaw. More recent data indicate a survival rate of 60–80 percent at established centers (Alikani & Cohen 1990; Edwards & Handyside 1990; Trounson 1990). Although knowledge about methods for freezing and thawing is improving (Fugger et al. 1991), the optimal scenario of freezing six or more embryos for leisurely transfer over a period of months has yet to be realized.

Does freezing actually benefit the patient physically? No injuries such as uterine infections from the transfer of thawed embryos have been reported, but neither does the evidence demonstrate that freezing significantly reduces the physical stresses from IVF for patients. The pregnancy rate remains low. For example, the 2124 transfers in 1989 resulted in 11 percent clinical pregnancies and 8 percent births (Medical Research International 1991, 20), although a report from one program shows a higher pregnancy rate than for embryos that have not been frozen (Edwards & Handyside 1990, 831). Pregnancies are not evenly distributed across centers. Only 10 of the 110 clinics reporting data in 1989 accounted for 56 percent of the pregnancies, for example (Medical Research International 1991, 20).

Moreover, use of frozen embryos may still result in multiple pregnancies, with 23 sets of twins from 172 deliveries born in 1989; spontaneous abortions occurred in 24 percent of the pregnancies (Medical Research International 1991, 20), although it appears that the use of thawed embryos is not correlated with greater miscarriage rates than for fresh embryos (Trounson 1990, 702–703). Due to the attrition rate of frozen embryos, the patients may undergo the rigorous initial IVF cycle only to be spared, at most, one repeat cycle.

Does freezing benefit patients emotionally? Physicians presume that patients build defenses against disappointment when embryos are stored, but some women do just the opposite and "enhance" the embryos by thinking of them as babies. Patients may develop attachments to their embryos during regular IVF, as indicated by their naming the embryos, asking for the petri dishes in which the embryos were fertilized as mementoes, acting and feeling pregnant after the embryos are transferred to their uteruses, and mourning the embryos' loss if they do not implant. Freezing has the capacity to enhance rather than diminish such bonding.

Bonding poses problems if clients need to stop embryo freezing prematurely. Couples in freezing programs are warned that they may divorce or lose a spouse and therefore need to agree about what should be done with their embryos in such an event. They are also asked to accept the consequences of failure of freezing equipment, which would result in loss of the embryos. They are not, however, necessarily prepared for unexpected reasons for discontinuing freezing, as when the wife has a hysterectomy, is prematurely menopausal, or develops other medical problems precluding a pregnancy. Additionally, the costs of freezing might become excessive for the couple, or they may have a multiple birth after the initial IVF cycle, adopt a child, or decide the strain of trying to circumvent infertility is so great they will stop the process.

Anecdotal evidence suggests that the presence of frozen embryos is not necessarily like money in the bank, with more being better, for clients who find they must decide what to do with spare or unneeded embryos. Will the couple experience remorse or guilt by asking for the destruction of their embryos? If donation is an option, will they later regret donating their embryos to other couples? It is not clear whether couples can easily carry out the decisions they had earlier agreed upon when the need to discontinue freezing is at hand.

Freezing also increases the patient's dependence on IVF as the answer to infertility in a way that can be emotionally unhealthy. Nurse coordinators have written of the need to counsel patients about resolutions to infertility treatment other than a pregnancy and birth, such as adoption or acceptance of infertility (Garner 1987, 305–311). Freezing interferes with closure on infertility for women who want to adopt or move on to other life goals but who find they cannot terminate the effort because of stored embryos. It also locks patients into treatment at the clinic where their embryos are stored even if they lose confidence in the program or feel pressured, either by clinic staff or by their own desires for pregnancy, to continue to try IVF.

Embryo freezing places women and men in the role of pioneers in uncharted psychological waters. By bidding technicians to judge embryos for their "freezability," the procedure opens embryos to evaluation and, in effect, encourages patients to evaluate their own self-worth (already assaulted by the legacy of infertility) by the number and quality of embryos they have stored. The embryo's appearance (regular or irregular? favorable or unfavorable?) is a strong predictor of its ability to survive the freeze and thaw (Trounson 1990, 701–702). Self-recrimination, which is already underway during IVF when women evaluate themselves on the basis of the number of follicles or eggs they produce, can be extended and broadened by embryo cryopreservation. Embryo freezing also prolongs the experience of being a "patient" inasmuch as a genetic part of the couple is in the hands of an infertility clinic. This can add to couples' feelings of vulnerability and dependence by causing them to worry about embryos stored in a laboratory (fearing damage to the embryos or a mix-up of ampules).

The financial benefits of freezing are also questionable. Freezing can save couples thousands of dollars in start-up costs if a sizable number of embryos are frozen and survive the freeze/thaw and if pregnancy rates are higher than for regular IVF. However, as noted, these conditions are usually only imperfectly met. Moreover, even if survival and implantation rates were high, freezing would save couples money only if it put them ahead of insurance coverage. If the couple has access to insurance coverage that pays most of the estimated $8000 for each cycle but still refuses reimbursement for freezing embryos, then the couple will pay out-of-pocket for the preparation, storage, and thawing of embryos. Freezing will place couples behind insurance coverage unless cryopreservation is explicitly included as part of an IVF protocol or unless couples are given a maximum benefit level for IVF to be spent at their discretion (for examples of state laws regarding IVF and insurance, see U.S. Congress 1988, 148–155).

Moreover, couples are billed for freezing irrespective of the outcome. If the machinery malfunctions, or if the couple donates the frozen embryos to other couples or to the hospital for study, or asks that they be discarded, the couple will still have paid for preparation and storage costs, which can run over time to hundreds or thousands of dollars.

Reservations about the physical, emotional, and financial benefits of embryo freezing raise questions about whether it is always in the best interests of patients and couples and how, if it poses harms as well as benefits, freezing can be practiced in a way that truly serves their needs. Should not their interests be an integral part of the criteria used to set up and administer freezing programs? What ethical obligations do practitioners have to their patients and to couples in deciding how to administer such programs?

Clinical Policies

Expediency, medical hunches, and the need to guarantee the program's future play a large role in how policies are made in pioneering freezing programs. Policies of innovative centers are passed to other centers in a lateral modeling through discussions among colleagues or through contracts with or workshops sponsored by well-known embryologists who pass on their program's consent forms and policies. Directors of IVF clinics state they make decisions primarily on the basis of their own discretion or the judgments of the IVF team (Bonnicksen & Blank 1988). In making decisions about embryo freezing practices, however, directors whom I interviewed spoke of the importance of modeling:

> We got input from the University of Washington. I was at UCLA so we used that. We also used Houston; one member of our staff is from there. The nitty-gritty was based on these three programs.

> We modeled our program after Fairfax, Virginia. It was modeled after Australia. We used the Virginia program because it was the most academic and had a large program geared to this research. The consent form was modeled after the program in Cleveland. It was a more exhaustive form. Lawyers, philosophers, and others were involved with it. I was impressed with the careful scrutiny.

> Tacoma, UCLA, Virginia—we got copies of the consent forms of everyone else and we'll take the best of them all (quotes from Bonnicksen 1989, 38-39).

Although lateral modeling helps standardize policies across centers, a careful weighing of the physician's obligation to patients threatens to become lost in the effort to do what is expedient, efficient, and effective in other centers. A global notion of presumed beneficence replaces an individualized search for demonstrated beneficence. Moreover, despite modeling, clinics vary in their approaches on a range of issues. Will a limit be placed on the number of years embryos are frozen? One center, for example, freezes embryos for a maximum of five years as a compromise between the two years proposed by some members of the hospital's ethics committee and the reproductive life cut-off favored by others. Other centers limit freezing time to avoid being in the "long-term storage business" or because they fear couples will move and abandon their embryos, leaving the program in an awkward legal position. Still others do not impose time limits in order to "keep our options open."

Most centers require couples to sign detailed consent forms stipulating the disposition of the embryos; at least, initially, some did not, arguing that such consent would be unenforceable in any event. Should clinics charge for the procedure before they achieve their first success? Some centers do not charge for freezing or charge only a nominal amount until a clinical pregnancy results. One center that recently started freezing, for example, charges a "freezing fee" of $300 and a "thawing fee" of $100 each time embryos are thawed and transferred. This is added to the costs of embryo transfer. The center reserves the option of starting a yearly storage fee if large numbers of embryos are stored. Other centers, however, charge $1000 or more for a one-time storage fee.

Should patients be able to donate extra embryos for research or to other infertile couples? Some centers do not allow donation of extra frozen embryos; others, in states with unclear embryo research laws, require donation as an alternative to discarding the embryos. Some centers give the option of donating extra embryos for research in accordance with the law; other centers do not have this option.

One may expect additional questions of disposition to arise when the genetic diagnosis of embryos becomes routine. Here one or two cells are removed from the embryos and examined for genetic or chromosomal defects.[4] If the biopsied cell is found to be normal for the tested conditions, the "parent" embryo will be transferred. One can expect clinics to want to freeze abnormal embryos for later study. If this is done, who will have responsibility for the abnormal embryos? What options will be given to patients about the disposition of those embryos?

The physician's obligation in administering embryo freezing programs is to identify the patient's interests and integrate those interests into decision making. This requires modesty about freezing's benefits for individual patients. It also requires a recognition of the pressure of unresolved societal dilemmas about working with human embryos that have implications for the needs of patients.

Freezing as an Option

Is it ever in the patient's interest for the clinic to present freezing as a normal part of the IVF protocol rather than as an option? Directors report that over 90 percent of patients with spare embryos elect freezing, which indicates that freezing is presented in a way that encourages patients' participation in the protocol (for example, by stating "our policy is to freeze embryos in excess of four"). Yet this leads to concern about how detailed the information given to patients about the risks and uncertainties of the procedure actually is. An examination of consent forms confirms that, at least in writing, patients are given the most general information. They may see in writing, for example, that the risks are unknown, freezing has worked for animal models, and the benefits "we hope" are to increase the chance of pregnancy.

As data are collected, it is possible to state with some certainty, as appears on one consent form, that "[s]tudies with frozen-thawed human and animal embryos do not demonstrate an increased risk of abnormalities in offspring." Although a small number of abnormalities in fetuses and offspring has been reported (Medical Research International 1991, 20; Rizk et al. 1991), a link between freezing and deformity has not been demonstrated. It is thought that embryos damaged in the freeze/thaw will not cleave and will therefore not be transferred to the woman's uterus. Embryos that survive the freeze/thaw have been found to have the same viability rates as fresh embryos (Trounson 1990, 702).

It could be argued that generalized information (which in effect presumes the goodness of freezing) is more helpful than specific data that are too premature or sketchy to give accurate guidance. Some practitioners also contend that presenting freezing as an accepted part of IVF will save clients from the responsibility of making yet another decision in the already stressful IVF cycle.

The often expressed presumptions in IVF that the infertile patient is "desperate," "willing to try anything," and in need of urgent action due to her "ticking biological clock" seem to negate providing detailed information to her. Such views do not, however, justify withholding from clients detailed information about choices with respect to embryo freezing. The couple is not, in fact, in an emergency medical situation, and decisions need not be made under pressure if patients express their choices at the start of the IVF cycle. Moreover, the data are not so complex as to overwhelm most patients. While the legacy of infertility may indeed leave some women in psychological distress with feelings of diminished self-worth, depression, and anxiety, others exhibit high ego strength and a need to accumulate information about the procedures in which they participate (Freeman et al. 1985; Garner 1987). Where patients do perceive themselves as desperate, this ought to signal caution, not permission, about freezing and the desirability of conveying full information to the patient about the experimental nature of the procedure.

Another reason for full disclosure of information, even if that information is sketchy or seemingly not desired by the patient, is to check on unseemly incentives for offering freezing. There are many motives for freezing—enhancing a program's prestige, setting the stage for research, bringing in fees to be funneled back into the IVF program—and patients are needed to meet these goals. Hence, the exploitive dissembling that has occurred in regular IVF and the ambiguity over pregnancy rates (Blackwell et al. 1987; Soules 1985; Younger 1989) are repeated in freezing when directors give global success rates only and do not itemize success rates at each stage of the freezing procedure. If the program is too new to have figures, patients should be aware that generalized figures apply only to other centers.

Physicians must integrate into their protocols ways of enhancing the patient's choice about whether or not to freeze spare embryos (Ethics Committee . . . 1990, 60S). The information on freezing should be given at the beginning of the cycle (not later when there might be time constraints on decision making). It should cover full information about costs, including whether the storage fee is for each embryo or for all embryos, subject to periodic renewals, subject to cost-of-living adjustments, and inclusive of thawing and transfer fees. Most importantly, it should contain written information about risks and success rates at that particular center, including the average number of embryos frozen at the center per patient; the number surviving the freeze/thaw; the number of thawed embryos transferred to patients; the number of clinical pregnancies and births with thawed embryos; and comparisons of pregnancy, birth, and pregnancy and birth complications for fresh and thawed embryos.

If the center is too new to have such data, the director should provide global data and data from one or two middle-level centers (not just from the most successful centers). The patient should also be informed about freezing outcomes for women with situations similar to hers. Does embryo survival correlate with maternal age? Are some couples more likely to produce morphologically sound embryos than others? Where data are not available, patients should be advised that many questions about freezing remain unanswered.

The Meaning of the Embryo

Lingering questions about the nature of the human embryo affect communication within the IVF/freezing program. These questions suggest that the physician should recognize the broader societal context when making decisions about embryo freezing programs and should respect the differing perceptions of the embryo that intermix in the clinical setting. To clients, the embryo symbolizes hope and potential parenthood. It affirms the wife's femininity, the husband's masculinity, and the couple's potency. It is a powerful symbol with which clients establish emotional connections. It may be the closest thing to parenthood the wife and husband will ever experience.

To physicians and scientists, the embryo is a collection of cells with distinct properties relating to its stage of development (Tejada & Karow 1986). Its morphology is evaluated on its predicted ability to cleave, grow, and survive the freeze/thaw, and evaluations are made on this basis. One question, for example, is whether technicians should transfer the strongest embryos while they are fresh and freeze the weaker ones (this makes sense if most embryos do not survive the freeze/thaw) or transfer the weak embryos and freeze the strong ones (this makes sense if the strong embryos will survive and can be transferred to the woman at a later, presumably more receptive cycle when she has not been hormonally stimulated) (Testart 1987). The importance of the embryo's appearance in predicting success rates places technicians in the position of identifying the criteria for an embryo that "looks good" or "looks odd," and this adds another qualification to the embryo's "worth," although a correlation between appearance and implantation rates has not been conclusively demonstrated (Alikani & Cohen 1990, 715).

Freezing creates an ironic situation in which couples tend to personalize their embryos over time and physicians tend to depersonalize them as they evaluate the embryo's freezability. These different perspectives may reduce meaningful communication between patient and doctor because one is using subjective criteria for making decisions and the other objective criteria. In deciding the disposition of unwanted frozen embryos, for example, couples who develop attachments to their embryos (especially if they have had a child through an earlier IVF cycle) may "see" donation of embryos to other couples as akin to giving a child for adoption or "see" discarding the embryo as akin to abortion. A physician unaware of these perceptions may decide what choices to offer couples on the basis of expediency and with diminished sensitivity to their emotional attachments.

The legal dimensions of embryo freezing add another "personality" to the embryo. In 1984, the American Fertility Society advised that "concepti are the property of the donors" (American Fertility Society 1984, 12). After legal disputes, IVF programs integrated language about ownership and property into consent forms, stating, for example, that "each embryo shall be the joint property of both of you, as the wife and the husband, who are deemed to be the legal owners." Couples who freeze embryos are asked to provide for the disposition of their embryo-as-property in the event of death or divorce. On the one hand, this personalizes the embryo as a potential child by bidding the couple to take responsibility for it. On the other, it commercializes this responsibility by defining it as one between owners and property.

The varied meanings of the embryo and the amalgam of language used to describe embryos (clients naming them "twins" or "preemie"; doctors calling them "sets of tissues," "prezygotes," or "preembryos"; and consent forms referring to "property" and "owners") reveal the moral uncertainty still underlying activities involving embryos. This uncertainty is heightened by language referring to the embryo's destruction. Some centers are euphemistic (for example, "You should be aware that the embryo that is thawed and not transferred will not undergo further development") and others are blunt (embryos will be "destroyed" or "disposed of"). Some centers refer to "ethical methods" of embryo disposal, without specifying what these methods are. At least one gives couples the option of overseeing embryo disposal, as if in a ritual of death. All this conveys confused messages that hinder communication. If, for example, the embryo is a "mere" set of cells or property, why do program personnel hedge when talking about its destruction? If this is done to avoid arousing public attention, what is the effect on communication within the IVF center?

In sum, much uncertainty continues to underlie cryopreservation in IVF centers. Ethical dilemmas remain unresolved and misunderstandings arise from faulty communication. The patients will bear the brunt of techniques used before the moral meanings are understood in the public debate. It may be in the patient's interest for physicians to depersonalize the embryo and use scientific language to prevent unfruitful and probably disappointing bonding. However, this runs the danger of closing communication between physician and patient that would reveal the subjective but morally significant perspectives of patients.

Open and frank discussion among ethics committees, patients, nurse coordinators, and physicians is needed to resolve the question of the many meanings of the embryo. Although some ethics committees may be fastidious in their review of new protocols, other hospital committees may be likely to approve, with little critical thought, additions to IVF programs presented with excitement by the clinic directors. Said a member of an ethics committee whom I interviewed, "Had I wanted to nitpick, I would have been out of place." Another said of the freezing decision: "Our function was to document the process" of having consulted the community before making decisions about embryo freezing (Bonnicksen 1989, 39). Whatever is included in written material, clinics must develop a pragmatic and honest language that does not disguise the embryo (in itself an acceptable term) either by personalizing it (for example, calling it "little one") or depersonalizing it (by calling it "the prezygote"). Honesty is also served by forthright communication about what will be done with embryos no longer needed. False propriety does little good, as when consent forms state the embryos will be "disposed of ethically," but the method is unstated and staff members are unclear about what an ethical method of disposition is. If it means a passive act (exposing the embryo to the air so it will disintegrate) rather than an active move (washing it down the sink), this should clearly be included in the consent form by stating, for example, that unwanted frozen embryos will be exposed to light and will disintegrate in a given period of time.

Beneficent Embryo Freezing

The growing field of alternative conception owes its energy to mixed forces, including the demands of patients, scientists' yearning for discovery, physicians' interest in satisfying patients' needs, lucrative possibilities, and public fascination with technology. At a basic level, however, it is the physician operating in the infertility clinic who makes everyday decisions that affect whether the techniques will serve or detract from societal interests (Brody 1987). Where physicians adhere to traditional notions of virtue in presenting freezing in the clinical setting, they take an important step toward integrating it into society in a way that will promote its promise. However, when they make ad hoc decisions with the clinic's interests primarily in mind, overlook the emotional side effects of the technique, and presume the benefit of freezing, patient and societal interests are ill served.

With normalcy, demonstrated safety, and routine come a diminished will and inclination to question the ethical dimensions of embryo freezing. The subtle ethical quandaries that arise in freezing programs are in danger of being overlooked in the absence of highly visible crises. Already egg freezing is being presented as an innovation that, if its safety can be demonstrated, raises fewer ethical and legal issues (Friedler et al. 1988, 761; Trounson 1990, 706) and negates the need for the more problematic embryo freezing (Trounson 1986, 11). To see new techniques as a way of reducing dilemmas is to fail to question the virtue of the model already being built. Where dissembling, ambiguous language, untested presumptions, and narrow medical criteria combine in the clinical setting, there is reduced opportunity for enlightened debate about the value of freezing and its technological successors for society as a whole. Clinical interactions are gatekeeping interactions. They ought to be developed and refined on the basis of ethically defensible criteria in which the observed needs of patients play a central role.

Notes

1. Physicians are aware, however, that ethical issues still exist in embryo freezing, especially in regard to safety and the disposition of embryos. See, e.g., Ethics Committee 1990, 58S–61S.
2. In an Australian case the responsibility for two embryos "orphaned" after the death of the contracting couple was held to lie with the clinic. In a Tennessee case a divorcing couple contested the disposition of seven of their frozen embryos. The county court judge awarded the embryos to the wife, negating her husband's claim that he had the right not to become a father against his wishes (*Davis v. Davis* 1989). On appeal, however, the Tennessee Court of Appeals held the embryos to be joint property, and it granted the husband and wife equal voices in the disposition (*Davis v. Davis* 1990; see Shevory, this volume). In a third conflict, a couple who had one frozen embryo in a Virginia IVF clinic sought to have the embryo released and shipped to California to a clinic closer to their home. Disagreement about the disposition of the embryo led to a legal dispute resolved when a court ruled in favor of the couple, stating, among other things, that the embryo was their property and that the program had the obligation to return that property (*Jones v. York* 1989) (Robertson 1989, 9–10).
3. Although technically the "patient" in IVF is the husband and wife as a couple, for clarity in the following pages attention is directed to the female partner as the patient.
4. For information on biopsies, see Abstracts . . . 1990; Dokras 1990; Verlinsky, Ginsburg, et al. 1990; Verlinsky, Pergament, & Strom 1990.

References

Abstracts of the First International Symposium on Preimplantation Genetics. 1990. 14–19 September. Chicago. *Journal of in Vitro Fertilization and Embryo Transfer* 7(4):183–221.

Alikani, Mina, and Jacques Cohen. 1990. Human oocyte and embryo cryopreservation. *Current Opinion in Obstetrics and Gynecology* 2:714–717.

American Fertility Society. 1984. Ethical statement on in vitro fertilization. *Fertility and Sterility* 41(1):12–13.

Blackwell, Richard E., Bruce R. Carr, R. Jeffrey Chang, et al. 1987. Are we exploiting the infertile couple? *Fertility and Sterility* 48(5): 735–739.

Bonnicksen, Andrea L. 1989. *In vitro fertilization: Building policy from laboratories to legislatures*. New York: Columbia University Press.

Bonnicksen, Andrea L., and Robert H. Blank. 1988. The government and in vitro fertilization (IVF): Views of IVF directors. *Fertility and Sterility* 49(3):396–398.

Brody, Eugene B. 1987. Reproduction without sex—But with the doctor. *Law, Medicine and Health Care* 15(3):152–155.

Davis v. Davis. 1989. No. E-14496. Blount Co. Circ. Ct., Tenn. 21 September.

Davis v. Davis. 1990. Tennessee Appellate: LEXIS 642. 13 September.

Dokras, A., I.L. Sargent, C. Ross, et al. 1990. Trophectoderm biopsy in human blastocysts. *Human Reproduction* 5(7):821–825.

Edwards, R.G., and A.H. Handyside. 1990. Future developments in IVF. *British Medical Bulletin* 46(3):823–841.

Ethics Committee of the American Fertility Society. 1990. Ethical considerations of the new reproductive technologies. *Fertility and Sterility* 53(6) (Supp. 21) S–109S.

Freeman, Ellen W., Andrea S. Boxer, Karl Rickels, et al. 1985. Psychological evaluation and support in a program of in vitro fertilization and embryo transfer. *Fertility and Sterility* 43(1):48–53.

Friedler, Shevach, Linda C. Giudice, and Emmet J. Lamb. 1988. Cryopreservation of embryos and ova. *Fertility and Sterility* 49(5):743–764.

Fugger, E.F., M. Bustillo, A.D. Dorfmann, and J.D. Schulman. 1991. Human preimplantation embryo cryopreservation: Selected aspects. *Human Reproduction* 6(1):131–135.

Garner, C.H. 1987. Psychological aspects of IVF and the infertile couple. In *Foundations of in vitro fertilization*, ed. Christopher M. Fredericks et al. Washington D.C.: Hemisphere.

Jones v. York. 1989. No. 33455. E.D. Va.

Medical Research International. 1988. In vitro fertilization/embryo transfer in the United States: 1985 and 1986 results from the national IVF/ET registry. *Fertility and Sterility* 49(2):212–215.

Medical Research International. 1991. In vitro fertilization/embryo transfer (IVF-ET) in the United States: 1989 results from the IVF-ET registry. *Fertility and Sterility* 55(1):14–23.

Rizk, Botros, Robert G. Edwards, Umberto Nicolini, et al. 1991. Edwards' syndrome after the replacement of cryopreserved-thawed embryos. *Fertility and Sterility* 55(1):208–210.

Robertson, John A. 1989. Resolving disputes over frozen embryos. *Hastings Center Report* 19(6):7–12.

Soules, Michael R. 1985. The in vitro fertilization pregnancy rate: Let's be honest with one another. *Fertility and Sterility* 43(4):511–513 .

Tejada, Rafael I., and William G. Karow. 1986. Semantics used in the nomenclature of in vitro fertilization, or let's all be more proper. *Journal of in Vitro Fertilization and Embryo Transfer* 3(6): 341–342.

Testart, Jacques, Bruno Lassalle, Robert Forman, et al. 1987. Factors influencing the success rate of human embryo freezing in an in vitro fertilization and embryo transfer program. *Fertility and Sterility* 48(1) :107–112.

Trounson, Alan. 1986. Preservation of human eggs and embryos. *Fertility and Sterility* 46(1) :1–12 .

Trounson, Alan. 1990. Cryopreservation. *British Medical Bulletin* 46 (3): 695–708.

U.S. Congress, Office of Technology Assessment. 1988. *Infertility: Medical and social choices.* OTA-BA-358.Washington, D.C.: U.S. Government Printing Office.

Verlinsky, Yury, Norman Ginsberg, Aaron Lifchez, et al. 1990. Analysis of the first polar body: Preconception genetic diagnosis. *Human Reproduction* 5(7) :826–829.

Verlinsky, Yury, Eugene Pergament, and Charles Strom. 1990. The preimplantation genetic diagnosis of genetic diseases. *Journal of in Vitro Fertilization and Embryo Transfer* 7(1):1–5.

Younger, J. Benjamin. 1989. Truth in advertising. *Fertility and Sterility* 52(5):726–727.

Chapter 16

THROUGH A GLASS, DARKLY: LAW, POLITICS, AND FROZEN HUMAN EMBRYOS

Thomas C. Shevory

Introduction

The birth of the world's first test-tube baby, Louise Brown, in Great Britain in 1978 dramatically expanded the potential experiences that human beings may have in relationship to their own reproduction. Some control over reproductive events has of course been available in the past—with the technologies of birth control, abortion, and, more recently, interventions such as artificial insemination. But the first successful birth of a child conceived in a petri dish outside of her mother's womb was a watershed event. While this example of successful in vitro fertilization (IVF) provided hope for the treatment of infertility, its effects upon social relations were hardly foreseeable. And its promises for developing even more remarkable reproductive interventions in the future are extremely unsettling.

Not surprisingly, conflicts generated in the application of the new reproductive technologies have begun to appear in the courts, where they have on occasion generated much publicity. I question whether the courts will treat issues raised by these technologies so that the legitimate interests of women and men to assert reasonable control over their reproductive prerogatives will be protected. Legal discourse, because of the requirements of the adversary system and its case orientation, fragments analysis of complex policy issues. Yet the courtroom provides an arena in which to observe the redefinition of political and social relationships. By examining certain legal disputes we can gain understanding of how our politics are being shaped by advanced technologies, the complete impact of which is now very obscure.

In this analysis I focus on legal and political implications of embryo freezing, a process that is now often routinely part of IVF procedure. Specifically, I focus on the case of *Davis v. Davis* (1989), a "custody dispute" over seven frozen embryos that were created in the Fort Sanders Medical Center Fertility Clinic in Knoxville, Tennessee. I shall consider issues raised at the trial and the appellate court levels. In directing most of my attention to this one case, I am not primarily interested in a defending a different position than the one held by Tennessee Circuit Judge W. Dale Young, who decided and wrote the opinion in the case (although I adamantly disagree with the judge's decision and am skeptical as well about the appeals decision). Rather, I wish to consider how the shape of the arguments in *Davis* indicates changes in the politics of reproduction, given the advent of the new reproductive technologies.

After providing some background to the Davis case, I examine three crucial aspects of *Davis v. Davis.* First, I analyze the politics of language in the distinction between "preembryo" and "embryo" in terms of its genesis and its implications for women's control over their reproduction. Second, I expose the paradox in and question the validity and viability of the rights orientation toward procreation that is central in the argumentation in *Davis.* Lastly, I argue that the legal disposition of embryos as "property" will result in a balancing of interests that favors men at the expense of women. In making these last two arguments, I propose that, in disputes related to reproduction, women's unique contribution to reproduction should give them a presumption of control over embryos, either inside the womb or outside it.

During the IVF procedure drug-induced superovulation may allow clinicians to retrieve 10 or more mature eggs from a woman's ovaries. If most of these are successfully fertilized in the laboratory, the result may be too many embryos to introduce into her uterus. A balance must be struck between creating sufficient embryos to increase the chance of implantation yet few enough to prevent multiple gestation with its attendant risks (Price 1988). The discovery that healthy infants could be born from cryopreserved embryos seemed to resolve that clinical problem even as it introduced legal and social problems.

Hypothetically, embryos can be kept alive outside a woman's uterus for about 14 days (although the record is 9 days) or through the early blastocyst stage. This time limit has been accepted by the U.S. Ethics Advisory Board,[1] the Waller Committee,[2] and the Warnock Committee[3] as the point up to which experimentation and research can be ethically conducted. The ethical justification for the 14-day limit is based on the facts that after 14 days embryos can no longer be implanted, that the so-called "primitive streak" can then be discerned within the embryonic disc, and that differentiation of the embryo is then evident. Both the Warnock and the Waller committees recognized the time limits as somewhat arbitrary. (See Warnock 1985[4]; Waller 1984.) This distinction becomes a focal point for argumentation in the Davis case, although it was ultimately construed as immaterial by Circuit Judge Young. According to Elias and Annas:

> Until the basis of the 14-day limit is more clearly articulated and publicly accepted, it cannot serve as a legitimate regulatory boundary. Are we concerned with what the embryo *is*, what it looks like, or what it feels? Or are we concerned with what it *will be*, or what it will never have a chance to be, or with what it will look like or feel? Or is the focus of our concern something else entirely? (Elias & Annas 1987, 227.)

These questions may never be adequately answered. But criticism of the 14-day boundary comes from two quite opposite directions. On the one hand, researchers in a variety of fields would like to use later stage embryos for research. On the other hand, "pro-life" advocates see the 14-day mark as meaningless, since "life begins at conception." They thus usually wish to eliminate using embryos for research, and sometimes advocate eliminating IVF programs altogether (see Flynn 1984; Tiefel 1990; Waller 1984 dissent). The politics of this distinction will be discussed below.

Antecedents

Davis v. Davis was not the first dispute about the fate of in vitro embryos. In the United States, the first legal controversy was *Del Zio v. Presbyterian Hospital* (1978). In 1973, Dr. William Sweeney, a New York fertility specialist, with Dr. Landrum Shettles of Columbia Presbyterian Hospital, New York City, undertook the first in vitro fertilization procedure in the United States. Sweeney removed an egg from Doris Del Zio, a woman with badly damaged fallopian tubes, in one hospital; John Del Zio carried it by taxi across town to Columbia Presbyterian, where Shettles added John's sperm to it and placed it in an incubator. Shettles had not, however, asked his hospital's permission to undertake the procedure. Raymond Vande Wiele, chair of Columbia's Department of Obstetrics and Gynecology, removed the fertilized ovum from its incubator, thus destroying it. According to Sweeney, Mrs. Del Zio's reproductive organs were too damaged to permit removal of another egg (Andrews 1984, 155–157).

In 1974, the Del Zios filed suit against the hospital for the destruction of the embryo on the grounds of improper conversion of property and intentional infliction of emotional distress. In 1978, a jury found in favor of the Del Zios on the emotional distress claim but not on the conversion claim. Thus, this provided legal precedent supporting an economic value for the embryo but left ambiguous the claim that the embryo constituted the couple's "property." (For a complete discussion, see Andrews 1984.)

A second case involved a Los Angeles couple, Mario and Elsa Rios, who undertook IVF at the Queen Victoria Medical Center in Melbourne, Australia, in 1981 (Holden 1984, 35). Three eggs removed from Mrs. Rios were inseminated by an anonymous donor. One of the three resulting embryos was implanted in Elsa Rios's uterus unsuccessfully; the other two were frozen (Saharelli 1985, 1030–1033). In 1983, the Rioses died in a plane crash in South America. Their preserved embryos attracted considerable international attention when the press learned that the couple had a large fortune that might eventually become the subject of an inheritance dispute (Holden 1985; Smith 1985–1986, 27)

In 1984, the Waller Committee released its "Report on the Disposition of Embryos Produced by In Vitro Fertilization." They made 60 recommendations for policy in Australia, including, that freezing and storing of embryos be done in regulated hospitals, that hospitals not become large embryo storage facilities, that couples be adequately informed about the processes of cryopreservation, that clear agreement about the disposition of the embryos be reached before they are frozen, and that untransferred embryos not possess rights or claims of inheritance (Waller 1984, 33–34).

The Waller Committee placed considerable emphasis on "respect" for preimplantation embryos and hence included the recommendation that unclaimed embryos be placed in a pool to be offered to anonymous recipients, and only if there were no interested parties could the embryos be removed from storage and discarded. Although the Rios's embryos were apparently offered to another couple, their ultimate fate is undisclosed. They would probably not have implanted successfully and been carried to term considering the relatively primitive state of cryopreservation techniques at the time (Holden 1985; Saharelli 1985). Apparently, however, the lessons of the Rios case were lost on the Fort Sanders Medical Center Fertility Clinic, since the clinic did not determine the disposition of the Davis embryos in advance.

Davis v. Davis

On February 23, 1988, Junior Lewis Davis, age 30, filed for divorce from his wife Mary Sue Davis, age 28, in the Circuit Court for Blount County,

Tennessee. The Davises had been married since 1980. Junior Davis's original complaint alleged that Mary Sue Davis had been guilty of cruel and inhuman treatment toward him, but this allegation was eventually dropped. Satisfactory division of the couple's property was reached, except for seven cryopreserved embryos, which were and are now being stored at the Fort Sanders Medical Center in Knoxville, Tennessee. Mary Sue Davis had suffered damage to her fallopian tubes from five ectopic pregnancies and was thus able to conceive only through IVF (Opinion of the Court 1989, 4).

Mrs. Davis underwent six attempts to produce a child through IVF before the couple gave up and attempted an adoption. After the failure of the adoption, they returned to Dr. King's clinic for another try at IVF, this time with knowledge of the new technique of cryopreservation, which "offered Mrs. Davis much welcomed relief from the rigors of the full procedure each time in vitro fertilization was attempted" (Opinion of the Court 1989, 5). In December 1988, nine ova were aspirated from Mrs. Davis. After fertilization, two were introduced into her uterus without success. The remaining seven embryos were cyropreserved and subsequently became the subject of the custody dispute. Junior Davis wanted the embryos destroyed, while Mary Sue Davis expressed a desire to have them implanted. On September 21, 1989, the Tennessee Circuit Court for Blount County found in favor of Mrs. Davis's right to custody (Opinion of the Court 1989, 5). Junior Davis appealed the case. Mary Sue Davis remarried and expressed her desire to "donate the embryos so that another childless couple may use them" (Opinion of the Court 1990, 2). On September 13, 1990, the Court of Appeals of Tennessee Eastern Section ruled in favor of "joint custody" (Opinion of the Court 1990).

Most interesting about *Davis* is not its narrow legal findings nor the precedential authority that it may establish. *Davis* is most significant as a *political* event. The arguments offered in *Davis* indicate ways in which the "symbols of IVF" can be "tracked" (to paraphrase Bonnicksen 1989, 11). By examining the argumentation on the disposition of these embryos in this Tennessee circuit courthouse, we begin to sense how the new reproductive technologies affect the meaning of some basic legal and political conceptions of privacy and property rights. Thus, the focus here is mainly on the briefs and opinion of the controversial circuit court decision, although it is analyzed in light of the appeals decision that followed.

Political Definitions of Embryonic Development

Many theorists in both the social and the natural sciences have analyzed the political significance of scientific language. *Davis* provides an exceptionally rich example of the intersection of forces of science and political interest through its attempts to conceptualize and control a nominally medical definition, i.e., of what constitutes an embryo and, indirectly, human life or personhood.

At the outset of his circuit court brief, Junior Davis's attorney, Charles M. Clifford, claimed that a "preembryo" was not a person (Brief for the Defendant 1989, 1–2). To support this argument he cited both *Roe v. Wade* (1973) and *Webster v. Reproductive Services* (1989). Both cases hold that a first trimester fetus (to use the language of the court in *Roe*) is not a person under the Fourteenth Amendment, and so, certainly, by implication, neither would an embryo be one nor would a preembryo. Why then did not Mr. Davis's attorney simply use the term "fetus," or even "embryo"? If the language of *Roe* was sufficient to control the case, why introduce a new concept? In fact, the plaintiff's attorney was implying that the closer the conceptus is to conception, the farther it is from any legal status of personhood, an argument drawn from *Roe*'s "trimester analysis," which makes a rough division of "fetal rights" that correlates with the temporal distance from conception.

More is at stake here, however, than simply a legalist distinction based on precedent. *Roe* was decided five years before IVF had a live human birth. The current distinction between "embryos" and "preembryos" was generated in response to recommendations of national ethics committees and to political pressures. After the Warnock Report recommended its 14-day limit for embryonic research, MP Enoch Powell, a member of Britain's Conservative Party, introduced a bill into Parliament—the Unborn Children Protection Bill—that would have entirely banned human embryo research and would have, in effect, stopped the clinical practice of IVF as well (Spallone 1989, 48). In reaction to such political pressures, the British Medical Research Council (MRC) and Royal College of Obstetricians and Gynaecologists (RCOG) in 1985 established a committee called the Voluntary Licensing Authority (VLA) to regulate IVF (Spallone 1989, 52).

The VLA was charged with the task of overseeing IVF clinical practices and research with human embryos. Early in its work, the VLA began to use the term "preembryo" because of the political pressures from British anti-abortion forces and in line with the Warnock Committee views on the status of early embryos. The Warnock Committee had itself been an indirect response to fears by researchers that conservative political forces might attempt to interfere with their activities. The term "preembryo," in other words, is a "scientific" term invented for a discrete political purpose.[5] Spallone characterizes the situation:

> The coining of the term pre-embryo was a political act. The 'pre-embryo' explanation from scientists has been tailored from the scientific 'facts'

> to accommodate the fourteen-day time limit, not vice versa. The word pre-embryo was invented for the purpose of human embryo research. It was taken up by the media, by scientific journals, by the medical and science bodies formalising their regulations on IVF/human embryo research, and by the lobby group Progress whose aim is to promote 'human embryo' research through the public understanding of the scientific issues (Spallone 1989, 53).

In the United States the American Fertility Society (AFS), a professional organization of physicians and researchers involved with infertility, adopted the term preembryo, in its 1986 "Ethical Statement on *In Vitro* Fertilization," (Ethics Committee . . . 1986) and reaffirmed its use in 1990 in a further ethical statement. It has been defended by University of Texas law professor John A. Robertson, a member of the Ethics Committee of the AFS, who testified on behalf of the plaintiff in Davis.[6] Pushing the distinction between embryos and preembryos are clinicians and researchers and the infertile couples who provide much financial support for IVF. Feminist analysts of the new reproductive technologies, however, do not support the distinction precisely because it protects fertility researchers and clinicians, and not women's reproductive rights.[7]

Moreover, the distinction between embryos and preembryos could be interpreted to support the contention of "right to lifers" that preembryonic and *post*-preembryonic entities deserve legal entitlement. The Warnock Report suggested that human preembryos be granted a moral status "higher" than animals,[8] while also asserting that it was acceptable for researchers to do experiments with them. Is research on preembryos compatible with the concept of respect? What about embryos proper? If the preembryo deserves respect, then does not the embryo proper deserve more respect, and perhaps legal protection? Researchers, having granted respect to preembryos, as a strategy to fend off conservatives and protect their research prerogatives, have made a significant concession to them, a concession that can then be turned to support legal arguments protecting concepti. This is exactly what happened in *Davis* because even though Mrs. Davis won the first round of the case, she did so on grounds that are clearly antithetical to reproductive choice.[9] The same arguments can then be turned against the researchers. A de facto moratorium on funding for fetal research by the United States Government has existed since 1980 when the Ethics Advisory Board disbanded (U.S. Congress 1988, 178). Moreover, 23 states have laws prohibiting fetal or embryo research. Although no states have outlawed IVF clinics (Caplan 1986, 246), that is a conceivable outcome of recent actions at the state legislative level on restricting abortion rights.

Whatever else he did, the circuit judge in *Davis* clearly recognized inconsistency in the arguments supporting Junior Davis's position. Judge W. Dale Young cited several passages in the report of the Ethics Committee of the American Fertility Society in which that committee recommended showing "respect" or "profound respect" for the preembryo (Opinion of the Court 1989, 11). Moreover, he pointed out that expert witnesses' usage of the term preembryo seemed artificial.[10] Thus, the judge turned the fertility society's own language on preembryos toward his inclination to preserve what he considered their full human rights. At the same time, he rejected the recommendations supporting research on preembryos because the court was not legally bound by them. He simply selected those aspects of the report that tended to support his position, that the embryo had a right to life. This use of selected guidelines from an ethics committee established considerable credibility for his position.

Reproductive Rights

In the Davis trial the rhetorical defense of women's reproductive rights comes from a very odd quarter—three amicus curiae briefs submitted by R.D. Hash, a local pro-life attorney. When the case opened, J.G. Christenberry, attorney for Mary Davis, based most of his argument in her defense on the disposition of marital "property." Christenberry used *Roe v. Wade* (1973) to buttress his contention that the embryo was not a person under law; it was property (Brief for the Defendant 1989, 9). However, attorney Hash recognized that the interpretation of *Roe* in *Planned Parenthood of Missouri v. Danforth* (1976) was more central to the claims made by Mary Davis for control over the embryos. Taken as a whole, Hash's briefs, strongly supporting Mary Davis, espouse a "right to life" position. Because *Danforth* held that spousal consent provisions of a Missouri abortion statute were unconstitutional under *Roe v. Wade*,[11] Hash argued that if a woman has an absolute right to terminate a pregnancy during the first trimester, then she has an absolute right to *continue* the pregnancy if she so desires. According to Hash:

> The State cannot delegate authority to any particular person, *not even the spouse*, to prevent abortion during that period. It follows then if the mother has the exclusive right to determine if she wants to abortion [sic], she has the right not to elect that remedy, and to allow full gestation and birth, and she has that right without interference from the State or her spouse (Hash 1989 3).

Hash is correct here in seeing the implications of *Roe* and *Danforth* for the case, although his line of reasoning, i.e., that the positive implies its negative, is questionable. It is ironic that an attorney representing "pro-life" forces should rely upon *Roe* as precedential authority. But a reading of Hash's arguments shows clearly that he is concerned with the reproductive rights of Mary Davis only insofar as they are consonant with the preservation of the embryo, which he regards as a complete human being. If Mary Davis sought to discard the embryos and if Junior Davis sought to have them implanted in another woman, doubtless Hash would have joined in support of Mr. Davis's position.[12] This irony in the trial record speaks to concerns already raised by several legal scholars about the utility of rights discourse for substantially advancing social justice.

Both legal realist and critical legal studies approaches to the analysis of law argue that the ideology of legal discourse, with its pretense of dependence upon determination of precedents and the application of them to discrete cases, is largely an elaborate fiction. "Law is simply politics by other means" (Kairys 1982, 17). Clearly, what is occurring in *Davis* is not a dispassionate application of legal principles to a highly exceptional set of facts, but rather it is a political discourse that deprives women of control over their reproductive processes while nominally defending them. This discourse depends upon an implied covenant among the parties involved to pretend that the arguments are legal and therefore can be disconnected from the political consequences that they imply. Hash has no obligation to make his defense of *Roe* consistent with his defense of the embryos' "rights to life," even though a complete argument in defense of Mary Davis's claim would require exactly that and would move him toward considering the actual interests that women have in such cases to maintain some control over reproduction.

Mark Tushnet (1984) argues that rights discourse is essentially "indeterminate," i.e., that it does not provide a stable means to allocate claims fairly or equitably in the various legal and political contexts in which it is often advanced. Tushnet argues, correctly I believe, that "the language of rights is so open and indeterminate that opposing parties can use the same language to express their positions . . . that it can provide only momentary advantages in ongoing political struggles" (Tushnet 1984, 1371). The Davis frozen embryo dispute provides an excellent example not only of how rights are used by each side to the dispute, but also of how complex and ironical such usages can become, as when Hash uses the privacy rights in *Roe* in defense of Mary Davis's right to control the disposition of the embryos.

Rights are especially indeterminate or unsettled in a context of rapid technological change. In *Davis*, for example, the new techniques of cryopreservation gave Judge Young an opportunity to establish a precedential "right to life." And disputes regarding the implications of this technology, along with the political context generated by "pro-life" forces during the 1980s, offered him a modicum of credibility in asserting this position.

On Distinguishing Inside from Outside

The right to reproductive choice for women has generally been associated with rights to bodily integrity, a central aspect it has been argued of the right to privacy as in *Roe*. This powerful argument for bodily control has been significant in the abortion debate. IVF, frozen embryos, and possibly even more complex reproductive technologies in the future, however, have the capacity to separate women's bodies to a greater and greater extent from reproduction. Indeed, these technologies are already having an impact on discourse of reproductive rights. Tushnet notes that two choices are made when a woman has an abortion: (1) the fetus is removed from the woman's body, and (2) the fetus is destroyed. Since originally the second decision was determined by the first, the status of the fetus (or embryo) apart from the woman's decision to have an abortion was a nonissue. But techniques that sustain fetuses in intensive-care nurseries make the distinction between abortion and embryo death less valid. Tushnet describes rights implications flowing from this distinction:

> If the choices were independent, there would no longer be a right to *reproductive* choice in the sense that interests us today. No one would care about a woman's decision merely to *remove* a fetus from her body, because that act would not have the consequence (i.e., the death of the fetus) that troubles many people today. If the removal of the fetus had some caretaker available to it, the mere act of removal would be morally inconsequential (Tushnet 1984, 1366).

Tushnet's point here is not to endorse this position but to demonstrate how technological innovation can alter the rhetoric of rights. Fairly widespread interest exists, in fact, in the potential policy consequences of separating reproductive processes from women's wombs. Much, for example, has been made of technological changes that have broadened the scope of "fetal viability" (see Callahan 1986; Engelhardt 1980; Wikler 1978).

Christine Overall's feminist analysis of reproductive issues (which she sees as firmly grounded in a tradition of rights discourse) emphasizes this distinction between abortion and fetal death. Overall argues that while a woman has no right to kill an embryo or fetus, she still has choice on the issue of abortion. "For to say that a person has no right to do something does not preclude her doing it, on occasion, and being morally right in doing so" (Overall 1987, 76). This is reinforced by the principle that "the embryo/fetus has no right to occupancy of its mother's (or anyone else's) uterus" (Overall 1987, 77).

The separation of woman from fetus provides for a new language of competing rights. And the location of the embryo can become of central importance because even though the location itself does not endow rights, "from the perspective of a woman experiencing pregnancy, the location of the embryo/fetus is naturally of the utmost importance, and that fact must be taken account of" (Overall 1987, 76). In fact, within a rights perspective, location becomes central because the potential rights conflict (between woman and fetus) can be dissolved by removal of the embryo or fetus from the woman's uterus. Women, from this perspective, have no special claim upon determinations of embryonic disposition because the fact that they may be involuntarily inhabited by embryos is merely the result of a natural accident that can now be "corrected."[13]

This sort of analysis, however, does not consider the power relationships differentiating men from women at this time. Rather than being seen as historically situated, men and women are cast as equal, autonomous actors, each with some claim to rights. Once the woman's special claims to reproductive participation are dissolved by exploiting the distinction between inside and outside the womb, she has no presumption to disposition; she and her husband can be seen as having equivalent interests in distributing procreation rights or disposing of property.

In an odd twist, the Tennessee Appeals Court, in a barely coherent opinion attempted to "balance" the procreation rights of Mary and Junior Davis. The court relied upon *Skinner v. Oklahoma* (the 1942 forced sterilization case) to argue that implantation of the fertilized ova by Mary Davis was *a violation of Junior Davis's right against forced procreation*. The reasoning was as follows:

(a) *Skinner* protects against forced sterilization.

(b) Forced sterilization is the equivalent of forced procreation.

(c) Allowing Mary Davis to implant the embryos is the equivalent of forcing Junior Davis to procreate.

(d) Ergo, implanting the embryos is a violation of Junior Davis's constitutional rights.

In the words of the court, "Awarding the fertilized ova to Mary Sue for implantation against Junior's will, in our view, constitutes impermissible state action in violation of Junior's constitutionally protected right not to be burdened with a child where no pregnancy had taken place" (Opinion of the Court 1990, 4). Thus, while the appeals court denied Judge Young's "pro-life" position, it awarded "joint custody," thereby "equalizing" the reproductive claims of each party (Opinion of the Court 1990, 6). In fact, since no implementation directive was specified (nor is one readily conceivable), the actual disposition of the embryos awaits further appeal. But the appeals court decision demonstrates the difficulties and dangers of invoking rights-based arguments to defend women's procreative prerogatives. Two significant problems of rights analysis are considered here.

First, a number of feminists have noted the apparent distrust, if not contempt, medical practitioners and scientific researchers hold for the capabilities of women's wombs. Corea (1985) interprets the enterprise of genetic and fertility research as driven by the fears and desires that men harbor toward women's reproductive processes. Spallone (1989) shows how the language of fertility researchers like Steptoe and Edwards favors the interests of scientific understanding and technological control over the legitimate concerns of women to protect their own health. She makes a strong case that "'basic' research on genetic mechanisms exists totally independently of women's health issues" (Spallone 1989, 107). Suspicion about women's reproductive capacities also drives the concern for "prenatal abuse," i.e., that women who improperly care for their own health are endangering the life and health of the fetuses they carry. As Overall states, the focus on "prenatal abuse" "seems to be connected to certain attitudes toward women, according to which the female body is a threat to the embryo/fetus: the pregnant woman cannot be trusted not to abuse it, pass on defective genes to it, or even kill it, let alone to protect it from environmental harm and give birth to it safely" (Overall 1987, 89). Given this, a rights analysis that balances competing claims on the disposition of frozen embryos is unlikely to be resolved in favor of women.

The second problem with a rights approach to defending women's reproductive prerogatives is its institutional association with the court system. Courts, as *Davis* indicates and as recent events at the national level make clear, are becoming increasingly hostile to the claims of women to maintain a protected reproductive sphere. And abortion is only one aspect of the hostility of courts to women's claims in relation to embryos or fetuses. Courts have been on the forefront of the movement to protect fetuses from their mothers insofar as women are deemed a threat to both their own lives and those of the fetuses they carry. To a certain extent at least, during the 1970s, and to some extent the 1980s, courts were the institutions most likely to give women some control over their own reproductive capacities. However, with changes in federal and state court memberships (the legacy of the neo-conservative revolution), no longer will this happen. Insofar as a rhetoric of rights implies actions taken in court, it is likely that those who favor women's control over their reproductive functions will lose out to political institutions that will be hostile to their claims. The circuit and appeals decisions provide evidence that this is the case.

Embryos as Marital Property

Finally, let us examine the property claim in this case. Rights claims are often connected to property claims in a very fundamental way in liberal societies, but the property claims in *Davis* are sufficiently distinguishable in this case to warrant separate treatment. The assertion of a reproductive right is different from the assertion of a marital property claim. Moreover, property arguments could become important in future cases on the disposition of embryos and other contested biological materials, although the property claims were ignored by the Tennessee judiciary in *Davis*.

Mary Davis's attorney, Christenberry, rested most of his argument, somewhat tentatively to be certain, on the assertion that the embryos *were* a form of marital property, to which Mary Davis had the strongest claim for possession. He states as follows:

> Looking together at the views of courts and commentators on this question, the consensus seems to be moving toward a finding that frozen embryos, while perhaps not property in the traditional sense, are much closer to being "property" than to being "persons." The clearest demonstration of this is not what the sources say, but in what they do not say. If frozen embryos were truly persons, one would logically expect strong criminal sanctions for their destruction, and the placement of a strong legal and moral duty upon physicians and parents to ensure that all embryos have a maximum chance at developing into babies. But few sources advocate these things (Brief for the Defendant 1989, 13).

Christenberry argued that the embryos are a kind of "quasi-property."[14] The strength of Mary Davis's claim on the embryos was then grounded, according to Christenberry, in the significance of her contribution to the creation of the embryo. "The woman's contribution is much greater because the process involved in removing egg cells from her body is much more discomforting than a sperm donation process" (Brief for the Defendant 1989, 14).

Christenberry is correct that the burden of producing eggs for IVF is greater than that of producing sperm, but the word "discomfort" is hardly adequate to characterize Mary Davis's experiences in the pursuit of pregnancy. First, she suffered several ectopic pregnancies before she turned to IVF, each of which could have seriously injured or even killed her. She then underwent six laparoscopies in the pursuit of IVF, each of which requires a general anesthesia (each in turn with 1/10,000 chance of death). Moreover, each of her laparoscopic surgeries followed potent hormonal treatments to induce superovulation, which can, in and of themselves, be physically dangerous (Holmes 1988; Spallone 1989, 59; U.S. Congress 1988, 118). So, while Mary Davis's attorney did not make the case as effectively as he might have, had the court hinged its decisions on property and the effort in producing it, doubtless the case would been decided in favor of Mrs. Davis.

Robertson has described the process of egg removal as "moderate"; he rejects what he calls the "sweat equity" position that presumes women should generally be awarded custody. "[T]he difference in bodily burdens between the man and woman in IVF is not so great (especially with transvaginal aspiration of eggs) that it should automatically determine decisional authority over resulting embryos" (Robertson 1989, 7).

In the case of Mary Davis who had laparoscopic egg removal, Robertson is clearly wrong. With new methods of egg retrieval and embryo freezing techniques, the burdens for women who undergo IVF will diminish only trivially. Although the disposition of embryos ought to be grounded in a utilitarian weighing of contributed effort by each party in the dispute, a court, unfortunately, is bound to do this weighing arbitrarily on any given occasion. We should at least hold open the possibility, then, that distinctive aspects of the woman's contribution to reproduction cannot be entirely disclosed by the fairly crass and potentially capricious weighing of costs and benefits that Robertson, for example, seems to endorse.

Weighing "psychological distress" might be a more gender-neutral and thus fairer means of determining disposition. The argument is that men and women could both undergo psychological stress from the idea of having unwanted progeny brought into the world; thus, in general, neither sex is injured by invoking such a test. The appeals court, in fact, used this criterion in favor of its decision to award joint custody. "It would," the court stated, "be . . . repugnant to order Junior to bear the psychological, if not the legal, consequences of paternity against his will" (Opinion of the Court 1990, 6).

But a "psychological distress test" should not necessarily favor the party who wants to discard the embryos. One can easily imagine some women and men who would be equally troubled at having potential future offspring destroyed. In other words, in a simple application of "greatest happiness" or "unhappiness" principles, *not* allowing the embryos to be implanted could cause as much distress as allowing them to be implanted.

I argue that the presumption for the disposition of embryos ought to heavily favor the woman. Not only is the woman's contribution to generating the embryos greater than the man's, but also the relationship between women and the embryos they carry and the children they bear is quite different. This relationship can be both empowering and disempowering to women. Bearing and raising children can contain women in a "separate sphere" of domesticity. Maintaining the fiction that men and women operate on equal terms to the reproductive process can also be a covert means of depriving women of control over their reproductive functions. General rules in favor of either preserving or discarding embryos can implicitly subvert women's reproductive prerogatives. At the very least, the hidden consequences of such rules need to be examined very carefully before they are adopted by legal scholars or courts.

Conclusion

Feminist commentators who criticize the new reproductive technologies may be correct to argue that they subvert women's control over reproduction in subtle but powerful ways. The new technologies may seem liberating, and they may ultimately *be* liberating, but given the current political and cultural context within which they operate, the discourse that they encourage will tend to reduce women's control over their unique contributions to human reproduction.

Ethics committee guidelines were not drawn to protect the reproductive rights of women; rather they support the work of fertility clinicians and researchers. The rhetorical defense of those interests provides an additional opening for conservative judges (and others) who are interested in asserting control over women's reproductive processes.

Given such a context, reliance on the notion of reproductive rights in courts of law, as a strategy to maintain control over the politics of reproduction, will likely be extremely disappointing. In this examination of the disposition of frozen embryos in *Davis v. Davis*, I have demonstrated the indeterminacy of rights analysis in one field where rapid technological change is occurring. The rhetoric of rights may be more indeterminate in some fields than others, but when indeterminacy exists, that rhetoric's usefulness in advancing substantive rights is suspect. The problems of rights indeterminacy are particularly apparent in cases involving women's reproduction since the application of balancing of rights will tend to discount a woman's unique contribution to human reproduction.

Notes

1. A 1975 law required the creation of an Ethics Advisory Board (EAB) within the U.S. Department of Health, Education, and Welfare. In June 1979, the EAB issued a report on scientific and ethical aspects of IVF, which approved research and recommended federal funding. Their recommendations have never been accepted (Caplan 1986, 102).

2. The government of Australia convened the Waller Committee, or Committee to Consider the Social, Ethical, and Legal Issues Arising from In Vitro Fertilization, to study the implications of the Rios case (Waller 1984). (See discussion of this case under "Antecedents.")
3. The British Parliament established the Warnock Committee, or Committee of Inquiry into Human Embryology, in response to the birth of Louise Brown (Warnock 1985).
4. The Warnock Committee specifically rejected the utilitarian view that the cutoff point for experimentation ought to be when neural development reaches the point when an embryo might "feel pain," in favor of a more rule-oriented position, i.e., that the beginning of differentiation should determine that point (Warnock 1985).
5. David Davies, a former editor of *Nature*, posits that the term "preembryo" was developed for political reasons. (Davies 1986, 208) And embryologist J.D. Biggers (1990) has recently characterized the "partition" of prenatal life as "arbitrary." Clifford Grobstein has defended its scientific validity (1988, 346–347).
6. In 1986, Robertson made the distinction between embryos and preembryos in a footnote, but he thought the term "preembryo" to be too "cumbersome" for customary usage, and used "embryo" throughout the article (Robertson 1986, n45), as he did in a later *Hastings Center Report* article (Robertson 1989). Yet according to the summary of witnesses' testimony at the Davis trial, Robertson testified on the moral status of the "preembryo." This very ambiguity is evidence of the political context of the usage of the term. The plaintiffs pushed the concept of a preembryo for two reasons, first: *re* concerns about the sympathies of Judge W. Dale Young, which turned out to be well-founded, to a "pro-life" position; second, *re* Junior Davis's own reservations on the moral status of embryos. According to the summary, "It is Mr. Davis' position that the embryos do not constitute life, but he firmly believes the embryos have the 'potential for life'"(Opinion of the Court, 1989, B4).
7. Corea and Spallone reveal the insensitivity toward their female subjects that borders on misogyny in the writings of Steptoe and Edwards (Corea 1985, 104–120; Spallone 1989, 16–32).
8. For example, the Warnock Committee stated, "[W]e were agreed that the embryo of the human species ought to have a special status and that no one should undertake research on human embryos the purposes of which could be achieved by the use of other animals or in some other way. The status of the embryos is a matter of fundamental principle which should be enshrined in legislation. *We recommend that the embryo of the human species should be afforded some protection in law*" (Warnock 1985, 11.17, emphasis in original).
9. Wurmbrand, for example, argues that the respect due embryos is such that the state has a legitimate, if not compelling, interest, in protecting them. Thus, the state can legitimately require that all frozen embryos be implanted in some recipient once they have been conceived, either the woman who produced the eggs or an anonymous recipient. She relies heavily upon Robertson's analysis (Wurmbrand 1986, 1091). Although Robertson does not endorse this position, clearly the discourse of respect has taken on a life of its own, from the Warnock Committee to *Davis v. Davis*.

10. Judge Young pointed out that Dr. King, director of the Fertility Center, never used "preembryo" in his notes on the status of Mrs. Davis. Moreover, referring to Robertson's *Hastings Center Report* article (1989), he states, "It is very curious that this very scholarly paper does not reflect the very fine distinction between 'preembryo' and 'embryo' made by Professor Robertson throughout his testimony at the trial" (Opinion of the Court 1989, 13).
11. In *Danforth* the court stated: "The obvious fact is that when the wife and the husband disagree on this decision [to terminate pregnancy], the view of only one of the two marriage partners can prevail. Inasmuch as it is the woman who physically bears the child and who is the more directly and immediately affected by the pregnancy, as between the two, the balance weighs in her favor" (*Planned Parenthood of Missouri v. Danforth* 1976, 805).
12. In fact, when, in June 1990, Mary Davis announced that she preferred to have the embryos anonymously donated, Hash submitted a petition to the trial court for him to be appointed as "guardian" to the embryos (Hash 1990, 1, 4).
13. Tushnet considers three rights-based arguments that could give women control over embryos or fetuses even after removal from the uterus. First, the "property-based" argument gives a person a right to control over his or her body parts (such as a spleen, for example) even after it has been removed. (But Overall would argue that embryos and fetuses do have competing rights once removed, unlike spleens.) Second, the "psychological argument" is that a woman should not be faced with the psychological burden of knowing that she has progeny in the world. "She may not want to worry for the rest of her life whether a person she saw on the street, who vaguely resembled her grandmother, might be her daughter." (Of course, a proximate psychological burden also exists for the father.) Third, a woman may have a property-right over her genetic heritage (Tushnet 1984, 1368–1369). (Here again, a man could presumably make the same claim.)
14. That the defendant's attorney would take such a position seems odd strategically since Mary Davis might make a much stronger claim for possession of the embryos if the court construed them as "life." On the other hand, he may have felt that, if the judge took a "pro-life" position his client would have no chance of winning, so that he had better defend the property claim. Moreover, the "right to life" argument was likely to be overturned on appeal.

References

Andrews, Lori B. 1984. *New conceptions*. New York: St. Martin's Press.

Andrews, Lori B. 1986. The legal status of the embryo. *Loyola Law Review* 32: 357–390.

Biggers, J.D. 1990. Arbitrary partitions of prenatal life. *Human Reproduction* 5(1): 1–6.

Bonnicksen, Andrea. 1989. *In vitro fertilization: Building policy from laboratories to legislatures*. New York: Columbia University Press.

Brief for the Defendant. 1989. *Davis v. Davis*, Blount Co. Circ. Ct., Tenn. 21 Sept.

Callahan, Daniel. 1986. How technology is reframing the abortion debates. *Hastings Center Report* 16 (1):33–42.

Caplan, Arthur L. 1986. The ethics of in vitro fertilization. *Primary Care* 13(2):241–253.

Clifford, Charles M. 1989. Brief in support of plaintiff's statement of issues. *Davis v. Davis*. Blount Co. Circ. Ct., Tenn. 14 July.

Corea, Gena. 1985. *The mother machine: Reproductive technologies from artificial insemination to artificial wombs*. New York: Harper & Row.

Davies, David. 1986. Letter to the editor. *Nature* 320:208.

Del Zio v. Presbyterian Hospital. 1978. No. 74 Civ. 3588. S.D.N.Y.

Edwards, Robert, and Patrick C. Steptoe. 1980. *A matter of life*. London: Hutchison Press.

Elias, Sherman, and George J. Annas. 1987. *Reproductive genetics and the law*. Chicago: Year Book Medical Publishers.

Engelhardt, H. Tristam, Jr. 1980. Viability and the use of the fetus. In *Ethics and public policy*, ed. Tom L. Beauchamp and Terry P. Pinkard. Engelwood Cliffs, N.J.: Prentice-Hall.

Ethics Committee of the American Fertility Society. 1986. Ethical considerations of the new reproductive technologies. *Fertility and Sterility* 46(3)(Suppl. 2): 1S–94S.

Ethics Committee of the American Fertility Society. 1990. Ethical considerations of the new reproductive technologies. *Fertility and Sterility* 53(6)(Suppl. 2):15–109S.

Flynn, Eileen P. 1984. *Human fertilization in vitro: A Catholic moral perspective*. New York: University Press of America.

Grobstein, Clifford. 1988. Biological characteristics of the preembryo. *Annals of the New York Academy of Sciences* 541: 346–348.

Hash, R.D. 1989. Final supplemental brief of amicus curiae. *Davis v. Davis*. Blount Co. Circ. Ct., Tenn. 21 Sept.

Hash, R.D. 1990. Petition to appoint a guardian/alternate temporary custodial parent and/or for change of temporary custody. Blount Co. Circ. Ct., Tenn. 20 June.

Holden, Constance. 1984. Two fertilized eggs stir global furor. *Science* 225(4867):35.

Holmes, Helen Bequaert. 1988. In vitro fertilization: Reflections on the state of the art. *Birth* 15(3):134–145.

Kairys, David. 1982. Legal reasoning. In *The politics of law: A progressive critique*, ed. David Kairys. New York: Pantheon Books.

Opinion of the Court. 1989. *Davis v. Davis*, Blount Co. Circ. Ct., Tenn. 21 Sept.

Opinion of the Court. 1990. *Davis v. Davis*, Ct. App. Tenn., E. Sec. 21 Sept.

Overall, Christine. 1987. *Ethics and human reproduction*. Boston: Unwin Hyman.

Ozar, David T. 1985. The case against thawing unused embryos. *Hastings Center Report* 15(4):7–12.

Planned Parenthood of Missouri v. Danforth. 1976. 428 U.S. 52.

Price, Frances V. 1988. Risking high multiparity: Multiple gestation and assisted reproduction. *Birth* 15(3):157–163.

Robertson, John A. 1986. Embryos, families, and procreative liberty: The legal structure of the new reproduction. *Southern California Law Review* 59(5): 942–1041.

Robertson, John A. 1989. Resolving disputes over frozen embryos. *Hastings Center Report* 19(6):7–11.

Roe v. Wade. 1973. 410 U.S. 113.

Saharelli, Joseph J. 1985. Genesis retold: Legal issues raised by the cryopreservation of preimplantation human embryos. *Syracuse Law Review* 36:1021–1053.

Skinner v. Oklahoma. 1942. 316 U.S. 535.

Smith, George P. 1985–1986. Australia's frozen "orphan" embryos: A medical, legal, and ethical dilemma. *Journal of Family Law* 24 (1):27–41.

Spallone, Patricia. 1989. *Beyond conception: The new politics of reproduction.* Westport, Conn.: Bergin & Garvey.

Tiefel, Hans O. 1982. Human in vitro fertilization: A conservative view. *Journal of the American Medical Association* 247: 3235–3242.

Tushnet, Mark. 1984. An essay on rights. *Texas Law Review* 62(8):1363–1403.

U.S. Congress, Office of Technology Assessment. 1988. *Infertility: Medical and social choices.* OTA-BA-358. Washington, D.C.: U.S. Government Printing Office.

Waller, Louis, et al. 1984. *Report on the disposition of embryos produced by in vitro fertilization.* Australia: Committee to Consider the Social, Ethical, and Legal Issues Arising from In Vitro Fertilization. August.

Warnock, Mary. 1985. *A question of life: The Warnock report on human fertilisation and embryology.* Oxford, Eng.: Basil Blackwell.

Webster v. Reproductive Services. 1989. 492. U.S. 490.

Wikler, Daniel. 1978. Ought we to save aborted fetuses? *Ethics* 90(1):58–65.

Wurmbrand, Marci Joy. 1986. Frozen embryos: Moral, social, and legal implications. *Southern California Law Review* 59(5):1079–1100.

PART IV

PSYCHOSOCIAL DIMENSIONS TO THE SEARCH FOR FERTILITY THROUGH IVF

Chapter 17

IN VITRO FERTILIZATION: THE CONSTRUCTION OF INFERTILITY AND OF PARENTING

Elizabeth Bartholet

Introduction

I am a woman who has experienced in vitro fertilization (IVF).[1] I "chose" to do so, of course. Indeed, I fought my way into IVF programs in the early days when places were scarce and when people who were single and over 40, which I was, were officially excluded. I was thrilled to be allowed to participate, as I was determined to have another biological child. I wanted to repeat what had for me been the quite wonderful experience of pregnancy, birth, and child rearing involved with my first child. I knew almost nothing about adoption. But I did know that it would be extremely difficult. I thought it might be impossible. And I had a lot of fears —fears of what I knew, and what I thought I knew, and most of all of what I didn't know. I pursued an IVF pregnancy in three different programs in three different states. After many failed IVF attempts I moved on to adopt.

I was one of the lucky IVF patients, because I *did* move on to adoption and to parenting. Few IVF patients ever become parents through the treatment

---

This essay is a modestly revised version of a paper presented June 4, 1990, at the Fourth International Interdisciplinary Congress on Women, in New York City, as part of a panel on IVF including papers presented by Williams and Holmes.

process. And it is not clear how many who might have been interested in adopting will have the will, the energy, the resources, or the ability, once they have stopped IVF, to get through the many barriers that society puts in the way of becoming an adoptive parent.

As a biologic *and* adoptive parent, I am acutely conscious of the ways in which these forms of parenting are exactly the same. And I am acutely conscious of the special qualities involved in a parenting relationship that is *not* the product of biology. I cannot imagine life without these two particular children born in Lima, Peru, from the body of another woman.

I look back in amazement at the person I was, traversing the country from one IVF program to another, in search of an infertility "fix." And I wonder at the role society plays in structuring the meaning of infertility and of parenting.

Linda Williams's chapter "Biology or Society?" raises questions as to whether women's pursuit of IVF should be seen as the exercise of choice or as the product of social conditioning. My own experience has left me intensely aware of the complexity of women's "choice" in connection with issues of fertility and parenting. It had seemed to me natural to pursue biologic parenting, as it seems to many. And my IVF pursuit felt like choice. I had a sense of excitement and even empowerment because, although my chances for success were slim, I was at least pursuing something that I really wanted to do. I had little sense of resentment at the burdens of the IVF process, despite the fact that I found IVF an extremely arduous, life-dominating experience, involving some eight unsuccessful attempts in programs spread from California to Massachusetts. Helen Holmes and Tjeerd Tymstra's chapter on "Dutch Women and In Vitro Fertilization" reveals that my uncomplaining attitude is quite common among IVF patients. I quit IVF when I did in part because I ran out of money, as insurance coverage was then essentially unavailable. What I understood at the time to be a financial constraint on my freedom of choice, I understand now as my liberation—liberation from IVF and from the obsession with reproduction and biological parenthood. I was freed up to move on to adoptive parenthood. Now that I have moved on, I am able to look back with some greater understanding of the forces to which I was subject and the problems for women inherent in the IVF process.

IVF and the Construction Process

The current pursuit of IVF is largely the product of social conditioning that makes women think of themselves in terms of fertility and think of parenting in terms of biological parenthood. At the same time the experience of IVF reinforces for women and for society as a whole this sense of the centrality of fertility to personhood and of biology to parenthood. The relationship is a circular one.

IVF as Product of Construction

The social conditioning at issue is all-encompassing. It includes the way in which women are taught that their identities are necessarily wrapped up in fertility, pregnancy, childbirth, and mothering. One important piece of the problem is that infertility is treated as a medical problem suited for medical solutions rather than as a social problem for which a range of social solutions should be considered. Infertile women tend to get onto a medical track as soon as infertility is suspected and to stay on it until they "give up" or admit "defeat." Alternatives to medical treatment are rarely considered until *after* medical options have been exhausted. Once on the medical track, women are led into the world of IVF treatment by their doctors, who tend to advise only about medical options. And women are lured into IVF treatment by the increasingly aggressive advertising of the IVF clinics. An advertisement published recently in the *Boston Globe* reads:

> Before you let go of the dream, talk to us.... There's no other perfume like it, the smell of a newborn: a milk scent, warm-scent, cuddle essence. Her skin, a kind of new velvet. Toes more wrinkled than cabbage, yet roselike. Tender, soft, totally trusting; a blessing all your own. That dream might still come true for you . . . (Fertility Center 1989).

Needless to say, no one is selling child-free life or adoptive parenthood in this way. Indeed the adoption world pushes people away with a variety of discouraging messages—there are no children to adopt, the process will take years, prospective parents may be disqualified as unfit on the basis of any of a myriad factors, the children may suffer from "genealogical bewilderment" or "the adoption syndrome." Adoption is constructed as the choice of "last resort."[2]

IVF as Agent in Construction

As Lene Koch's chapter "The Fairy Tale" emphasizes, IVF is not simply the product of the social conditioning process to which women are subject — it functions as an active agent in that process. IVF treatment reinforces the sense that it indeed *is* essential to achieve a fertility fix that will enable reproduction. The IVF process takes over the life of the woman going through it. The statistics are such that it only makes sense to start down the IVF path if you are prepared to keep going for at least three or four tries. The treatment process is so intensive that it is almost impossible to get through it *without* focusing most of your life energies on the attempt to become pregnant. Each

IVF failure reinforces the sense of loss and inadequacy involved in the infertility struggle. And each IVF failure is likely to reinforce the felt need finally to overcome infertility, to fix the medical problem, to repair the inadequate body, and to achieve personhood through pregnancy. Since IVF almost always comes at the end of an already long period of infertility treatment, lives that have been put on a fertility fix hold for two or five or ten or more years, are put on hold for yet longer. And, of course, there is generally no logical end to IVF treatment since most IVF failures occur at the implantation stage, and the reason for failure at this stage is almost always a mystery. An important part of the felt compulsion to make repeated IVF attempts is the sense that in the numbers game that IVF seems, next time might always be the time that your number comes up.

IVF reinforces the sense that reproduction is essential not simply to personhood but to parenthood, since the two concepts become merged in this context. The ironic and sad fact is that the IVF pursuit may as a practical matter mean that women who actually want to parent, and not simply to overcome infertility, are precluded from becoming parents through adoption. By the time women give up on the IVF pursuit and move on with their lives, they may discover that by virtue of their age their options in the adoption world are severely constricted. In any event, they may no longer have the financial or emotional resources for another uphill battle to parenthood. A related piece of the picture here is that society has constructed the institution of adoption in a way that *makes* adoptive parenthood an uphill battle.

Thoughts on Reconstructing Infertility and Parenthood

Feminists in Western countries have generally been more vocal in voicing their concerns with IVF than they have been in formulating concrete advocacy positions that might bring about change. Although I have no detailed agenda to propose at this point, I do have some thoughts as to directions for change. I am convinced that it is important that feminists get themselves organized for advocacy efforts. There are powerful forces pushing in the direction of expanded use of IVF. The number of IVF clinics is growing apace, and in a few short years IVF has gone from being perceived as a wildly improbable and highly experimental procedure to a standard part of the infertility treatment process. It is already late to be thinking about taking effective action, but we are in a better position to act today than we will be tomorrow.

My own tentative advocacy positions fall into three categories:

1. We should oppose certain currently popular IVF regulatory proposals.
2. We should advocate other IVF regulatory proposals.

3. We should develop advocacy programs designed to change the socialization process surrounding issues of infertility and parenthood, and to change the institution of adoption.

Forms of IVF Regulation That We Should Oppose

The major regulatory move of the day in the United States is toward mandated health insurance coverage. Several states in the last few years have passed legislation requiring insurance companies to provide reimbursement for IVF. Some private companies have moved on their own to broaden insurance coverage to include IVF. A support group organization called RESOLVE that sees itself as representing the interests of infertile people, has made mandated insurance coverage a major legislative priority. Many feminists have taken the position that IVF should be more generally accessible to those of limited means and thus have advocated the expansion of insurance coverage to include IVF, as well as the expansion of Medicaid and other schemes for free medical care for those not covered by insurance. Many countries other than the United States already provide free access to IVF treatment as part of their nationalized health care systems. The arguments for expanded coverage in this country are generally based on familiar ideas of social justice and the importance of maximizing women's choices.

I see expanded insurance coverage and other proposals to subsidize IVF treatment as extremely dangerous developments. Making IVF cost-free would represent an extraordinarily significant green light for expansion of the technology in this country. The fact that IVF costs as much as it does is a major deterrent preventing women who enter IVF treatment from investing years in repeated attempts or continuing without limit. And the cost, of course, prevents women of more limited means from entering into IVF treatment at all.

It is arguable that IVF is so inherently problematic that access should never be expanded by making it cost-free. In any event, it seems clear that *in the current context* this society should not give such a green light to IVF. The following considerations are key.

- The system as a whole is already massively biased in favor of reproduction and biological parenthood and against adoptive parenthood. By system here I mean the structure of laws, regulations, and policies that surround adoption and make it as difficult and expensive as it is; the fact that our society provides a variety of tax deductions and other financial incentives that encourage reproductive parenting and almost no financial reimbursement for adoptive parenting; and all the factors discussed in the next two sections. If society is to weigh in with a bias it should be in the direction of encouraging people to parent the children who already exist and need homes. We should, in any event, not act to increase the bias in the direction of high-tech reproduction.

- Health care resources are already allocated disproportionately for fancy treatments that benefit the most privileged, while basic health needs of the poor are neglected. At a time when pregnant poor women are getting wholly inadequate prenatal care, and a large percentage of the country's infants and young children are suffering from inadequate health care and poor nutrition, it makes no sense to expand our resources for high-tech infertility treatment for the benefit of those who are privileged enough to seek out the opportunity to parent but unwilling to parent the children already waiting for homes.
- Given the current conditioning to which infertile women are subject, and the absence of real choice discussed above, expanded coverage does not serve women's interests.

Forms of IVF Regulation That We Should Advocate

We should be pressing for forms of regulation that would ensure that IVF "consumers" are provided with better and more accurate information about the pros and cons of IVF treatment and provided with better protection against the risks inherent in the treatment process. At the moment there is essentially no such regulation in the United States. We rely on the medical profession to self-regulate, and self-regulation has not worked adequately to inform and protect IVF patients and the public at large, as the following examples indicate.

- IVF practitioners have systematically disseminated massive disinformation regarding the likely success of IVF treatment, thereby misleading both IVF patients and policy makers. Among the problems have been the widely repeated claims that 15–20 percent or even 25 percent success rates are typical or are to be expected, when the truth is that even in the better, more established clinics the chances that any IVF treatment cycle will produce a live baby are 8–10 percent (see generally U.S. House 1989).
- The IVF medical establishment has failed to create on its own initiative a system capable of providing adequate information regarding success statistics. Only recently did IVF practitioners agree to keep a registry of *named* rather than anonymous clinics with their success statistics, and this was done only as the result of pressure from a U.S. congressional committee and the implicit threat that if the profession didn't act on its own, Congress might move in to impose regulation (U.S. House 1989).

Even now clinics are under no *mandate* to submit their statistics, in connection with their identity, to the registry.

- The IVF medical establishment has not taken adequate steps to ensure that appropriate research is conducted or to mandate essential guarantees with respect to health and safety issues. For example, only recently have any research studies even been *initiated* that will track IVF patients and their children to assess any long-term health risks associated with the intensive hormone treatment, the numerous ultrasounds, and the other practices associated with the IVF process. In addition, little effort has been made to control the quality of IVF services provided in the private IVF clinics, despite the fact that many of these clinics have long been known to engage in a range of highly questionable practices (U.S. House 1989).

Accordingly, we should be advocating regulation that would at a minimum:

1. Mandate the conduct of appropriate research and the collection and dissemination of appropriate information regarding health and safety risks, success statistics, and the like, so that consumers and public policy makers can make better-informed choices.
2. Mandate the establishment of minimum standards to govern IVF clinics, relating to such matters as staff credentials, lab facilities, and systems for providing counseling and adequate information regarding success statistics and other matters.
3. Mandate the monitoring, perhaps through a licensing system, of IVF clinics, to ensure that they satisfy minimum standards, and to identify new issues to bring to the attention of policymakers.

Other Advocacy Programs We Should Be Promoting

The kinds of recommendations listed above, however, do little to solve the real problem. That problem is that, conditioned as women are to feel that they must resolve issues surrounding infertility with a medical fix, they will likely continue to plunge eagerly into IVF treatment if they can find, or others will provide, the money to pay for it, *even if* they have access to appropriate information about the risks and about the limited prospects for success. Although a new regulatory structure would provide some needed protections for IVF patients and the children they bear, the fact remains that IVF in anything like its present form, with its burdens on the women involved and its limited prospects for success, is not a good solution for women dealing with infertility.

Something must be done about the conditioning process itself. The problem here, of course, is that a myriad different societal forces are responsible for women feeling the way they do about themselves, about their fertility, and about the need for and nature of the parenting experience.

I offer the following proposals as ways to get started on the project of reconstructing infertility and parenting. We should advocate the provision of counseling for infertile women at the point that they first suspect infertility and think that they want to do something about it. This counseling should be designed to help them work through feelings about infertility and feelings about the various child-free and parenting options open to them. In addition, we should advocate that this form of counseling be made a precondition to entry into IVF treatment, with the counseling provided by entities operating independently of the IVF clinics and outside of the traditional medical establishment. And we should advocate a substantial restructuring of the institution of adoption. We should focus not simply on notions of rights and empowerment for women, but also on notions of connection with and responsibility for others. Adoption should be opened up as an option, not only because this would serve the real parenting interests of many infertile women, but also because it would simultaneously serve the equally real and often quite desperate needs to receive parenting experienced by existing children.

Notes

1. For a description of in vitro fertilization see the first several paragraphs in Williams's essay. I use IVF throughout my essay to refer both to the classic in vitro fertilization procedure and also to medical technologies such as GIFT (gamete intrafallopian transfer) and ZIFT (zygote intrafallopian transfer), which involve a similar although not identical treatment process, with relatively similar emotional and physical costs for the patient, as well as relatively similar prospects for success.
2. In a forthcoming book with the working title *Children by Choice*, to be published by Houghton Mifflin, I challenge current ways of constructing adoption.

References

Fertility Center, New England Memorial Hospital. 1989. Advertisement. *Boston Globe* 21 March:92.

U.S. House of Representatives, Committee on Government Operations. 1988. *Medical and social choices for infertile couples and the federal role in prevention and treatment.* Hearing, 14 July. Washington, D.C.: U.S. Government Printing Office.

U.S. House of Representatives, Committee on Small Business. 1989. *Consumer protection issues involving in vitro fertilization clinics.* Hearing, 9 March. Serial No. 101-5. Washington, D.C: U.S. Government Printing Office.

Chapter 18

BIOLOGY OR SOCIETY? PARENTHOOD MOTIVATION IN A SAMPLE OF CANADIAN WOMEN SEEKING IN VITRO FERTILIZATION

Linda S. Williams

Introduction

For most women who wish to have children, achieving a pregnancy is relatively simple. But this is definitely not true for everyone. It is estimated that 10 to 15 percent of all married couples in North America are infertile (Hepworth 1980; National Center . . . 1985). Prior to the late 1970s, only three solutions were available to infertile couples who wished to become parents—they could undergo infertility testing and treatment, they could adopt a child, or if the husband was the infertile partner, they could attempt artificial insemination with donor sperm. Today, many infertile couples have an additional option—they can try to become parents through in vitro fertilization (IVF), commonly known as the "test-tube baby" procedure.

In vitro fertilization was originally developed to enable women whose fallopian tubes are blocked to bear children because IVF procedures bypass the tubes. A woman's ovaries are stimulated with strong fertility drugs to produce multiple eggs, which are surgically removed. Her partner then produces a sperm sample by masturbation, and the eggs and sperm are combined in a glass dish. If fertilization occurs, the resulting human embryos are inserted into the woman's uterus. If they implant in the uterine wall, a pregnancy will begin. The woman will give birth nine months later if she does not miscarry, but the implantation failure/miscarriage rate per embryo transfer can be as high as 85 percent (Wagner & St. Clair 1989).

A single IVF attempt lasts approximately three weeks. It involves surgery, plus repeated ultrasonography and blood drawing. The fertility drugs that are essential to the procedure can produce a wide range of distressing and potentially dangerous side effects. IVF is also emotionally stressful, since it may fail at any point in the procedure and the attempt will be canceled. It is also very expensive: most North American and Australian clinics charge $3000 to $6000 per attempt; most couples make several attempts. IVF also has low success. Recent research has shown that an IVF attempt produces a baby approximately 10 percent of the time at the best clinics (Wagner & St. Clair 1989).

The technology that has made in vitro fertilization possible also permits, for the first time in human history, access by doctors and scientists to human eggs, and second, the production of human life outside women's bodies. Because of this technology, attempts may be made to use human eggs and human embryos in genetic engineering, postconception sex selection, human cloning, and the development of artificial wombs. Future use of such technologies would create a world in which the process of human reproduction would be further radically and perhaps irrevocably changed, especially for women. Thus in vitro fertilization is the key technology in a wide array of new reproductive possibilities.

No matter how potentially useful or dangerous a new reproductive technology may be, it cannot exist without a market. A market for IVF exists to a large extent because some women want children so much that they are willing to undergo the emotional, physical, and financial costs for the low chance of becoming biological mothers. Women who undergo IVF are often described, and indeed sometimes describe themselves, as desperate to have children at any cost. Their strong desire to become biological mothers is usually seen as "natural" and unproblematic, a desire taken for granted by the general public and doctors and scientists who develop IVF. Usually missing from the public discussion on IVF is any analysis of how a desire for children might be *socially constructed*. In other words, to what extent does our society *create* a market for IVF by placing so many important meanings on fertility that to be infertile indeed becomes an unbearable problem. This essay describes a portion of the results of an exploratory study that was undertaken specifically to examine the parenthood motivation of couples seeking IVF and the extent to which it was socially constructed.

Literature on Couples Seeking In Vitro Fertilization

Information about couples seeking IVF is found in both the popular press and scholarly papers. The popular literature includes books by couples (Brown & Brown 1979; Tilton et al. 1985) or by supporters (Singer & Wells 1985; Walters & Singer 1982; Wood & Westmore 1984) and articles in news or popularized science magazines (Clark 1982; Eagan 1987; Gold 1985; Greenwalt 1988; Levin 1987; Seligman 1987; Wallis 1984). This literature often describes couples' strong desires for children, but the source of this motivation and the reasons for its strength are rarely examined or even questioned.

A large scholarly literature attempts to evaluate the psychological state of IVF participants prior to, during, and following IVF so that counseling assistance can be provided. These studies recognize that the parenthood motivation of these couples is extremely strong; however, they generally do not attempt to examine the source of this motivation or its social aspects (see Alder & Templeton 1985; Appleton 1986; Bombardieri & Clapp 1984; Fagan et al. 1986; Freeman et al. 1985; Freeman et al. 1987; Given et al. 1985; Haseltine et al. 1985; Hearn et al. 1987; Leiblum et al. 1987; Mahlstedt et al. 1987; Seibel & Levin 1987; Stewart & Glazer 1986).

A small body of sociological and/or feminist literature examines women's and couples' experiences with IVF and discusses some of the social aspects of the use of this technology. Crowe (1985) interviewed 16 women in an Australian IVF program concerning their attitudes toward motherhood and infertility and their IVF experiences. She found that most of the women adhered to the dominant ideology of the importance of motherhood for women and had experienced strong external social pressure to bear children. These findings were echoed by Klein (1989) in her study of 40 Australian women who tried IVF. Koch (1989, 1990) interviewed 14 Danish IVF participants and found that attempting IVF allowed these infertile women to adopt the socially acceptable identity of an *involuntarily* childless woman in a pronatalist society (my emphasis), since IVF represented their "last chance" at biological motherhood. Holmes and Tymstra (1987) surveyed 78 current and potential clients of a Dutch IVF clinic by mail to determine motivation for participation, reaction to treatment, and subjects' views on current ethical and social issues concerning IVF. They found that IVF patients placed an extremely high value on motherhood but that the genetic origin of a child and the experience of giving birth seemed relatively unimportant. Bonnicksen (1988) interviewed 25 women who had undergone IVF, but she dealt with consumer issues only.

To the best of my knowledge, only three studies have included both women who have undergone IVF and their male partners. Lorber and Greenfeld

(1990) conducted separate telephone interviews with 20 IVF couples to understand the social meaning of IVF as a medical experience and to determine its latent function. They did not attempt to determine the parenthood motivation of the couples they interviewed. Callan and Hennessey (1986) interviewed 77 Australian IVF couples to examine their perceptions of infertility treatment, IVF, and attitudes toward adoption. Parenthood motivation was not investigated. The third sociological study of IVF couples is my own research, which will be described below (Williams 1988).

Ontario Study

I interviewed 22 women who had applied for or undergone IVF in the province of Ontario, Canada, between 1984 and 1987. The husbands of 20 of these women were also interviewed separately, for a total sample of 20 couples and 2 individual women (N = 42). All interviews were taped and transcribed. The purpose of this qualitative study was to examine the parenthood motivation of couples seeking in vitro fertilization to determine to what extent this motivation and, hence, the market for IVF, are socially constructed. Respondents were located through contact with an infertility support group (N = 7), advertisements in IVF clinics (N = 2), a letter to a local newspaper (N = 22), a radio announcement (N = 4), and personal contact and word of mouth (N = 7).

The women in this sample were highly educated. Only 5 of the 22 women had no postsecondary education whatsoever. Three women were homemakers, 3 had quit their jobs to be available for infertility treatments including IVF, 4 did wage work part time and 10 full time, and 2 were graduate students. The incomes for 10 of the 12 women who worked full time at wage labor or were graduate students ranged from $17,750 to $56,900 Canadian dollars, with a mean of $32,465.

All but 2 of the 22 women had experienced at least one IVF attempt. Of the group, 16 were childless, having no biological or adopted children, 3 had an adopted child, and 3 had at least one biological child. The parenthood motivation of the childless women is the focus of this essay.

Results

Two types of parenthood motivation were found in the childless respondents in this sample. The first type of motivation, which I call personal, describes those motivations that seem to come from *within* the individual and are influenced by their own lived experience. I subdivide these reasons into two categories: the pleasures of parenthood and the advantages of parenthood. The pleasures of parenthood included such things as a strong liking for children, a desire to watch a child grow and to contribute to its development, a desire to give love and nurturance to a child, and a wish to recreate oneself in the present or leave something of oneself behind in the future.

Some of the stated advantages of parenthood were the belief that a child would make life more meaningful and "keep you young." Children were also seen as a potential source of emotional support in one's old age. Other personal factors, such as a strong bond with one's spouse, a previous abortion, and the psychological effect of undiagnosed infertility, also played a role in the parenthood motivation of some childless persons.

The second type of motivation, the one that is the focus of this essay, derives from the social meaning of parenthood. Jean Veevers (1973) believes that the social meanings of parenthood and non-parenthood revolve around six central themes, which she defines as follows:

1. Morality—Desire for parenthood is a *religious obligation*; being a parent is being *moral*.
2. Responsibility—Desire for parenthood is a *civic obligation*; being a parent is being *responsible*.
3. Naturalness—Desire for parenthood is *instinctive*; being a parent is *natural*.
4. Sexual Identity and Sexual Competence—Desire for parenthood is *acceptance of gender role*; being a mother is *proof of femininity* and of *sexual competence* as a woman; being a father is *proof of masculinity* and of *sexual competence* as a man.
5. Marriage—Desire for parenthood is the *meaning of marriage*; being a parent *improves marital adjustment* and *prevents divorce*.
6. Normalcy and "Mental Health"—Desire for parenthood is a sign of *normal mental health*; being a parent contributes to social *maturity and personality stability* (Veevers 1973, 293).

The respondents in my study mentioned three of the above six themes—marriage, sexual identity, and naturalness, as influences on their desire for parenthood, with 12 of the 16 childless women stating at least one.

Reproduction and Marriage

Two important and interconnected social themes emerged from the childless women's views on the connections among parenthood, marriage, and becoming a family.

Parenthood as an Expected Part of Marriage. The ideological connection between being married and having children has long been recognized by sociologists. As Busfield has stated, "On the one hand it is expected and regarded as desirable that those who marry will have children; and on the other it is expected that those who want children will marry" (Busfield 1974, 14, quoted in MacIntyre 1976, 158). Four of the women in the childless subgroup saw marriage without children as inconceivable. Moreover, the existence of certain conditions within the marriage, i.e., the fact that it was strong and that the couple was financially secure, served to strengthen this expectation. Their comments also showed, to a certain extent, an awareness that the connection between marriage and having children is a social construct. Sandra[1] said:

> "I don't know what originally made me decide to have children. Probably partly society because after you've been married for a while you start looking in that direction, if you're going to have kids or if you're not going to have kids. The fact that I figured that we had a very good marriage and we had given it a good length of time. 'Cause I was very aware of the fact that marriages don't last a lot of the time. And I don't know, it was just sort of something I guess I started thinking about and then Gary started discussing. Not discussing a lot, but just sort of references here and there, and we decided that, yup, that would be something that we would like to do."

Later in her interview Sandra added, "Probably because everybody else had kids."

Children as the Essential Element in Family Formation. Even more important than the connection between marriage and children was the desire to be a family, and becoming a family was clearly equated with having children for five of the childless women. Mary said:

> "I think of us as a couple. It's strange that I'm making that differentiation. I don't know. No, I think of us as a couple. When I say family, I take in the whole nuclear family, you know, my mother, my father, my sister, my grandmother. But just the two of us I think of as a couple."

Since creating a family was vitally important to these women, having children therefore became necessary to attain that goal. Several women used the phrases "having a family" or "starting a family" when they talked about trying to become pregnant, phrases that are commonly used in our culture to describe a couple who are having their first child. The notion that a married couple without children does not constitute a family is perhaps one of the most deeply ingrained of all cultural ideas concerning families and one that played an important role in the reproductive thinking of many couples in this study, whether childless or not.

Reproduction as Part of the Female Role

No other role is as socially prescribed for women in virtually all cultures as that of mother. The fact that infertile women often do experience feelings of guilt or inadequacy over their supposed failure to fulfil this role expectation has been observed by many writers, as expressed especially succinctly by Barbara Eck Menning, who is herself infertile.

> "Infertility hurts. I know . . . I am an infertile woman. There was a time, some years ago, when I was not able to say those words at all, much less think of myself as an infertile *woman.* The words seemed mutually exclusive. I could be either infertile or a woman but not both" (Menning 1977, xi).

In an attempt to find out to what extent the women in this sample saw reproduction as part of their femininity, all of the women were asked: "Some people feel that having a child is part of being a woman. Do you see it as being an important part of your femininity or your womanhood, however you define that?" Nine of the 14 childless women stated that they did not see having a child as an important part of their femininity. As one woman said:

> "I never felt less a woman because of infertility. I just felt that it was a medical problem. Like some people have diabetes, or some people have multiple sclerosis, or whatever. This was just a problem that I had, or that we had, we didn't know. I never really felt that it interfered with my self-image as a woman."

Five of the 14 childless women, however, did see a definite connection between reproduction and femininity. When I asked that question of Marilyn, who was sterile from two ectopic pregnancies, she replied:

> *Marilyn*—"To a degree, yes. I think I felt that way more so when I knew that I couldn't at the time [of her second ectopic pregnancy]. When I felt that something had been taken away from me, I really felt that I'd been . . . it's almost as if a man were being castrated. It's been removed from you. That's it, you're finished. I'm taking away your reproductive organs. Anyway you want to look at it, I couldn't have a child. . . . I used to get hell [from my friends. They'd say] "You're a bright person. Why do you feel that way?" And I said if you take it down and you look at it on paper and you look at it logically, there's nothing wrong and nothing's changed. But, I've changed, in that there's something that I can't do, and it's something that bothers me. . . . And in that time I think I felt less and less, not as a person, but less and less as a woman . . . because there was something I couldn't do now that other women could."

However, now that a few years have passed since Marilyn's ectopic pregnancies she feels differently about the connection between her femininity and reproduction.

> "Now I look upon it as, what's happened, happened. It's a learning experience. Nothing I would really wish on my own worst enemy. But I haven't changed. I know I am a woman. I know I satisfy my husband. I know I satisfy myself in the things I do. Maybe I'm making up for it in some other way as opposed to having children. I see that more clearly. I think for the first six or seven months afterward I didn't see that at all."

Other women made the following statements about what they saw as the connection between motherhood and femininity:

> *Frances*—"It's important for me. But if you generalize to women in general, I wouldn't say it's important for every woman, no. If they don't have any children and that's their choice, that's fine by me. Yeah, it's important to me. [In terms of feeling like a woman?] Yeah, I feel something's missing. Like I haven't, you know, done what I'm supposed to do or something. You know, your conscious mind says you shouldn't feel that way but you do. I do.
>
> "I guess it's just the way you're brought up. My mother, like I say, that was her whole life, that I ever saw, was her family and her children. . . . Most of my friends if their mothers did work, it was part time. So it was kind of like all the role models I had were mothers that stayed home with their families. So I got to see that was the way it should be, kind of thing."

> *Connie*—"To a certain extent. It fulfills a need that's inside of you from the time I think you're a little girl. You always hear, 'Wait until you grow up and have children of your own.' . . . In some women there's a certain need that they need to have that . . . I have that need, and I need it, so therefore I'll go out and get it. And I'll fight for it."

> *Debra*—"I want to have a child because I keep thinking, 'Why do I have these organs?' That's part of it."

The connection between motherhood and femininity for these women was very complex, and that complexity is clearly demonstrated by Judy's comments below. Her ambivalence and uncertainty about the extent to which she sees motherhood as a part of her femininity are obvious.

> *Judy*—[asked about the discovery of her infertility] "I don't feel good about myself. I feel less of a woman sometimes. I sometimes think Howard [her husband] might think of me as less of a woman, even though he says he doesn't. I have to believe him, but I don't, sort of thing.
>
> [When asked about the connection between her femininity and womanhood] "I think [I saw a connection] more so when I was first going

> through this. I really, I think, really did feel less of a woman. Yeah, but I think I'm feeling better about that now. I think I'm still a woman regardless of whether I give birth or not. I don't think it's affected my self-image as part of being a woman. . . . I guess being a woman and being a person in some ways have to be the same. Fulfilled and being happy. Part of that definition for me is having my own child. So part of that is giving birth, which is what a woman does."

Thus we see that for 5 of the 16 childless women in this study the connection between motherhood and femininity was very real indeed; however, several themes emerged that show that this connection was neither simple nor straightforward, but fraught with ambiguity.

For most of these women the belief that they would grow up and have children seems to have been taken for granted. Moreover, this idea seems to have been ingrained very early in life, as expressed by Connie's comment, "Wait until you grow up and have children of your own." This childhood socialization led them to believe that motherhood was not only to be expected, but would also be a major source of personal happiness and fulfillment. As Judy said, "It was what I expected to do . . . fulfilling myself was going to be having little babies around, and spend time with them."

For Frances, these ideas were supported by the example of her own mother and the mothers of her friends whose lives were largely focused on home and family. She states quite clearly that these women were her role models and that she saw having babies and staying home with them as "the way it should be."

Although these women accepted the notion that giving birth "is what a woman does," they also recognized that any inadequacy they felt as women for not being able to do so was irrational, and several of them were obviously aware of the social origins of this idea. Frances and Connie also took pains to point out that they also recognized that childbearing was a *choice* for women and not a requirement. Debra's remarks add a further complicating note of biological determinism to this analysis, for she saw the simple fact that she possessed reproductive organs to mean that she was meant to reproduce.

The one conclusion that can definitely be made from examining these comments is that although a clear connection between motherhood and femininity did exist in the minds of these childless women, it was often complex and ambiguous. What is perhaps surprising, given the prevalence of the motherhood mandate for women in our culture even today, is that so few of the childless women expressed these beliefs. Several reasons are plausible. First, the notion that women ought to bear children and that doing so is an essential part of womanhood may be so much a part of some women's "taken-for-granted" reality that they may not be able to recognize this factor in their motivation for parenthood, or that they are affected by it on any level. As Bem and Bem (1970) have pointed out, the idea that a woman's primary role in life is to become a mother is often so thoroughly inculcated in young girls that it becomes a "nonconscious ideology," and *not* bearing children therefore becomes literally unthinkable.

Second, these women may be leery about admitting that they espouse traditional views. As seen in the disclaimers of Marilyn and Judy above, women who said they did *not* make this connection may actually have held such views, but they have recognized their irrationality in this day and age and simply chosen to deny to an interviewer that any such connection existed in their minds.

Third, a connection between motherhood and femininity may simply *not* have been very important to most of the childless women in this sample. This hypothesis gains some weight because many of these women were highly educated and most worked outside the home for exceptionally good wages. Since persons of higher socioeconomic status tend to hold less conservative views on gender stereotyping than others (Mackie 1983), it is perhaps not surprising that many women in my sample do not see a strong link between motherhood and femininity.

Reproduction as Natural or Instinctive Behavior

As pointed out above, Veevers has identified naturalness as one theme comprising the social meaning of parenthood. According to Veevers (1973) there are two components to this theme: one is the idea that a desire for parenthood is instinctive; the second, that a desire for parenthood is natural. Until the advent of effective contraception, most married couples did in fact bear children, whether they wanted them or not. This simple fact contributed to the idea that childbearing is natural or instinctive human behavior. According to Veevers:

> When a particular kind of behavior is distributed ubiquitously in human societies, there is a tendency for social scientists as well as laymen to attribute the cause of that behavior not to social learning but to human nature itself (Veevers 1973, 295).

The purpose of this essay is not to discuss whether parenthood is a natural or instinctive phenomenon. As Veevers has pointed out, whether or not this explanation of the desire for parenthood is valid, "it constitutes an important element in the social meaning of parenthood to the extent that people *believe* (my emphasis) that it is valid" (Veevers 1973, 297).

The notion that a desire for children was natural or instinctive was mentioned by 4 of the 16 childless women interviewed. Three women invoked the

Freudian concept of the maternal instinct to help explain why they wanted to have children. One woman, however, did not see this desire as a *maternal* instinct, but rather as something very real and strong that exists in both sexes. Janice said:

> "You know, some people say if you're biologically a woman you really want to have children, and I don't think it's more a woman or a man. I think there's something inside you."

The notion that a desire for children is natural and instinctive might also be considered a nonconscious ideology (Bem & Bem 1970). This ideology affects infertile women in two ways. First, the fact that the ideology is nonconscious may make it almost impossible for these women to recognize that the idea that childbearing is "natural" is itself a social construct. This lack of recognition in turn makes it difficult for them to examine and perhaps deal with the social pressures that may be influencing their reproductive decisions. Second, the notion that childbearing, and hence a desire for children, is natural and instinctive helps justify and legitimize heroic measures such as IVF.

Conclusion

This essay has briefly outlined the extent to which a motivation for parenthood was socially constructed among the childless women who sought IVF in a recent Canadian study. Motivations that prompted some of these women to seek parenthood did not only come from within themselves, but were also influenced by notions that parenthood is an essential part of marriage and family formation, that parenthood is part of the female gender role, and that having children is natural and instinctive. In 12 of the 16 childless women, the desire for parenthood did indeed appear to be socially constructed, at least in part.

This finding is significant within the context of in vitro fertilization since a lack of understanding of the role that social factors play in parenthood motivation reinforces the continued construction of infertility as a medical problem only. This construction serves to legitimize the medical "solution" of IVF for some infertile women, helps to create a market for IVF, and fosters its further growth and development.

No matter how potentially useful or dangerous a new reproductive technology may be, it cannot continue to exist without a market, a market that, in the case of IVF, is both internally and externally constructed. Since this technology and others that it may spawn have the potential to change radically the social relations of human reproduction, it must be examined within its entire social context, and not simply as a medical phenomenon or ethical problem, as is usually the case.

Notes

1. All names of women interviewed used in this essay are pseudonyms.

References

Alder, E., and A.A. Templeton. 1985. Patient reaction to IVF treatment. *Lancet* 1:168.

Appleton, Tim. 1986. Caring for the IVF patient—counselling care. In *In vitro fertilization: Past, present, future*, ed. S. Fishel and E.M. Symonds. Oxford, Eng.: IRL Press.

Bem, Sandra D., and Daryl J. Bem. 1970. Case study of a nonconscious ideology: Training the woman to know her place. In *Beliefs, attitudes, and human affairs*, ed. Daryl J. Bem. Belmont, Calif.: Brooks/Cole.

Bombardieri, Merle, and Diane Clapp. 1984. Easing stress in IVF patients and staff. *Contemporary Ob/Gyn* 24:91–99.

Bonnicksen, Andrea. 1988. Some consumer aspects of in vitro fertilization and embryo transfer. *Birth* 15(3):148–152.

Brown, Lesley, and John Brown, with S. Freeman. 1979. *Our miracle called Louise*. London: Magnum Books.

Busfield, J. 1974. Ideologies and reproduction. In *Integration of the child into a social world*, ed. M.P. Richards. Cambridge, Eng.: Cambridge University Press.

Callan, Victor J., and John F. Hennessey. 1986. IVF and adoption: The experiences of infertile couples. *Australian Journal of Early Childhood* 11:32–36.

Clark, Matt. 1982. Infertility: New cures, new hope. *Newsweek* 6 Dec.:102–106, 108–110.

Crowe, Christine. 1985. 'Women want it': *In-vitro* fertilization and women's motivations for participation. *Women's Studies International Forum* 8:547–552.

Eagan, Andrea Boroff. 1987. Baby roulette. *Village Voice* 25 Aug.:16–21.

Fagan, Peter J., Chester W. Schmidt, John Rock, et al. 1986. Sexual functioning and psychologic evaluation of in vitro fertilization couples. *Fertility and Sterility* 46:668–672.

Freeman, Ellen W., Andrea S. Boxer, Karl Rickels, et al. 1985. Psychological evaluation and support in a program of in vitro fertilization and embryo transfer. *Fertility and Sterility* 43:48–53.

Freeman, Ellen W., Karl Rickels, Jane Tausig, et al. 1987. Emotional and psychological factors in follow-up of women after IVF-ET treatment: A pilot investigation. *Acta Obstetrica et Gynecologica Scandinavica* 66:517–521.

Given, Jeannette E., Georgeanna S. Jones, and David L. McMillen. 1985. A comparison of personality characteristics between in vitro fertilization patients and other infertile patients. *Journal of in Vitro Fertilization and Embryo Transfer* 2:49–54.

Gold, Michael. 1985. The baby makers. *Science 85* April:26–27, 29–38.

Greenwalt, Julie. 1988. Thankful for five tiny blessings. *People Magazine* 15 Feb.:92–100.

Haseltine, F.P., C. Mazure, W. De L'Aune, et al. 1985. Psychological interviews in screening couples undergoing in vitro fertilization. *Annals of the New York Academy of Sciences* 442:504–522.

Hearn, Margaret T., Albert A. Yuzpe, Stanley E. Brown, and Robert F. Casper. 1987. Psychological characteristics of in vitro fertilization participants. *American Journal of Obstetrics and Gynecology* 156:269–274.

Hepworth, H. Philip. 1980. *Foster care and adoption in Canada.* Ottawa: Canadian Council on Social Development.

Holmes, Helen Bequaert, and Tjeerd Tymstra. 1987. In vitro fertilization in the Netherlands: Experiences and opinions of Dutch women. *Journal of in Vitro Fertilization and Embryo Transfer* 4:116–123.

Klein, Renate. 1989. *The exploitation of a desire: Women's experiences with in vitro fertilization.* Geelong, Australia: Deakin University Press.

Koch, Lene. 1989. *Ønskebørn. Kvinder og reagensglasbefrugtning* (The wish for a child. Women and in vitro fertilization). Copenhagen: Rosinante.

Koch, Lene. 1990. IVF—An irrational choice? *Issues in Reproductive and Genetic Engineering* 3:235–242.

Leiblum, Sandra R.. Ekhehard Kemmann, Daniel Coblurn, et al. 1987. Unsuccessful in vitro fertilization: A follow-up study. *Journal of in Vitro Fertilization and Embryo Transfer* 4:46–50.

Levin, Eric. 1987. Motherly love works a miracle. *People Magazine* 19 Oct.:39–43.

Lorber, Judith, and Dorothy Greenfeld. 1990. Couples' experiences with in vitro fertilization: A phenomenological approach. In *Advances in Assisted Reproductive Technologies*, ed. S. Mashiach et al. New York: Plenum Press.

MacIntyre, Sally. 1976. Who wants babies? The social construction of "instincts." In *Sexual division and society: Process and change*, ed. D.L. Barker and S. Allen. London: Tavistock.

Mackie, Marlene. 1983. *Exploring gender relations: A Canadian perspective*. Toronto: Butterworths.

Mahlstedt, Patricia P., Susan Macduff, and Judith Bernstein. 1987. Emotional factors and the in vitro fertilization and embryo transfer process. *Journal of in Vitro Fertilization and Embryo Transfer* 4:232–236.

Menning, Barbara Eck. 1977. *Infertility: A guide for the childless couple.* Englewood Cliffs, N.J.: Prentice-Hall.

National Center for Health Statistics. 1985. *Fecundity and infertility in the United States, 1965–82. Advance data from vital and health statistics.* No.104. DHHS Pub. No. (PHS)85–1250. Public Health Service. 11 Feb. Hyattsville, Md.: U.S. Department of Health and Human Services.

Seibel, Machelle M., and Susan Levin. 1987. A new era in reproductive technologies: The emotional stages of in vitro fertilization. *Journal of in Vitro Fertilization and Embryo Transfer* 4:135–140.

Seligmann, Jean. 1987. The grueling baby chase. Test-tube fertilization: Much hope, much hype. *Newsweek* 30 Nov.:78–82.

Singer, Peter, and Deane Wells. 1985. *Making babies: The new science and ethics of conception.* New York: Scribner.

Statistics Canada. 1987. *Family incomes. Census families, 1985.* Catalogue No. 13–208. Ottawa: Ministry of Supply and Services Canada.

Stewart, Sandra, and Greer Glazer. 1986. Expectations and coping of women undergoing in vitro fertilization. *Maternal-Child Nursing* 15:103–113.

Tilton, Nan, Todd Tilton, and Gaylen Moore. 1985. *Making miracles: In vitro fertilization.* New York: Doubleday.

Veevers, Jean E. 1973. The social meanings of parenthood. *Psychiatry* 36:291–310.

Wagner, Marsden G., and Patricia A. St. Clair. 1989. Are in-vitro fertilisation and embryo transfer of benefit to all? *Lancet* 2:1027–1029.

Wallis, Claudia. 1984. The new origins of life. *Time* 10 Sept.:40–44,49,51.

Walters, William, and Peter Singer, eds. 1982. *Test-tube babies.* Melbourne: Oxford University Press.

Williams, Linda S. 1988. Wanting children badly: An exploratory study of the parenthood motivation of couples seeking in vitro fertilization. Ph.D. dissertation, University of Toronto.

Wood, Carl, and Ann Westmore. 1984. *Test-tube conception.* Winchester, MA.: Allen & Unwin.

Chapter 19

THE FAIRY TALE AS MODEL FOR WOMEN'S EXPERIENCE OF IN VITRO FERTILIZATION

Lene Koch

A number of studies have explored women's experiences with in vitro fertilization (IVF) treatments (Crowe 1985; Klein 1989; Koch 1989; Williams 1988, 1990). This research could moderate the enthusiasm of those who claim that IVF is an unproblematic solution to the problem of infertility. In addition to the important documentation that only a minority of the women on IVF programs actually give birth to a healthy child, these often feminist studies have shown that IVF technology triggers a number of physical, social, and psychological problems that accompany the frequently prolonged treatment. From my study (Koch 1989), including semistructured interviews with 14 women in a Copenhagen IVF program, two important theses emerged:

1. IVF as a reproductive technology to a certain extent transforms women's consciousness about their reproductive possibilities and creates a new framework within which decisions are made. It turns out that these decisions (about entering, staying on, and eventually leaving an IVF program) are not made on a rational basis. The information that women receive about their chances of success is itself inaccurate; therefore their views are not based on objective information but rather on a magical belief in success, which arises from a variety of factors,

including the woman's own self-confidence, random information, and her wishful perceptions.

2. IVF is a process that is experienced in very different terms by the two main parties, the woman and the doctor. The difference in perspective includes different views on the purpose of the treatment and the condition being treated. The woman's experiences are made in a social system—the hospital—where all activities are structured in accordance with the traditions and views of the medical profession. Yet the woman enters this system with her own perspective on her condition and the treatment she is about to receive. During the treatment, situations often occur in which the woman experiences a clash between the two points of view.

The Problem and Its Treatment: Two Perspectives

From the woman's point of view, involuntary childlessness constitutes a unity of bodily, psychological, and social problems: the condition is often caused by a physical defect, such as blocked tubes; it is often a burden on her personal relationships and on her social role in a society that considers motherhood a vital part of femininity. Because in our society primary attention is given to the biological side of infertility, this aspect is the one most often treated by medical doctors. This one-sided definition of infertility as a physical defect contrasts with the woman's holistic experience of infertility as a unity of diverse elements. For the woman, childlessness is an existential problem, a human crisis that requires much more complex help than the purely medical.

To the doctor, however, infertility is a medical and, increasingly, a technical problem. Consequently, the treatments offered by health authorities are based on a limitation of the concept of infertility to a purely medical problematic. Only rarely is psychological or social counseling offered, in spite of the fact that most IVF patients express the need for such counseling and in spite of the fact that many members of the hospital staff acknowledge the need for such counseling. This conflict can be defined as a difference in logic. Doctors most often practice a narrow therapeutic logic: to put it bluntly, they treat diseases, not patients. More important to the woman is the logic of caring; what she needs, as an involuntarily childless person, is someone who cares for her as an individual. If her infertility is not cured with existing medical technology, she is still in need of professional care. When the women in my study realized that the problem of infertility was being reduced to a medical problem, several regretted this reduction in human worth.

These different logics may be illustrated in many ways, the most obvious having to do with the perception of the problem treated: the doctor seeing the job as one of bypassing the natural function of the tube artificially. If pregnancy results, the doctor is successful. Since the establishment of pregnancy shows the medicotechnical ability to imitate nature, pregnancy is counted as success in the international medical literature. But pregnancy may result in abortion or be extrauterine. For the woman, success is the birth of a healthy child.[1]

Textual Analysis as a Method of Understanding Women's Experience

During the interviews the women in IVF treatment told me the stories of their infertile lives. Often these stories were given the form of the classical narrative: the women described their wish for a child, the various types of treatment they had gone through, the ordeal of IVF and ultimately the sad or happy ending of their story. In these life stories as it were, the women invested with meaning the various elements of the experience they went through. In structuring their experience as narrative they obviously made sense out of their lives, even though frequently the results were futile and their efforts seemed pointless. The fictionalization of life made facts livable and created a coherence in life that was otherwise characterized by traumatic and meaningless experiences. Since the medium for this communication was language, such interviews can be seen as "text" in a literary analytical sense, i.e., a mass of data that requires textual analysis to yield the information that the respondent seeks to communicate.

Modern structuralism, drawing ultimately on Ferdinand de Saussure's (1985) original theoretical work on linguistic structures, has sought to systematize the structures we use when we narrate fictional or factual stories. Using the analogy of grammatical analysis in which surface structures (the infinite variety of sentences that we produce daily) are derived from a common deep structure of language, Klaus Jensen (1989) attempted to establish a grammar of narrative deep structures. Particularly in the study of traditional folk tales, which often follow very similar structural patterns, Vladimir Propp (1984) demonstrated a basic narrative structure. Using the Russian folk tale as his model, Propp suggested that in these tales a very limited number of role types interact according to very specific conventions. Later other structuralists, with A.J. Greimas (1972) as the most influential in literary structuralist research, developed these ideas further.

Greimas's actant model has proved very useful for the analysis of the experience of women in IVF programs. In fact, the women themselves often interpreted IVF treatment as a fairy tale—an excellent model for the experience of IVF. Every woman's experience is made up of the same elements—only the results are not adventurous for all. An additional reason to compare women's participation in IVF programs with a myth or a fairy tale is given by those research results that show that reason, cognitive knowledge, or rational calculations are *not* what govern the decisions of these women—neither initially when treatment is begun nor finally when treatment is ended. Rather faith, hope, confidence, and the opposites of these feelings (doubt, anxiety, or suspicion) are dominant. Just as the fairy tale is listened to over and over again, because it reflects one's own fantasies and holds promise of a utopian condition that we all long for, the IVF cycle is repeated again and again. The infertile woman sees no other alternative. The most unrealistic solution appears most credible. Simultaneously, the most realistic possibilities for action seem most remote and unreal. The adventure is seductive but rarely meets one's expectations.

Greimas's Actant Model

In the actant model a distinction is made between the actors or characters of the story and the actants or deep structural positions of the narrative. Each character in the story enters into relations with a number of others. The protagonist of the fairy tale (often a prince) who occupies the subject position of the model has an object (often a princess) who is the goal of the striving. This striving is called the "project," and the relation between subject and object is illustrated by the project axis or axis of desire of the model. On his way through the story the prince may encounter helpers (good fairies or animals) and opponents (evil witches or dragons). This is the axis of conflict, where good and evil are defined and where the stronger will decide the outcome of the project. Ultimately, the prince will win the princess and become the recipient of his object. The donor of the desired object might be the old king, and this relation takes place along the axis of communication. The three dyads—subject and object, helper and opponent, and donor and recipient—constitute the positions of the model. The actant model thus consists of six major positions and three major axes.

Interestingly, the same character may occupy more than one position in the actant model. An analysis may reveal that an actor (i.e., a woman in the IVF program) is both her own helper and her own opponent—this may indicate that a person contains unresolved personal conflicts.

Figure 19–1

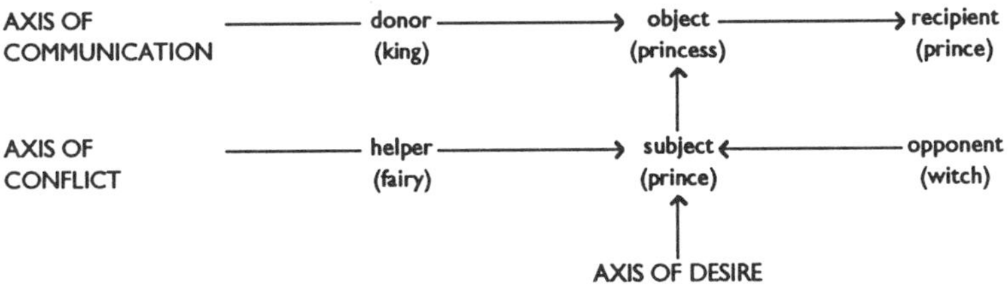

Let us look at the model applied to the personal stories of the women in the IVF treatment, as they were narrated in the interviews.

The Infertile Woman as Subject

For a woman in IVF treatment, a child is usually the primary object of her desires: however, to resolve her infertility, to try everything possible, or simply to receive care or attention may be other objects. The woman is the would-be recipient of the child and in almost all instances she *perceives* modern reproductive technology or medical science (not herself) as the donor of the child. This role may also be occupied by the individual doctor or by the public health services as such. A number of factors are perceived as helpers. The criteria for inclusion into an IVF program vary from country to country, but in many publicly financed programs a number of social criteria apply: for one, patients must live in either marriage or a stable heterosexual relationship of some duration. This means that heterosexuality will help realize the woman's project. If a woman wants to continue pursuing her object, a secure economic situation is an obvious advantage, since money is the precondition to further treatment in the private health sector. Stable personal relationships are recognized to be important by all the women with whom I spoke.

The opponents are often difficult to identify. Many women stated that they felt their own bodies were the main opponents to obtaining a positive result. Several identified related opponents: some women had become infertile after the use of an IUD or through other iatrogenic factors that enabled infections in the tubes. In this instance medical technology was considered an opponent. For some, infertility was caused by infections after an induced abortion. Here the woman's previous sexual practice or an abortion clinic was the opponent. The fact that the biological condition of the infertile woman has to be overcome is of great importance for the subjective experience of women who undergo IVF treatment. The woman may express a feeling of guilt that she had abused her body in her earlier life, and she may be burdened by the feeling of powerlessness this creates toward the doctor and the treatment itself.

Most women in the survey felt frustration that they had no impact on the result of the treatment. In the model this means that the woman is not her own helper. She can do nothing to further the project except subject herself to the treatment and hope and wait. Although brief, this outline on using the fairy-tale model to analyze women's experiences reveals some of the underlying structures that influence women's behavior during treatment and especially shows how women are led into certain patterns of powerlessness and inaction.

The Doctor as Subject

Since doctors' experience of IVF has not yet been documented through interviews or otherwise, texts that directly illustrate their perspective do not exist. Their perspective, however, may be deduced from articles in scientific journals, from their position in the medical profession, and from the structure of the medical establishment. Therefore, I go further, both in using an expanded concept of "text" that includes social structures and scientific documents and in employing the model as an imaginative tool rather than simply as a method of textual analysis. To include whatever "text" is at hand to understand the differences between the parties, I must place the doctor in the position of the subject. What is the doctor's role in the system that makes the woman a passive patient? Can an analysis of this role illuminate the frustrations she experiences in IVF and increase our understanding of the conflicts that appear?

In attempting to complete the model with the doctor as subject, I have to consider what the doctor's project actually is. The international medical measure of success in IVF is the pregnancy rate achieved; thus to make women pregnant is definitely part of the doctor's project. But the individual doctor has therapeutic and research ambitions that reach beyond any immediate desire to make infertile women pregnant. Scientific knowledge, prestige and recognition in the community of scientists, and eventually the possibility of controlling human reproduction are also vital objects of the doctor's ambition.

Furthermore, the doctor is his or her own donor. Individual qualifications and abilities in research and therapy are decisive for achievement. Production of scientific results and publications will determine whether the doctor reaches this part of the desired object: recognition, prestige, and control. But what happens to the woman in this version of the model? She also becomes the doctor's helper: her contribution of body, eggs, and uterus are necessary instruments for carrying out the doctor's project. If she becomes pregnant, the doctor becomes successful. Other helpers may be included: the economic support of the medical industry (sponsors) such as pharmaceutical firms and equipment manufacturers and the level of technological development. Among the opponents we find the religious and feminist groups' criticism of IVF treatment and its various spin-offs, such as egg donation and freezing—criticism that IVF is immoral or is too experimental.

When I make the doctor the subject of the model, I demonstrate that the woman's cooperation is vital to the chances of reaching the doctor's object. She is an indispensable helper in the project. Opposed to this is the role of the woman in the version of the model where *she* is the subject. As we saw, she is not even her own helper; rather, she is powerless in her attempt to fulfill her own project. The fact that women are indispensable if IVF doctors are to achieve their object is not clear to most women undergoing IVF treatment. They perceive themselves as powerless and of no importance in the larger context. They most often express the feeling that they ought to be grateful that the doctors want to help them, but they do not realize that they are actually helping the doctors. At the extreme, they may even bring a doctor success while they themselves fail.

This contrasting of the two versions of the model, with woman and doctor as subjects, respectively, illustrates that the woman's feeling of powerlessness is certainly not justified. It is a product of a certain structure that organizes the health system of which IVF is a part. She is, in fact, potentially powerful because she is a necessary resource in the development of a new medical technology. This insight can be phrased differently: the woman is the doctor's helper as the doctor is hers. Although this reciprocity might create a stronger feeling of equality between the two, certain factors prevent it from occurring. Not only is the hierarchical structure of the medical system important, but especially the widespread belief that the doctors' only interest is to heal patients. The fact that medicine has a double purpose—to heal and to control—has been documented by several researchers, but its mention still seems to be taboo in medical circles and is very rarely brought to the attention of patients. In this medical system the woman is fixed in her powerless position subjectively and objectively. The fundamental structural difference between doctor and woman is never obliterated: she remains a passive helper, a patient in the literal sense of the word, while the doctor is the active subject for his or her own aspirations. The doctor, not the patient, is the true hero of the adventure.

The Doctor as Hero

The doctor figures as the heroic protagonist of the adventure, as the giver of the child and of marital happiness, because the wish for a child has been constructed as a biological need. Human biology is the domain of medicine. The gap between the wish for a child and the biological definition of infertility can only be bridged by the doctor. The doctor, hand in hand with science, which in our culture is a representative of hope, progress, and success, may close the gap between the unhappy couple's desire for a child and their happiness. When childlessness is viewed in this unilaterally biological way, other possibilities than reproductive medical technology disappear from the perspective.

The heroic role of the doctor is supported by both the medical system and the social and cultural context. One factor, however, is often overlooked, which may be the most important one in the discussion of IVF. The doctor's project and the woman's have great similarities and are in fact symmetrical. It is no surprise that these projects coexist so easily. They are characterized by the same focus on medical and biological solutions to infertility, and for that reason the doctor and the woman have mutual interests. The almost universal cultural acceptance of the biological definition of infertility gives strength to the specific interpretation of reality that the models described above represent. The problem is how—and whether—this can change.

Accepting Life Without a Child

A number of studies have shown that childlessness may be considered a psychological crisis (Lalos 1985; Sundby & Guttormsen 1989). They show that the precondition for escaping the crisis unscathed is to accept that life without a child is one part of the human condition. And since only a minority of the women who seek IVF actually leave with a child, it seems reasonable to deal with the necessity that many couples accept infertility as an alternative basis for a good life. If this basis is accepted, the woman actually obtains new possibilities of action as well as ways to influence her own situation, possibilities that were absent in the version of the fairy-tale model just discussed.

In this—utopian—situation the infertile woman places herself not just as the passive receiver of experiences but as the active subject of her own life. The important difference is the conscious change of object. If she can make the object of her striving a satisfactory life, *with or without* a child, she has changed away from the focus on the child as the only acceptable result of the process. In order to receive her new desired object, she must accept the biological side of her infertility. This project only she can complete. To utilize the fairy-tale model, the helpers here can be a sense of reality, a redefinition of female identity, or the ability to grieve one's infertility constructively. Such processes are described in psychological crisis theory. The opponents can be unrealistic expectations about the chances of success in the IVF program and a traditional feminine ideal, which is perhaps the most persistent opponent to the acceptance of infertility. To accept her body as infertile would free the woman from a compulsory seeking of IVF treatment and make her an active and independent actor, whether or not she chooses to make use of the medical system. A natural consequence of this is to change the doctor's place in the system as well. Most important of all, treatment of infertility might come to be based on a broader understanding of the concept of infertility, one that accords with the experience of women.

Conclusion

I have tried to document the uses of textual analysis in the interpretation of data produced in qualitative interviews of IVF candidates. IVF may be seen as a story, a fairy tale, a line of events that can be viewed from more than one perspective. In a patient-doctor relationship like the one we encounter in IVF treatment, textual analysis reveals the differences between the perceptions, experiences, and interpretations of the parties. We gain insights into subjective factors that make different experiences out of the same event—and consequently gain insights into factors that prevent constructive communication between doctor and patient. These insights drawn from a large mass of interview data show the importance of doing a serious evaluation of subjective experiences. People act according to what they believe and according to the fiction that they create out of their lives. For this reason, if none else, knowledge about people's subjective views is important. To avoid the risk that a researcher translates subjective statements into views that he or she can manage, a textual approach is important. Different contexts will give different meaning to the utterances of individuals. To be able to read the text, i.e., to hear the fairy tale behind the narrative of the respondent, may therefore be one of the most important qualifications of the qualitative researcher.

Notes

1. Here I ignore the fact that some women felt that IVF was worthwhile even though they did not give birth to a child, e.g., because they now felt that they "had done everything possible." For a detailed discussion of the "rationality" in women's choice of IVF, see Koch 1990.

Acknowledgments

I am grateful to Henrik Zahle, Kirsten Drotner, and Signild Vallgårda for their comments.

References

Crowe, Christine. 1985. 'Women want it': *in-vitro* fertilization and women's motivations for participation. *Women's Studies International Forum* 8(6):547–552.

Greimas, A.J. 1972. *Semantique structurale* (Structural semantics). Paris: Larousse.

Jensen, Klaus Bruhn. 1989. Discourses of interviewing: Validating qualitative research findings through textual analysis. In *Issues of validity in qualitative research*, ed. Steinar Kvale. Lund: Studentlitteratur.

Klein, Renate. 1989. *The exploitation of desire. Women's experiences with in vitro fertilisation. An exploratory survey*. Geelong, Victoria: Deakin University Press.

Koch, Lene. 1989. *Ønskebørn. Kvinder og reagensglasbefrugtning* (The wish for a child. Women and in vitro fertilization). Copenhagen: Rosinante.

Koch, Lene. 1990. IVF: An irrational choice? *Issues in Reproductive and Genetic Engineering* 3(3):235–242.

Lalos, Ann. 1985. Psychological and social aspects of tubal infertility. Umeå Medical Dissertions, 152 Umeå.

Propp, Vladimir. 1984. *History and theory of folklore*. Manchester, Eng.: Manchester University Press.

Saussure, Ferdinand de. 1985. *Cours de linguistique general* (Course in general linguistics), ed. Charles Bally and Albert Sechehauge. Paris: Payot.

Sundby, Hanne, and Gro Guttormsen. 1990. *Infertilitet*. (Infertility) Oslo: Tano.

Williams, Linda S. 1988. It's gonna work for me. *Birth* 15(3):153–156.

Williams, Linda S. 1990. Wanting children badly: A study of Canadian women seeking in vitro fertilization and their husbands. *Issues in Reproductive and Genetic Engineering* 3(3):229–234.

Chapter 20

DUTCH WOMEN AND IN VITRO FERTILIZATION: SURVEY RESULTS AND REACTION TO A MEDICAL EMERGENCY

Helen Bequaert Holmes and Tjeerd Tymstra

Research Goals

People who experience a medical technology ought to be asked their views on the ethical issues involved and on the policies appropriate for deploying that technology. But they rarely are, and affected *women* are even less likely to be included in the ethical debate.

Therefore, when we surveyed participants in the first in vitro fertilization (IVF) program in the Netherlands, our first goal was to determine the views of the actual participants on public policy and ethics questions. A second goal was to discover these women's reactions to specific aspects of the treatment.[1] Finally, a somewhat incidental third goal was to explore their motivations for taking part. The results demonstrate the complex relationships between humans and modern medical technology.

Methods

In 1985 we distributed a questionnaire about IVF to 113 Dutch women. We set out to approach women in six groups: (1) those with a baby or twins conceived via IVF (16 women), (2) those still trying IVF after one or more unsuccessful attempts (17 women), (3) those who had tried and then quit the program (20 women), (4) some of those on the waiting list (40 women), (5) infertile women who had decided against IVF (7 women, the only respondents to our magazine and newspaper advertisements for women with these views), and (6) a control group of fertile women (with two or more children delivered at home by a midwife) (20 women).

Women in the first four groups (called hereafter "clients") were previous or potential participants in the first and largest Dutch IVF program at Dijkzigt Hospital, which is affiliated with Erasmus University in Rotterdam. Here experimentation started in 1979, with the first live birth in 1982. At the start of our survey 18 babies had been born: 14 singletons and two sets of twins. The first Dutch IVF baby outside the Dijkzigt program arrived during the course of our study.

The bulk of this questionnaire was a series of statements and simply asked for a choice among: "strongly agree," "agree," "it depends/ undecided," "disagree," or "strongly disagree." Some examples of the statements are: [first goal] "Dutch health insurances should pay for IVF"; [second goal] "The most unpleasant part of the treatment was anesthesia for laparoscopy"; [third goal] "Raising a child is an experience that all women should have." (Of course, questions relating to the second goal were sent only to the women who had experienced IVF.) Space was also allotted to invite women to respond to some open-ended questions.

The director of the Dijkzigt program, Dr. A.Th. Alberda, hand-addressed and mailed our questionnaires to current, former, and prospective IVF participants, with a letter urging them to respond. A low-key, empathetic man, Alberda assured us that clients would recognize his handwriting and be certain to open these envelopes. For the 20 fertile women, a member of the Groningen midwives collective posted the questionnaires. We saw names and addresses of no participants, except the seven who responded to our advertisements.

In conducting this research, we followed research guidelines that Holmes had developed to meet certain feminist concerns:

First, we protected anonymity. Not only did we not know the names of the respondents, but—contrary to mainstream principles of sociological research—we also did not request any personal or demographic data. Although standard scientific research uses statistical analysis on differences in responses to see whether they are due to factors such as religious background, income level, or what-have-you, we wished to encourage responses by not asking for personal information. Furthermore, in this small group some people might be easily identifiable through their unique combinations of characteristics.

A scientific argument against doing statistics with such demographic variables is that only with large numbers will results have significance. The surveyed groups, furthermore, must be truly random samples. For example, are infertile Catholics a true sample of all Catholics? And one cannot be completely certain that any significant difference found is really due to the analyzed variable instead of some factor not considered.

Second, we tried to make responding to our questionnaire a beneficial, positive experience. Providing both a checklist *and* a chance for open-ended responses caters to different personalities. The questionnaire was fairly short and attractively designed. Language throughout was noncoercive, for example: "If there are still matters that you'd like to share with us about IVF, . . ."

Third, we honored the respondents by making them the *first* to get a research report. Since we did not know who had responded, in August 1985 mailing labels from Dijkzigt Hospital were used to send a report (in the form of an informal three-page letter) to *everyone* who had received our questionnaire from Dijkzigt Hospital or from the midwives collective. In that mailing, each was invited to send her name if she wished also to receive copies of any reports we would put in medical journals.

Results

From all groups except the patients who had left the program we obtained an excellent return: 80 to 88 percent. Here we present selected results of particular interest.[2]

Policy and Ethics Questions

The most verbiage and the liveliest phraseology was inspired by our statement, "Dutch health insurances should pay for IVF." Among the clients, 98 percent wanted the government to fund IVF. One comment volunteered was, "The government should wake up to [our] grief and misery." Another stated that if the government does not fund IVF, then it is discrimination for it to fund abortion. Waiting for funding of IVF to start, one said, was "hell."

In response to our ethical questions about extending IVF beyond the partners' sperm and eggs, a large majority of the IVF clients (77 percent) approved donor egg; a majority (61 percent), donor egg and sperm together; and half (49 percent) donor womb (now called surrogate gestation). Fewer (approximately half) fertile women approved each of these options, resulting in a statistically significant difference for the first (donor egg) question. On some questionnaires we found inconsistencies probably due to emotional involvement in the technology. For example, one woman who had written in the open-ended section, "We need a child of our own to give meaning to our lives," in the checklist nevertheless approved donor egg and sperm, donor wombs, and combinations.

Despite the general attitude of approving technological extensions of IVF, both clients and fertile women were strongly against the development of an artificial womb and against payments to surrogate (gestational) carriers.

Reactions to Treatment Steps

Groups 1 and 2 who had been treated at Dijkzigt Hospital were very satisfied (100 percent and 80 percent) with their experiences in the hospital and the considerate handling of their treatment. To friends with the same problem, 97 percent would recommend IVF; 86 percent would return for another treatment; 79 percent would have another treatment to give doctors experience with IVF even if they could not have a baby.

As has been found in other surveys of IVF participants (in other countries[3]), the most unpleasant part of the treatment was not a clinical procedure, but "waiting to see if I was pregnant": 69 percent said "agree." Along this line, one respondent wrote that the physical part of IVF was not as miserable as the psychological part. One of the few negative comments was that more information should have been provided, especially about the side effects of clomid.

Motivations

In this category we found several significant differences between the clients and fertile women. Although a majority in both groups agreed that a "right to a child of one's own was a fundamental human right" and that they had "always wanted to have children," a higher (and statistically significant) percentage of the clients agreed: "right to a child," 79 percent versus 59 percent; "always wanted," 90 percent versus 65 percent. About one-third of the clients versus one sixth of the fertile women believed that raising a child and pregnancy-and-childbirth are experiences "that all women should have," although many women in both groups selected "undecided" for these two statements.

Women Who Chose Against IVF

Our efforts to learn whether there were any *different* views held by women in affected groups who had decided *against* IVF were in the main unsuccessful. In contrast to 80 or 88 percent, *zero* percent of the women who had quit the Dijkzigt program (our group 3) responded. We doubt that they received their questionnaires.

Of the seven infertile women who responded to our newspaper requests (our group 5), four accepted IVF: one of these will participate when success rates get higher; the second worries about extensions such as cloning; the third has no partner at the moment; and the fourth, the only one writing no comments, responded like most of the waiting-list women.

The others, who would make no use of the technology, used dramatic language that revealed how IVF had changed their world also. One commented that it is a typically Western method of problem solving and said that infertile women should accept their condition and get on with their lives. The second echoed that view and recommended, "Let's scrap the whole IVF!" And the third said she might try IVF to learn whether her husband's sperm would fertilize her eggs, but only if success rates improve and women's health is not risked. "We mustn't get roped in by doctors who developed the test-tube baby for their own honor and glory, not to help women," she said.

IVF Grassroots Activism in the Netherlands

In 1985, Dutch IVF patients formed a support-and-lobbying group, the Nederlandse Vereniging voor Reageerbuisbevruchting (NVRB) (Dutch Society for Test-Tube Fertilization) (Bout 1990; de Wit 1989; Overbeeke & de Witte 1988). Since then they have been active in running informational meetings, publishing a newsletter (subsidized by the pharmaceutical firms Organon Nederland and Pharma Import/Serono), and lobbying the government to provide insurance coverage and set up more IVF centers. Women comprise the majority of the founders and the continuing leadership. This group had some 2000 members in 1988 (Overbeeke & de Witte 1988) and continues to flourish.

They also managed to get a hearing by the national health council; perhaps their relentless lobbying helped lead in March 1986 (shortly after our research), to government subsidy of IVF at 5 approved sites, all of which had already been attempting IVF. Then for three years women who met certain specifications (blocked tubes or endometriosis) were permitted up to three attempts at those 5 sites. Meanwhile another 25 other hospitals were also trying IVF, a development the press called "wild growth."

The Hepatitis Exposure

In early 1988, 172 women undergoing IVF at Dijkzigt Hospital were exposed to hepatitis B virus when the culture fluid used for embryo development contained virus-contaminated human blood serum. Of these 172, some 25 contracted hepatitis and an additional 30 tested positive for the virus. The hospital tried to contact all exposed women for testing and vaccination. Later it was announced that the hospital's insurance company would make settlements on an individual basis. The inspector of public health for South Holland investigated the incident, made an official report, and required certain changes in the blood procurement procedure (Alberda et al. 1989; Drogendijk 1989; Holmes 1989).

The NVRB too sprang into action. They ran seminars for both infected and uninvolved patients and reported developments in their quarterly newsletter. They monitored on site the hospital's response and soon found themselves forcing accountability on the hospital. When they wished to learn the names of exposed women, how many actually contracted hepatitis, and how severe their cases were, the hospital would not cooperate. Therefore, they devised a questionnaire (de Gruyter 1988; Quint 1989) that they distributed to their own membership and to patients in the IVF clinic waiting room. From this they learned that three women have chronic hepatitis, which means that eventually (perhaps after many years) they are very likely to die from liver failure or cancer.[4] Most other women have recovered, although some still have arthritic pains. No babies contracted hepatitis (Alberda et al. 1989; Drogendijk 1989).

More confrontations with the hospital occurred about insurance. NVRB felt that the individually worked-out settlements were much too small. Dijkzigt Hospital's insurer would not reimburse housecleaning help or wages lost when sick women could not work. Particularly annoying was the insurer's insistence on train ticket receipts when women who gave birth were required to bring their infants to Rotterdam for tests and vaccination (Quint 1989).

One interesting outcome of the hepatitis incident was that public demand for IVF did not decrease; in fact, even at Dijkzigt it increased (Holmes 1989). The press brought attention to IVF and incidentally showed that some couples were indeed getting babies. Other hospitals than Dijkzigt took the occasion to state that such an infection could never occur in *their* facilities (de Wit 1989).

Probably sobered by the hepatitis crisis and to stem the "wild growth" of IVF centers, the government in 1989 decided to license only 12 laboratories and, without putting IVF in the regular national health insurance, to subsidize three treatments per couple at these approved centers. The unlicensed centers, however, still continue (de Wit 1989; Helmerhorst & Keirse 1990). The NVRB continues enthusiastically to foster IVF in the Netherlands, although they now strongly insist on quality control (de Wit 1989; Gruyter 1988).

Discussion and Conclusion

Our survey, our perusal of newspaper accounts of the hepatitis incident, an interview with the treasurer of NVRB, and Tymstra's further survey of IVF clients (de Zoeten et al. 1987) give insights on participants' attitudes toward IVF. Here we share four conclusions.

First is the clear faith in technology, a modern, ubiquitous Western faith. Perhaps the Dutch have a stronger than average dose of it because, of course, most of them live below sea level—an impossible feat without technology. With IVF such faith means a belief that every infertile woman can have the baby to give meaning to her life, with more centers, a little more money, and a few more attempts.

Second and noteworthy is the imperative character of the IVF technique. Working with de Zoeten (1987), Tymstra found in a survey of 80 women on the Dijkzigt waiting list, strong agreement with the following statements:

1. "With a two-percent success rate, I would choose IVF." (65 percent agreement)
2. "I wish to make use of the IVF method because I might be sorry later if I don't seize the chance." (80 percent agreement)
3. "Now that the IVF method exists I feel that I should make use of it; then at least I will have tried everything possible." (92 percent agreement) (de Zoeten et al. 1987; Tymstra 1989)

The reactions to the latter two statements illustrate "anticipated decision regret," a factor that strongly influences many people to "choose" to use a medical technology (Tymstra 1989).

A third matter deserving attention is the almost overwhelming satisfaction expressed by Alberda's patients—at least those who got our questionnaire. Most likely he did indeed treat them well. Woolley et al. (1978) have shown that patients are satisfied even with failed treatments if they experience good doctor-patient communication. Yet the extremely small amount of dissatisfaction worldwide, even among IVF patients who fail to get babies and even among those who say they have been treated as experimental material, requires some explanation.

Several factors may contribute to this unreasonable satisfaction: (1) Almost all IVF patients are given a diazepam tranquilizer at one or more points in the treatment cycle. This produces a feeling of euphoria during the procedure and some memory loss afterward. (2) Patients may hesitate to complain because they fear they may then be forced to leave the program. This factor may have caused our group 3 to fail to respond. (3) An IVF patient and her body is the center of attention while her uterus and body fluids are being closely monitored. Everyone likes to be fussed over, and our bodies are ourselves. The (apocryphal?) story is told of the IVF patient who, after taking home a healthy baby, still phoned the clinic each month to report the day her menstrual period started. (4) A further factor is addiction to doctors, either to a specific doctor or to being doctored. (5) A sort of masochism may be involved: if one does not produce babies as befits a true woman, then one should suffer and keep on suffering until one actually does become a true woman.

A fourth insight gives a nuanced and complex picture of patient involvement in ethics and policy making. We still hold that those most affected should be involved in setting policy and analyzing ethical issues. We believe this even though patients will be hedonistic, always tipping the scale in their own self-interest; even though they will want the newest and most intricate biomedical technologies; even though they will demand a disproportionate share of medical resources. But, because of their own self-interest, they may be the first to recognize safety issues and clinical abuses. If they band together in groups, they will be partners with doctors only to a point—the partnership will break down whenever doctors are perceived to be serving their own advantages instead of patients' needs.

In sum, the shift from blind advocate to alert, knowledgeable watchdog can be easily made. Concerned advocates of patient well-being should encourage and foster these women's strengths to set policy in the world of IVF.

Notes

1. For a description of the series of clinical procedures that comprise IVF, see Williams, this volume.
2. For the set of questions asked and more detailed results, see Holmes and Tymstra 1985, 1987.
3. For reference to surveys of IVF participants in four other nations, see the first four citations in Holmes and Tymstra 1987. See also Klein 1989; Koch, this volume, and Williams, this volume.
4. One of these three women gave birth and is so pleased that she has not asked for an insurance compensation (Quint 1989).

Acknowledgments.

We thank Dr. A.Th. Alberda and Professor Dr. G.H. Zeilmaker of the Dijkzigt Hospital and Erasmus University for the opportunity to carry out this research and J.

Jansen Verplanke of the Biology Center at the University of Groningen for facilitating our work. HBH presented a much briefer version of this paper at the Fourth International Interdisciplinary Congress on Women, New York City, 4 June 1990.

References

Alberda, A.Th., H.C. van Os, G.H. Zeilmaker, et al. 1989. Hepatitis B-virusinfectie bij vrouwen behandeld met in vitro-fertilisatie (Hepatitis B infection in women treated with in vitro fertilization). *Nederlands Tijdschrift voor Geneeskunde* 133(1):20–24.

Bout, Willeke. 1990. Geschiedenis van de N.V.R.B. (History of the N.V.R.B.) *NVRB Nieuwsbrief* 6(4):28–32.

de Gruyter, D. 1988. Verslag van de vervolg enquete m.b.t. de hepatitis-B affaire Dijkzigt (Report on the follow-up questionnaire about the Dijkzigt hepatitis incident). *NVRB Nieuwsbrief* 4(4):10–11.

de Wit, G. Ardine. 1989. Diffusion of medical technology: A case study on in vitro fertilization. Dissertation. University of Limburg, Maastricht.

de Zoeten, M.J., Tjeerd Tymstra, and A. Th. Alberda. 1987. Waiting for IVF: Motivations and expectations of women who entered an IVF programme. *Human Reproduction* 2(7):623–626.

Drogendijk, A.C. 1989. Hepatitis B-epidemie bij vrouwen die behandeld werden met in vitro-fertilisatie (Hepatitis B epidemic in women who were treated with in vitro fertilization). *Nederlands Tijdschrift voor Geneeskunde* 133(1):7–9.

Helmerhorst, F.M., and J.N.C. Keirse. 1990. In vitro-fertilisatie in Nederland (In vitro fertilization in the Netherlands). *Nederlands Tijdschrift voor Geneeskunde* 134(43):2077–2080.

Holmes, Helen Bequaert. 1989. Hepatitis—Yet another risk of in vitro fertilization? *Reproductive and Genetic Engineering* 2(1):29–37.

Holmes, Helen Bequaert, and Tjeerd Tymstra. 1985. In vitro fertilisatie in Nederland (In vitro fertilization in the Netherlands). *Medisch Contact* 40:1341–1344.

Holmes, Helen Bequaert, and Tjeerd Tymstra. 1987. In vitro fertilization in the Netherlands: Experiences and opinions of Dutch women. *Journal of in Vitro Fertilization and Embryo Transfer* 4(2):116–123.

Klein, Renate. 1989. *The exploitation of a desire: Women's experiences with in vitro fertilization. An exploratory survey*. Geelong, Victoria: Deakin University Press.

Overbeeke, George van, and Joke de Witte. 1988. *Reageerbuisbefruchting in Nederland: Aspecten van in vitro fertilisatie* (Test tube fertilization in the Netherlands: Aspects of in vitro fertilization). Amsterdam: Vrij Universiteit Uitgeverij.

Quint, Gerard. 1989. Treasurer of NVRB, interviewed by HBH, 14 April.

Tymstra, Tjeerd. 1989. The imperative character of medical technology and the meaning of "anticipated decision regret." *International Journal of Technology Assessment in Health Care* 5(2):207–213.

Woolley, F. Ross, Robert L. Kane, Charles C. Hughes, and Diana D. Wright. 1978. The effects of doctor-patient communication on satisfaction and outcome of care. *Social Science and Medicine* 12A:123–128.

PART V

NEW PERSPECTIVES ON CONTRACT PREGNANCY

Chapter 21

SCRUTINIZING SURROGACY

Hilde Lindemann Nelson

The term "surrogate mother" is conceptually so confused that I expect it to fall out of use. A surrogate, someone who acts on another's behalf, in this instance is said to be giving birth to a child on behalf of another woman. From the point of view of the child she bears, however, a surrogate would be the woman to whom the child is turned over for care—the woman who performs maternal functions on behalf of the birthgiver. Of the host of confusions surrounding the practice, its nomenclature is perhaps the only one that can be resolved by fiat: let us adopt Laura Purdy's usage, and call the arrangement whereby a woman deliberately bears a child for others to rear *contract pregnancy.* We can all agree that the woman within whose womb the fetus grows to maturity is the birthgiver. We can also agree that the man who provides the sperm and intends to rear the child is the father. Finding a name for the other woman—the one to whom the child is to be turned over at birth—is less easy. We might call her the contracting mother, except that often it is her husband rather than she herself who makes the contract with the birthgiver. Perhaps we had better call her the social mother.

There are two kinds of contract pregnancy. The vast majority of them have involved nothing fancier than turkey-baster technology, whereby the birthgiver is inseminated with the contracting father's sperm—now often called "traditional" contract pregnancy. Bill Handel, the attorney who heads Beverly Hills' Center for Surrogate Parenting Inc., estimates that there have been 4000 births by this method in the United States since the late 1970s (Kasindorf 1991). Perhaps another 80 births have been of the gestational variety: after the social mother's eggs are extracted from her ovaries and inseminated in vitro with her husband's sperm, the resulting embryos are transferred to the birthgiver's uterus. Of course, donor sperm could be used, but then the intending rearing father would not have the legal status generally enjoyed by genetic fathers.

The social mother's legal status can also be called into question, particularly in cases of "traditional" contract pregnancy, as the essay in this collection by Ruth Lucier and her colleagues points out. Robert Moschetta, for example, contracted for a baby with Elvira Jordan without telling her that he was considering divorcing his wife Cynthia. On learning of the impending breakup, Jordan refused to release the baby for adoption, although she did allow the Moschettas to take the child home, providing they sought marital counseling. Six months later, when Robert Moschetta filed for divorce, he triggered a three-way custody battle that promises to be both baroque and prolonged. It is not clear whether he or Jordan will eventually win custody, but what does seem certain is that Cynthia Moschetta will not; the Orange County (California) Superior Court judge who heard the case ruled that Moschetta cannot be the baby's mother because, according to the Reuters account of April 8, 1991, she "has no biological or blood relationship to the child" (Efron 1991).

Gestational contract pregnancy has so far affirmed the claim of the social mother, but only because her genetic ties to the baby are held to be more significant than the gestational bond. In a second California case, Anna Johnson, hired by Mark and Crispina Calvert to gestate an embryo grown from their egg and sperm, sought near the end of the pregnancy to remain involved with the Calverts in rearing the child. But Judge Richard Parslow ruled that Johnson had no maternal rights over the child—this despite California's recognition in law that the woman who gives birth to a child is that child's mother—but rather was only the "foster parent providing care, protection, and nurture during the period of time that the natural mother, Crispina Calvert, was unable to care for the child" (Kasindorf 1991).

Anna Johnson is a black single mother with a four-year-old daughter. Elvira Jordan is a Latina with a seventh-grade education. Are they typical? The Office of Technology Assessment (U.S. Congress 1988) published a survey of "Surrogate Mother Matching Services" that indicates they are not. On average, women who agree to undergo a contract pregnancy are between

26 and 28 years old, 60 percent are married, and 90 percent are non-Latina whites. Two-thirds are Protestant, and one-third are Catholic. They are not especially well educated: fewer than 35 percent ever attended college and only 4 percent attended graduate school. But they are not poor. About 53 percent earned $15,000 to $30,000 a year, and another 30 percent were in the $30,000 to $50,000 income bracket, while 5 percent earned more than $50,000. Only 13 percent had household incomes of less than $15,000 a year. Indeed, many brokerages will not accept applicants who are on welfare or not "financially independent" (U.S. Congress 1988, 273). While these demographics might have shifted somewhat since the survey, the average fee has remained the same since 1984—$10,000. The typical broker's fee now surpasses that amount.

Who seeks to hire a contract birthgiver? The overwhelming majority—90 percent—are married couples in their late thirties or early forties, with homosexual couples comprising about 1 percent; at least one single man has fathered a child by contract pregnancy (having also sought to select sperm to increase the chances of the child's being male). The clients are generally well educated and affluent. At least half have been to graduate school, and another 37 percent are college educated. Some 64 percent enjoy household incomes of over $50,000, while an additional 28 percent earn $30,000 to $50,000 annually (U.S. Congress 1988, 269–270).

Such affluence should not surprise us, as contract pregnancies are expensive. In addition to the fees paid to the birthgiver and the broker, the fee for artificial insemination is about $2000 to $3000 (and in gestational contracts the IVF and embryo-transfer fees are considerably higher). The attorney's fee for drawing up the contract and arranging for adoption is another $5000. Adding in the hospital and medical bills, the cost of a contract pregnancy will come to between $30,000 and $50,000. The OTA estimates that, of all the fees and expenses for arranging such a pregnancy, only one dollar in four actually goes to the birthgiver herself (U.S. Congress 1988, 275–276).

No one knows the number of unpaid contract pregnancies that have occurred in the last decade or so, as these are arranged informally and without the services of a broker. The birthgiver in unpaid arrangements is often motivated by love or altruism to help an infertile relative or friend. While most of these come under the "traditional" category, a well-publicized gestational unpaid contract pregnancy is taking place at this writing. Arlette Schweitzer, a school librarian in South Dakota, became pregnant by embryo transfer with her own twin grandchildren, as her daughter was born with ovaries but no uterus (Plummer & Nelson 1991).

The majority of contract pregnancies, it is sometimes claimed, proceed to the satisfaction of everyone involved. To say this, though, is to say nothing about whether the parties ought to be satisfied. In the unpaid arrangements just mentioned, for example, Janice Raymond (1990) has pointed out that cultural and familial socialization of women might put such a heavy premium on feminine self-sacrifice as to extract the "gift" from the birthgiver by subtle (or less than subtle) forms of familial coercion.

The collection of essays here sets out to explore a variety of issues concerning contract pregnancy, from a number of very distinct perspectives. Under examination are not only the ethical concerns surrounding the practice, but also the historical and social values that have influenced its acceptability as well as cultural values that can be used to call it into question. How should we think about this form of assisted reproduction in the context of a liberal, democratic nation-state? What arguments have the courts found persuasive? What political obstacles might feminists encounter in their attempts to influence a country's public policy?

Laura Purdy, troubled by the appeals to nature that are used to argue against contract pregnancy and further troubled by the ease with which the desire for children is dismissed, considers the degree to which paid birthgivers might be harmed by the sexual and racial imbalances of power inhering in American culture and concludes on utilitarian grounds that contract pregnancies should be regulated rather than forbidden. In a society where each adult is afforded liberty to pursue her own interests as she herself defines them, the author can find no justification for banning the practice outright. (A similar line of argument was adopted by the majority of the Australian National Bioethics Consultative Committee, discussed below.)

Kelly Oliver examines the arguments used in "The Matter of Baby M" and other court cases: the father's right to procreate; treating semen, egg, and womb donors alike; women's freedom to use their bodies as they wish; the uncoerced nature of the birthgiver's agreement to relinquish the child; a couple's right to be related to their child genetically. She finds all such arguments wanting, yet she notes that even when the courts agree they are wanting, judges are likely to deny the birthgiver custody of the child, as the "best interests" of the child are presumed to lie with the more affluent father and his wife.

Ruth Lucier and her colleagues examine contract pregnancy from the perspective of traditional sub-Saharan African cultures, offering not so much ethical principles as community values to guide their discussion of the benefits and harms to the father, the birthgiver, the social mother, and the child, respectively. While the societies from which the authors draw their values have been and continue to be notoriously exploitative of women, the decision not to condemn *tout court* the cultural ground on which one stands may surely be defended. The values the authors have extracted from that ground are used to inform a cost-benefit analysis whose conclusion weighs against contract pregnancy, although if carefully and impartially monitored they deem it permissible.

Sarah Boone, like Ruth Lucier and her co-authors, weighs the practice of contract pregnancy from the perspective of African-American women's history and culture. But the segment of history she chooses is that of the slave woman in the antebellum southern United States, whose experience provides an analogy to the commodification of women and children in contract pregnancy. While present practice weakens the author's claim that the bulk of contract mothers is likely to come from the same socioeconomic rank as the slave woman, she is correct to point out that, like the slave woman, the contract birthgiver is legally alienated from her children, and her body lies open for use by men of social standing and power. For slaveowners, sexual coercion of female slaves was a natural extension both of male rights over female bodies and of white property rights over black bodies. In the light of that experience, Boone asks, is the ultimate value at work in contract pregnancy "really motherhood, parenthood, or even respect for autonomy rights? Or is it simply the perpetuation of a ruling caste?"

Heather Dietrich contributes a first-person account of the demise of Australia's National Bioethics Consultative Committee, which came to grief over the question of legalizing contract pregnancies. In April 1990, the committee issued a report recommending legalization with strict governmental control, to which the author and Sister Regis Dunne appended dissenting reports. A year later, in response to strong negative public outcry, the states' ministers of welfare and health refused to accept the majority report, proposing instead that such contracts be unenforceable and that third-party involvement in contract pregnancies be criminalized. In the same breath, the ministers recommended that the National Bioethics Consultative Committee be disbanded. The author's reflections on the ideology that informed the committee's deliberations, the reasons why her feminist voice on the committee was not well heard, and the implications of it all for Australian public policy serve as an important object lesson in bioethical politics.

Political, historical, social, philosophical, personal—here is a wide sampling of the languages in which the debate proceeds. There is more to say, of course. What it means to separate the gestational from the genetic or social strands of motherhood is a complicated question indeed—particularly as it must be set into the patchwork history of many different kinds of women, some of whom have moved through their daily lives with considerably more freedom than others. We have only just begun to understand the complexity of the imbalance of power between men and women in postindustrial America; we do not yet know the implications for our society, for our families, or for ourselves of taking motherhood apart.

References

Efron, Sonni. 1991. Surrogate mother says that couple deceived her. *Los Angeles Times* 10 Apr.:B1.

Kasindorf, Martin. 1991. And baby makes four. *Los Angeles Times Magazine* 20 Jan.:10–16, 30–33.

Plummer, Martin, and Margaret Nelson. 1991. A mother's priceless gift. *People* 26 Aug.:40–41.

Raymond, Janice. 1990. Reproductive gifts and gift giving: The altruistic woman. *Hastings Center Report* 20(6):7–11.

U.S. Congress, Office of Technology Assessment. 1988. *Infertility: Medical and social choices*. OTA-BA-358. Washington, D.C.: U.S. Government Printing Office.

Chapter 22

ANOTHER LOOK AT CONTRACT PREGNANCY

Laura M. Purdy

Introduction

It is not surprising that the practice now widely known as "surrogate motherhood" has excited so much interest, so many articles, even books.[1] The practice—even though it need involve nothing more high-tech than a turkey baster—invites us to reconsider some of the most fundamental human relationships and raises a host of issues and problems. What, if any, are the necessary and sufficient conditions of motherhood? Who should have the right to rear a child when biological mother and father do not live together? What are the grounds for claims to children, anyway? Is it wrong for women deliberately to bear a child for others to raise? And if not, should they be paid? The questions go on and on, and new twists like egg donation and contracted embryo gestation simply add more dimensions for moral philosophers and lawyers to ponder.

I have already argued elsewhere (and will not recapitulate the details here) that if stringently regulated with an eye toward women's welfare—a big "if"—contract pregnancy could offer significant benefits for them, and perhaps also for the babies (Purdy 1989a, 1989b). First, alleviating infertility can create much happiness for both women and men. Second, even where infertility is not the issue, there is often good reason to try to transfer burden or risk from one individual to another. Pregnancy may be a serious burden or risk for one woman, whereas it is much less so for another. Some women love being pregnant, others hate it; pregnancy interferes with work for some, but not others; pregnancy also poses much higher levels of risk to health (even life) for some than for others. Reducing burden and risk benefits not only the woman involved, but also the resulting child: high-risk pregnancies create, among other things, serious risk of prematurity, one of the major sources of handicap in babies. Society also benefits when expensive problems like prematurity are avoided. Furthermore, serious genetic diseases could be avoided by allowing some women to carry babies for others. Third, contract pregnancy makes possible the creation of nontraditional families, which can be a significant source of happiness to single women and gay couples. Fourth, contract pregnancy could be the lowest technology method of achieving these aims, uses the fewest medical resources, and could potentially be controlled mainly by women.

All these proposed advantages of contract pregnancy presuppose that there is some advantage in making possible at least partially genetically based relationships between parents and offspring. Although it is clear that we might be better off without this desire, I doubt that we will soon be free of it. This desire does not justify risking either women's or children's health; nobody's general well-being should be sacrificed to it, nor does it warrant huge social investments. However, it is something that, other things being equal, it would be good to satisfy as long as people continue to have anything like their current values (Purdy 1989a, 19–22).

Nevertheless, many objections to contract pregnancy have been raised. The transfer of risk and burden from one woman to another has been characterized as either contingently or necessarily involving class– or race-based exploitation. Another argument is that the practice degrades women because it reinforces the view of them as "brood-mares" and harms them by violating their maternal instincts. Furthermore, the practice is held to constitute morally undesirable baby selling, and to harm children by disrupting their sense of family. I believe that these objections are less well-founded than is generally recognized and have argued against them elsewhere (Purdy 1989a, 1989b). However, it also seems clear that there is more to be said about some of these issues. In particular, it would be helpful to look in more detail at ideals of motherhood, the moral status of infertility, and what I shall label "utilitarian worries."

Motherhood: Surrogate or Otherwise

One problematic aspect of the practice of women's bearing babies for others to rear, one that is indicative of the moral tangles lurking here, is what to call it. "Surrogate motherhood" seems inappropriate, both because it looks peculiar to call a woman pregnant with her own fertilized egg a surrogate and because it calls up undesirable associations with respect to motherhood. Sara Ann Ketchum (1989) attempted to resolve this problem by referring to the practice as "contracted motherhood" or "baby contracts." But the former creates similar assumptions about motherhood, while the latter seems to focus on the baby, leaving the woman invisible. Previously, I used "contracted pregnancy" which still seems to me the most accurate term; for simplicity's sake, I will shorten it to "contract pregnancy" (Purdy 1989a, 20).

This is not just a semantic issue. Contract pregnancy (along with new conceptive technologies generally) raises pressing new questions about the whole notion of motherhood. Because language both expresses underlying assumptions and contributes to future ones, the implications of our linguistic choices are not always trivial.

My concern about calling pregnant women "mothers" is that it suggests without argument that they have at least the same obligations toward their fetuses that they do toward their children. That conclusion, however, should not be accepted without further argument, given its bearing both on the morality of abortion and on women's legal duties toward fetuses they plan to carry to term (Purdy 1990). A related problem, as Mary Mahowald notes, is that "mother" suggests fetuses are separate individuals, with all the moral baggage implied by that claim (Mahowald 1990).[2] It would therefore seem preferable to reserve the term "mother" for women who nurture a child.

This move seems perfectly plausible until we ask whose child she is nurturing. Does the child in question have to be biologically hers? If so, that leaves out many women who are doing all the same things mothers do. If not, then what is the status of the woman who bore the child? As the furor over the Baby M case shows, these issues should not be decided by manipulating definitions or by tradition—but by solid argument. In the meantime, neutral terms are needed that do not prejudice the matter one way or the other. It follows that Patricia Spallone's assertion that "the woman who goes through pregnancy and gives birth is the mother" is also to be regarded as problematic (1989, 175).

Until recently such a claim would have been considered simply bizarre, for mothering just *was* the natural progression of pregnancy, labor, delivery, and nurturing. Of course, some unfortunate women and children did not fit this mold. Some women adopted children because they were unable to have their own; others married widowers or divorced men with children; still others got pregnant in inconvenient circumstances and gave up their babies for adoption. Likewise, some children lost their mothers and acquired "new" ones by dint of their fathers' remarriage or by being adopted. But these were peripheral cases—if not statistically, then psychologically. However, contemporary social conditions and scientific knowledge are, as Michelle Stanworth puts it, "deconstructing" motherhood: "motherhood as a unified biological process will be effectively deconstructed: in place of 'mother,' there will be ovarian mothers who supply eggs, uterine mothers who give birth to children and, presumably, social mothers who raise them" (1987, 16).

What are we to make of this development? First, it constitutes explicit recognition of the split between biological and social relationships already existing in human lives. And, it should be noted that splitting the two has often enhanced welfare: it has, among other things, permitted women unable to rear their children to give them over to others more able to do so, a practice that has often benefitted all. Of course, too, the outcome has often been less satisfactory, as where adoptive parents have been insensitive to the special problems faced by their children, or where prejudice based on race, class or sexual orientation has led the state to appropriate children unjustifiably. Second, by now distinguishing genetic and gestational components of biological motherhood, deconstructed motherhood also constitutes a new dimension of that split.

This fragmentation of the concept "mother" is deeply disturbing to some critics of the new conceptive technologies, including many feminists. "Motherhood," is, after all, an enormously complicated term because of its emotional associations. They fear its loss and see it as a way of reducing women's power as mothers, just as the power inherent in skilled labor is undermined when complicated industrial processes are broken up into smaller sections, each of which can be done by more easily exploitable unskilled workers. In reproduction, the threat inherent in this process is reinforced by the fact that such a division of labor entails relying on technology controlled mainly by men: it takes technology to get eggs out of women, as well as to fertilize them and put them back in. Thus the division of labor and reliance on technology render the new conceptive technologies dangerous terrain for women.

That these worries constitute sufficient grounds for rejecting them seems to me dubious, although they do suggest a need for extreme caution. I am more troubled at present by something else. I am grateful to the radical feminist critics of the new conceptive practices for their vigorous attention to new developments, even though I often disagree with their conclusions, for they bring to light dimensions of the issues that might otherwise remain hidden. But their positions, too, sometimes rest on inadequately articulated presuppositions that need to be brought out into the open. In particular, I have been increasingly concerned about the images of womanhood and motherhood upon which many of their criticisms of the conceptive technologies rest, images that draw much of their strength from a disconcerting appeal to nature that, as Stanworth argues, "ignores . . . the strenuous, and partly successful efforts of the women's movement to transcend the identification of women with nature" (1990, 299).[3] The image I question is that of ideal motherhood, constituted by a natural progression of pregnancy, labor, and child rearing.

Before going any further, note the invisibility of sex here. Mercifully, it is absent from this progression, although it is hard to see on what theoretical basis it has been excluded. Why do I say this? On the one hand, pregnancy must be preceded by sex, given radical feminist doubts about new conceptive technologies, as there is no other safe way to initiate pregnancy. On the other, surprisingly, pregnancy might have to follow sex. First, consider Stanworth's perceptive rebuttal to the radical criticism of infertile women's dependence on male-controlled technology: " . . . is it only infertile women whose attendance at medical clinics validates medical power, or is this an unintended side-effect of the use of many contraceptive or abortion or birthing technologies as well as of conceptive ones?" (1990, 293) In other words, it may be inconsistent to regard contraception and abortion as innocuous but conceptive technologies as dangerous! Feminists have rightly been quite outspoken about the defects of contemporary contraceptive technologies and about medical control of abortion, but rejecting them wholesale would leave us still worse off. Furthermore, this same point could be extended to any technology upon which we come to depend, such as clothes washers or optometry. Thus, if we are not to be reduced to some fairly primitive state, we must surely focus on bending technology to our needs rather than becoming Luddites. Second, some radical ecofeminist critiques reject the whole notion of controlling nature. They see our desire to do so as the source of most of our woes; a few have not flinched at extending that rejection to women's control over their bodies. The logical extension of concern about women's dependence on technology as well as ecofeminist attempts to locate in obsession with controlling nature the root of many of our problems obviously have disturbing implications for those of us who take it as given that the advantages of separating sex from reproduction are overwhelming, not only for heterosexual women, but also for lesbians.

Now the appeal to nature here arises from far different motivations than the transparently controlling versions promoted by such institutions as the Catholic Church (Raymond 1987). It seems to me to be compounded of a number of perfectly defensible motivations. First, although I do not subscribe to the extreme gender-polarized picture of human society that motivates the radical feminist rejection of the new conceptive technologies, women obviously do need to be on their guard toward a medical establishment whose track record on their behalf leaves a great deal to be desired. Second, celebrating the female bodily functions and activities that have been so devalued by most human societies is a good thing. However, it is essential to do this in ways that ensure that it does not become as constricting as more traditional views of the good life for women. This task is part of the more general enterprise of feminist ethics, which must find ways to validate connections and relationships without devaluing some of the choices that liberal theory rightly aims to protect.[4]

Such constriction can arise from surprising corners. Thus, for instance, consider the apparently progressive view that the primary obstacles to happy motherhood are social arrangements created by patriarchy and capitalism. The assumption is that if pregnant women had access to good prenatal care and guarantees of economic and social support for rearing their children, they would not have abortions or adopt out their children. Although women clearly need much more help than they are getting, and they do sometimes abort or give up their babies for such reasons, the way these claims are often asserted holds up a standard that could make it quite difficult for a pregnant woman who is *not* economically oppressed to refuse motherhood.

Even an unimaginably supportive society—especially one of the sort argued for by some radical feminists where abortion for genetic defect is frowned upon—will not take all the burden of motherhood from women. There will always be women whose other projects are incompatible with those demands, and it is surely best for both woman and child if such a reluctantly pregnant woman either aborts or lets others do the rearing. While the perfect contraceptive may considerably reduce this problem, it will not, given human imperfection, make it go away altogether. In any case, we do not want a society in which women cannot change their minds about a given pregnancy.

Surely, abortion should always remain a legal option, and it would be surprising were feminists to disagree about this. However, is it farfetched to worry about the possibility of an "ethic" that could, for all practical purposes, foreclose it as a real choice? To judge by statistics and news reports, such an ethic is already influential among poor women of color. Furthermore, similar attitudes are already apparent in many of my students who believe that although abortion ought to be available, they personally would never have one. Whether or not they do go on to have abortions, their attitude is significant and derives from a number of factors that will continue to be a factor in women's thinking. It reflects in part the intellectual strategy chosen by the national women's institutions leading the pro-choice movement that has emphasized the moral difficulty of abortion decisions, while affirming our right to make them. This strategy was chosen, I suspect, because of the philosophically demanding nature of the arguments in favor of abortion, arguments ill-suited for the emotionally charged political environment in which the abortion debate has had to be carried out. Worse yet, even absent that emotional element, few people in our philosophically unsophisticated society—whether inclined toward the pro-choice position or not—have the background or patience to work through the arguments in search of a sound position on abortion. Therefore, the potential for a negative view of abortion becoming widespread is real and, combined with the assumptions underlying the radical feminist critique, could be more coercive than even current pro-life rhetoric, since the latter does at least promote adoption as a moral alternative for unwanted babies.

Conversely, there will probably always be women who love being pregnant but who do not particularly enjoy child rearing. Surely, it would be regrettable if social pressure to live up to the idealized version of motherhood described earlier prevented them from providing infertile women with babies they could not otherwise have.

Infertility and Its Remedies

The natural image of motherhood implicit in the comments of some feminist critics of the new technologies is integral to their conception of a new and better society. Yet this image seems to leave out in the cold women who cannot conceive when they want to. Nor does it leave any remedy for single individuals or homosexual couples. What about them? One thing seems clear: in that better society there will not be many—if any—babies available for adoption. Nor should there be any of the pitiful older children now desperate for good homes, the handicapped, the racially mixed, the emotionally disturbed; they will all be cared for already.

The radical feminist answer is, in part, as Patricia Spallone rightly points out, that infertility will be much reduced due to better "primary health care for women, screening for pelvic inflammatory disease and cervical cancer, by securing a higher standard of hygiene and nutrition for poor women, by cleaning up the workplace from environmental hazards that cause infertility in women and men, and congenital health problems in infants" (Spallone 1989, 27). One might also add that infertility could quite likely be reduced still further by social policies that permit women to have babies at a time in their life which is now "too soon" for many professions.

What about those women who remain infertile despite all these improvements? Apparently, according to many radical feminists, they will have to grin and bear it: women do not really need babies to be fulfilled and their conviction that they do is just a consequence of socially promoted pronatalism. Yet this answer would not really be consistent with the more humane attitudes we all hope for in a better society, as that pronatalism would be gone, along with other patriarchal pressures. However, not only will there undoubtedly be a transitional period where the legacy of such pressures persist, but, more generally, the ease with which the desire for children is dismissed is troubling: I do not believe that the strong desire for children is merely an artifact of patriarchy. As a voluntarily childless woman myself, I am as aware as anybody that life can be fulfilling without a child of your own. However, as one who has also participated in parenting, I also know that—for better or worse—there is nothing else quite like it. It just will not do to tell people that they should adopt a Girl Scout troop instead. A special closeness arises from being a child's primary caretaker and a special thrill in witnessing the child's development into a human person. In addition, for some people, their ties to children are the strongest and most enduring human connections they will ever make. So long as we think human survival desirable, these interests are likely to unite into a wish to be involved in child rearing.

Now it is true that wanting X does not necessarily justify your having it; after all, going after it may be harmful to others so that their interests override yours. But rejecting women's desires as unreasonable or immoral without adequate consideration of possible compromises is a hallmark of traditional sexist attitudes toward women; it pains me to see it reproduced in some feminist thinking.

A cavalier attitude toward the infertile, despite ritual expressions of concern for them, seems to me implicit in the answers currently promoted for infertile women who want children. They are told that their desire for a healthy, genetically related baby is not "authentic" and that if they truly want to be parents they should be ready to adopt an older child, even if he or she is handicapped, emotionally disturbed, or of a different ethnic background (Stanworth 1990, 289).[5] It is also suggested that any attempt to create a new, genetically related child via conceptive technologies is so immoral as to override any standing the desire for such a child might have. These uncompromising and unsympathetic stands strike me as likely to obscure the important issues raised by radical feminist critiques.

Consider first that adoption is not necessarily the panacea it might seem. As Stanworth points out, "The description of infertility as a social condition of involuntary childlessness doesn't hold for all women. For some, pregnancy and childbirth are not only a route to a child, but a desired end in itself . . ." (1990, 293). This desire must surely count for something with those who want to validate women's experiences of gestation and labor.

She notes two other difficulties with adoption. First, "adoption and fostering are often subject to strict surveillance and regulation . . . not necessarily benign to women" (293). She defends her claim by describing some of the standards used to judge whether women should be granted a child:

> Their policies and criteria of assessment are framed against a conventional notion of parenting—and particularly, of motherhood—which will deter many would-be mothers. Adoption agencies in Britain may (and often do) refuse single women or those aged over thirty; may (and usually do) refuse those who are not heterosexual, whether married or not; may (and sometimes do) refuse women who have jobs, women who have had psychiatric referrals, women with disabilities, women whose unconventional lifestyles cast doubt—for the social workers at least—on their suitability as mothers (Stanworth 1990, 294).

Second, adoption may well mean taking a child from another woman: "The pressures that lead some women to surrender their babies for adoption are very like those condemned in the case of surrogate mothers, right down to the possibility of exploitation of women from subordinate ethnic communities or from poorer nations" (1990, 294). According to Stanworth, white parents in Britain can no longer easily adopt black children because of worry about the potential for exploitation of this sort. Such realism about the conditions and consequences of different remedies for problems like infertility is essential; all too often, the disadvantages of a disfavored solution are contrasted with the advantages of the favored one, where a more thorough assessment would suggest quite a different picture.

Even if a woman morally can adopt, reluctance to do so is often brushed off as prejudice by radical feminist critics of the new conceptive technologies. Thus, for instance, the desire for a young baby is, despite ample evidence of the importance of the early years for later development, discounted: infertile women should be ready to take on whatever painful legacy is left by inadequate care, just as they should be ready to take on the physical or emotional problems that might afflict a "hard-to-adopt" child.

As I have argued elsewhere, there are two points that need to be made about this position (Purdy 1989b, 44). On the one hand, raising difficult children is not a task to be undertaken lightly, for it can be so demanding as to require virtual abandonment of all other significant plans. It is easy for those who do not have to face such daily realities as high-priced, inaccessible medical care, incontinence, special equipment, full-time surveillance, lack of mobility, violent antisocial behavior, and the like to recommend that others should take them on. Nor should critics ignore the fact that, as society is currently organized, most of those left to cope with these problems will be women, not men. Is this the price radical feminists want to extract from their sisters who want to mother a child? "Normal" reproduction, too, is a kind of lottery, of course: fertile couples are not guaranteed normal children, although most get them. That some people are willing to devote their lives to difficult children is admirable and to be encouraged; asking those who might be excellent parents of a normal child to parent an especially demanding one may be, as things now stand, a recipe for misery and perhaps even child abuse. We, as a society, are not doing much to relieve such parents of the special burden they bear; providing this kind of help as a matter of course would undoubtedly also reduce the number of children given out for adoption as well as encourage adoption of those who are now given up. Our collective failure to render such help is unconscionable.

On the other hand, given our collective irresponsibility here, who are we to hold only the infertile responsible for difficult children? Why do we expect such supererogatory behavior of them without seeing that the same arguments apply to the fertile? Why, indeed, do radical feminists not argue that so long as there are homeless children, it is wrong for the *fertile* to have their own babies? As Stanworth rightly suggests, "Our critique of pronatalism and of reproductive technologies will be all the more persuasive when it ceases to distinguish so categorically between fertile women and infertile" (1990, 293).

Some of the same points could be made about accusations of racism. Undoubtedly, there are racist whites who look down on people of color and would not have such a baby in the house. Bigotry of this kind is obviously deplorable and ought to be eradicated as quickly as possible, but forcing black or Chicana children on such individuals is hardly in anyone's best interest. Furthermore, it is inaccurate to attribute all reluctance at interracial adoption to such base motives. As noted before, some situations might risk exploitation of poor women of color. In others, individuals might quite rightly fear serious difficulty for the children in question. For example, in a white rural area such a child would stand out in a very uncomfortable way. Although it could be argued that forging ahead despite that possibility is the only way to change racist attitudes, once again this position underestimates the probable cost to these pioneers and discounts other less traumatic ways of making social progress. Another problem with such adoptions is the identity issue the children would face as they grow up in what is still a racially polarized world, one where they may face discrimination from whites because of their color but where members of their own ethnic group might see them as "oreos."

Utilitarian Worries

These points should make it clear that some objections to unorthodox reproduction are more problematic than they might at first seem. The ideal of motherhood against which practices like contract pregnancy are measured contains its own Achilles heel, and the most obvious traditional approaches to infertility may often be unsatisfactory. Contract pregnancy and other conceptive technologies might still not be justifiable, however, if radical feminists' conception of reality were accurate.

Some such feminists argue that men, as a class, and for a variety of reasons, want to control women. Women, despite a long history of restriction, still largely control reproduction, and much of their power and perceived value is predicated on this control. The new reproductive practices show promise, however, of finally putting reproduction in men's hands, partly because it is men who control technology and partly because technology has a logic of its own that promotes hierarchy. Hence, even if certain conceptive technologies benefit particular women, they harm women as a class.

The most extreme versions of this picture suggest that what men really want is to eliminate the need for women altogether. Now this aim would clearly be shortsighted, for we generally still do more than our share of such tasks as child rearing for which men in general show little enthusiasm. Furthermore, unless we are also to believe that all men are latent homosexuals, we would be missed in other ways as well.

But do men want to control (as opposed to eliminate) women? It is undeniable that some men do want to control us; it is also undeniable that many men unconsciously act in ways compatible with such a desire. If nothing else, the widespread violence against women shows that men's attitudes toward women are less than egalitarian. Women's inferior social position is obvious from the statistics on work, income, and wealth; that most positions of power are occupied by men also supports this conclusion.

Now this is obviously not the place for a detailed examination of the radical feminist view of society, but deciding about contract pregnancy cannot wait until that issue is resolved. How, in the meantime, is it possible to proceed?

First, it seems to me that the situation is a good deal more complicated than the foregoing would suggest. On the one hand, individual men do not necessarily hold these negative attitudes. On the other, factors like class and race interact with gender in ways that would complicate this picture considerably, even if it were accurate. Some writers, like Maria Mies, implicitly recognize this fact when they reject the claim that if and when more women become technical experts we would have less to fear from technology. For instance, she asserts that "we can no longer pursue the biologistic fallacy that social conditions would change if as many women as possible were sitting at the control panels of power, in the privileged positions in politics, economics, culture, and in the ever more elitist and centralist world of the new technology." She goes on to say that "we must ask what policies, what aims these women represent. The existing technology is still an instrument of domination if women control it. If they do not want to fight patriarchy and capital at the same time, they will turn it against women, too" (Mies 1987, 41).

It will be no easy matter, given the ongoing and sometimes violent disagreement among feminists, to decide where this pessimistic view of human society intersects with reality. Despite the obvious hostility of substantial numbers of men, I am still unconvinced that the battle lines are so irrevocably drawn as the radical feminist picture would suggest. Furthermore, like Stanworth, I am convinced that even were it accurate, negativism about conceptive technologies is not necessarily the best coping strategy (1990, 295). She asks, for example, whether wholesale rejection of them

> is really the best way to protect women who have sought (and will continue to seek) their use. An implacable opposition to conceptive technologies could mean that any chance of exerting pressure on those who organize infertility services—for example, pressure for better research and for disclosure of information; for more stringent conditions of consent; for means of access for poorer women, who are likely to be the majority of those with infertility problems—would be lost. Would it be wise to abandon infertile women to the untender mercies of infertility specialists, when a campaign, say, to limit the number of embryos that may be implanted (and thereby to reduce multiple pregnancies, pressures for selective reduction, and so forth), or to regulate the use of hormonal stimulation, might do a great deal to reduce the possible risks to women and to their infants? (Stanworth 1990, 295–296)

Her general point, though well taken, still leaves unanswered the objection that it is not maltreatment of the infertile that is most worrisome, but the consequences for women as a group if the infertile, seeking to advance what they see as their own interest, make the overall situation worse. Among the objections of this type are that recourse to such practices as contract pregnancy, especially when money changes hands, promotes the view of women as breeders, exploits poor women, and is potentially racist in new and horrifying ways.

What evidence is there that letting women engage in contract pregnancies for money will cause deterioration in men's attitudes toward women? I believe that reasonable men who do not already have unfounded negative attitudes toward women will not be precipitated by the existence of paid contract pregnancy to the view that women are primarily breeders. However, we have little evidence one way or the other on this empirical issue; what *can* be said is that there is nothing about the practice itself that would justify any such judgment (Overall 1987, Chap. 6; Purdy 1989a, 24–30).

Is the assertion that contract pregnancy exploits poor women better founded? I have shown elsewhere that arguments so far given for this claim are unsuccessful. Neither Christine Overall's Marxist argument that it constitutes an especially degrading kind of alienated labor nor the standard liberal argument about appropriate protection from risk are persuasive (Overall 1987; Purdy 1989a, 24–26, 32–33). The latter, in particular, depends upon ignorance of the kinds of risks working-class people routinely face; it also depends upon a refusal to take seriously the fact that circumstances ought to make a difference in whether a given act is judged prudent or moral.

What needs to be shown here is that contract pregnancy is more exploitive than other services the rich now buy from the poor. The rich, by definition, have more money than the poor; that is why the rich dine in expensive restaurants that employ poor waiters, hire help to clean their houses, and procure for themselves a variety of other services the poor cannot afford. Of course, the gap between rich and poor ought to be smaller so that the poor can have greater access to some of these luxuries. That way, for example, more poor women at risk for health problems in pregnancy could avoid them just as their richer sisters can now do via contract pregnancy.[6] A more economically just society would not, by itself, necessarily provide women with appropriate protection from exploitation, although the pool of women who would submit to any indignity for money would be greatly reduced.

It is undeniable that the potential for exploitation in our own inegalitarian society is substantial, for poor women are much less able to protect their own interests than they would be in a better society. However, it does not follow from this that potentially exploitable but otherwise morally permissible practices should be banned altogether. One way to protect otherwise vulnerable individuals is to regulate them. With respect to contract pregnancy no one has yet shown either that it is not morally permissible or that such regulation is impossible.

Here, for example, the state could set a minimum wage for contract pregnancy and lay out a model contract prohibiting some of the conditions now routinely required of women. The now standard $10,000 for U.S. women *does* constitute exploitation, given the risk, discomfort, and responsibility that go with pregnancy: $20,000 would be a much fairer fee. Certainly, paying the woman and broker both the same wages as is now common degrades women and continues the unacceptable and insulting tradition of devaluing women's work. It would, in any case, be necessary to outlaw private brokers because their interests would too often conflict with those of the other participants.

Some would argue that upping the compensation for engaging in contract pregnancy is precisely the wrong response to the problem of exploitation. They suggest that, on the contrary, women should only be allowed to do it for free; otherwise they are selling babies or commodifying themselves. I have argued elsewhere against the accusation of babyselling and will not recapitulate those claims here (Purdy 1989a, 28–29). The commodification argument also seems to me naive, as it fails to show that there is any morally relevant difference between engaging in contract pregnancy and many other occupations. Furthermore, this argument seems to accept and promote the view that women can be respected for altruistic and socially useful actions only when they receive no monetary compensation, whereas men—physicians, scientists, politicians—can be both honored and well paid (Purdy 1989a, 30). Finally, women have until now been expected to do such reproductive labor for free. Seeing them paid for some of it might just remind us that it is socially valuable (Purdy 1989a, 34).

What about the accusation of racism? The last word here cannot come from members of the dominant group since we may be racist in ways that we, despite the best intentions, are unaware of. However, this fact does not relieve us of responsibility for attempting to evaluate such claims as best we can.

So against this backdrop, what can be said here? The case that surrogacy watchers have been waiting for happened in summer 1990. Anna Johnson, a black woman, bore a boy from the fertilized egg of Crispina and Mark Calvert; finding herself attached to him, she sued for (and was denied) visitation rights (Pollitt 1990, 842). Egg donation of this kind also raises the possibility of Third-World women of color being used as even cheaper incubators for white couples (Corea 1985, 215).

Now, is the practice of white couples hiring women of color to gestate their babies racist?[7] In the Calvert case, Katha Pollitt suspects that the Calverts deliberately chose Johnson to gestate the baby because they knew that no judge would find for a black woman who wanted to keep a white baby (Pollitt 1990, 842). If that were true, their behavior would indeed have been racist, although an interesting wrinkle here is provided by the fact that Crispina Calvert is herself Asian, not "white." The most despicable racism, however, would be on the part of a society that rewards racist individuals with judgeships, making the couple's parasitical racism possible.

The more interesting question here is whether the fact of using women of color in this way, whether in the United States or in the Third World, is, other things being equal, racist. Racism would be implicit in the judgment that they are "good enough" to gestate a child, but that their own "colored" eggs would not be acceptable. This position is clearly racist, and hiring women of color on that basis would also be clearly racist, although if the women benefitted anyway, the practice would not necessarily be wrong. However, whites hiring a woman of color need not be racist. After all, the main point here is to create a genetically related child; if one cares about this sort of thing, then having a child who is genetically related to both woman and man is better than having one related only to the latter. This point is reinforced by the fact that in traditional contract pregnancy, as critics point out, the wives of male clients have no genetic link to the children, and hence, according to the trend in recent court decisions, no claim on them (Pollitt 1987, 683; 1990, 842). So one could easily imagine that were the positions reversed, a black couple would also prefer to use their own egg. That they might not *would* be a symptom of the society's racism: the social rewards for light skin might lead them to prefer, after all, the white woman's egg. But it does not follow from this that it would always be racist for a white couple to use their own egg.

One might argue, too, that an attempt to avoid racist instances of the practice by banning interracial transactions could have racist consequences, just as legislation "protecting" the class of women from certain occupational choices turned out in many cases to be sexist: it might bar women of color from jobs they want and could, on balance, benefit from. A better solution would be to include in the regulation of contract pregnancy clauses that would take into account the special vulnerability of women of color.

Do the same sorts of considerations apply to foreign women of color? One major complication here is the fact that they would be paid less, although if they were paid wages comparable in buying power to what U.S. women ought to be getting, then they would not, other things being equal, be economically exploited. The danger here is that other things may be far from equal. There may be, for instance, far different cultural attitudes toward family, such that contract pregnancy "costs" them more emotionally; more concretely, factors like bad nutrition and health care due to extreme poverty pose special danger to women's welfare. Should this kind of contract pregnancy therefore be banned? Again, it is by no means easy to make the right decision in the context of a world saturated with class hierarchy, racism, and sexism. This background could lead women to accept conditions seriously detrimental to their own interest. Yet, if regulated to avoid these worst cases, contract pregnancy might help women better their circumstances within that context. Regulation would be still more problematic than in the United States, however, as it would require cooperation on the part of both our government and others with still worse records of protecting their citizens. Hence, the prospect of a morally tenable practice of contract pregnancy is substantially more dubious than at home. A truly well-informed decision here, nevertheless would, require the views of a spectrum of potentially affected Third-World women.

A Tenable Strategy

I have been proposing a series of solutions that attempts to maximize contract pregnancy's possible benefit and to minimize its possible harm. These ideas will no doubt infuriate both those who see the limits I propose as unreasonable fetters on freedom and those who disagree with my premise that there is substantial good to be derived from a carefully formulated reproductive policy that includes contract pregnancy. On the one hand, to have a tolerable society, individual freedom must quite often be limited in the name of the greater good, despite libertarians' belief to the contrary. On the other, since the burden of proof is on those who would limit freedom, such proposed limits require more searing scrutiny than contract pregnancy has so far received.

One of the most troublesome issues here is the extent to which we try to tailor our positions to what we perceive as contemporary reality, as opposed to some better future state. According to Maria Mies, "It is a historical fact that technological innovations within exploitative relationships of domination only lead to an intensification of the exploitation of the groups being oppressed" (1987, 42). However, I am unconvinced that fighting for morally desirable technologies is such an all-or-nothing prospect: I agree with Stanworth that it is both desirable and worth doing.

Consider one harmful potential of contract pregnancy: a major objection to it, argues Katha Pollitt, is that it could limit women's physical freedom. She adds:

> Right now a man cannot legally control the conduct of a woman pregnant by him. He cannot force her to have an abortion or not have one, to manage her pregnancy and delivery as he thinks best, or to submit to fetal surgery or a Caesarean. Nor can he sue her if, through what he considers to be negligence, she miscarries or produces a defective baby. A maternity contract could give a man all those powers, except, possibly, the power to compel abortion . . . (1987, 684).

Pollitt is certainly right that no contract containing such clauses should be written or enforced. This could be done either by banning contract pregnancy altogether or by fighting for model regulation that rules these sorts of things out. Given the foregoing, I think the latter should be first on our agenda. Not only would that go far toward making contract pregnancy a fair practice, but it would also help establish legal precedents for women's more general right to control their bodies in pregnancy. If, on the other hand, we concentrate on getting rid of the practice of contract pregnancy, we will not necessarily have made any progress at all on this latter important issue. The realities of class-, gender-, and race-based discrimination in this world mean that we cannot seek only to eradicate their symptoms, but that we must rather seek to win the most broadly based victories we can. Otherwise, like the Hydra, two frightening new heads may sprout for every one we chop off.

In conclusion, I think that the arguments against contract pregnancy do not show that it should be prohibited; they do show that it must be stringently regulated so as to protect the interests of the women who participate. This would include standardized contracts guaranteeing the kind of conditions I have suggested here, such as better pay, physical autonomy, and so forth. Such a model contract would also have to contain clauses on other issues I have not argued for here, such as full pay for stillborn babies and perhaps provision for women (whether they provided their own egg or not) to change their mind about keeping the baby or having visitation rights. In the absence of such protections, women will be exploited and abused, and the practice should be discouraged or banned.

In general, I think that in a better society, the call for contract pregnancy would be less, but so would the risks. In our own society the practice could have, as I have argued, substantial benefits to all parties. It is tempting to reject such technological and social innovations out-of-hand, partly, perhaps, to counterbalance the uncritical enthusiasm with which every dream-child of science seems to be received in many quarters. It is also all too easy to evaluate them solely from our own privileged perspective, forgetting that it may blind us to the kinds of choices daily faced by some of those about whom we are arguing.

Notes

1. See Helen Bequaert Holmes, "Contract Pregnancy: An Annotated Bibliography," Chapter 27 in this volume.
2. I argue that the usual assumptions about the implications of describing fetuses as part of their mothers do not necessarily hold, however (Purdy 1990).
3. Christine Pierce (1977) lays out beautifully the difficulties in any such claim.
4. I am not talking about promoting the purely contractual view of human relationships that leads to so much misery but about the kind of freedom from certain kinds of social pressure discussed by John Stuart Mill in *On Liberty*.
5. Comments such as these about adoption come with utter predictability from most of those who consider themselves socially progressive.
6. I am well aware that many—but not all—health problems endured by the poor are a result of poverty itself.

7. The whole notion of race is problematic as biologists now speak of genetic pools and breeding populations instead. Furthermore, the categories we routinely apply to the United States population are especially questionable, given the large amount of mixing that has occurred and the extent to which "blacks" and "whites" share a gene pool. Nonetheless, "race" is a socially constructed category that will continue to have some usefulness as long as distinctions in treatment are based on it.

References

Corea, Gena. 1985. *The mother machine*. New York: Harper & Row.

Ketchum, Sara Ann. 1989. Selling babies and selling bodies. *Hypatia* 4(3):116–127.

Mahowald, Mary. 1990. Fetal tissue transplantation and women. Paper presented at the meeting of the Eastern Division, American Philosophical Association, 27–30 Dec., Boston.

Mies, Maria. 1987. Why do we need all this? A call against genetic engineering and reproductive technology. In *Made to order: The myth of reproductive and genetic progress*, ed. Patricia Spallone and Deborah Lynn Steinberg. Oxford: Pergamon Press.

Overall, Christine. 1987. *Ethics and human reproduction: A feminist analysis*. Boston: Allen & Unwin.

Pierce, Christine. 1977. Natural law language and women. In *Sex equality*, ed. Jane English. Engelwood Cliffs, N.J.: Prentice-Hall.

Pollitt, Katha. 1987. The strange case of Baby M. *Nation*. 23 May: 667, 682–686.

Pollitt, Katha. 1990. When is a mother not a mother? *Nation*. 31 Dec.: 825, 840–844.

Purdy, Laura M. 1989a. Surrogate mothering: Exploitation or empowerment? *Bioethics* 3(1):18–34.

Purdy, Laura M. 1989b. A response to Dodds and Jones. *Bioethics* 3(1):40–44.

Purdy, Laura M. 1990. Are pregnant women fetal containers? *Bioethics* 4(4): 273–291.

Raymond, Janice G. 1987. Fetalists and feminists: They are not the same. In *Made to order: The myth of reproductive and genetic progress*, ed. Patricia Spallone and Deborah Lynn Steinberg. Oxford: Pergamon Press.

Spallone, Patricia. 1989. *Beyond conception*. Granby, Mass.: Bergin & Garvey.

Stanworth, Michelle. 1987. Reproductive technologies and the deconstruction of motherhood. In *Reproductive technologies: Gender, motherhood and medicine*, ed. Michelle Stanworth. Minneapolis: University of Minnesota Press.

Stanworth, Michelle. 1990. Birth pangs: Conceptive technologies and the threat to motherhood. In *Conflicts in feminism*, ed. Marianne Hirsch and Evelyn Fox Keller. New York: Routledge.

Chapter 23

THE MATTER OF BABY M: SURROGACY AND THE COURTS

Kelly Oliver

New reproductive technology has raised social, moral, and legal questions. Yet, one of the most publicized cases involved the low technology procedure that has come to be known as surrogacy. This so-called *Matter of Baby M* brought the controversy over the morality and legality of surrogacy into the public forum. The way in which this case was handled within the legal system is telling. Traditional contract law with its basis in liberal notions of rights and equality covers up central social issues that make surrogacy arrangements possible. In fact, the surrogacy contract would not take place if the parties to the contract had equal rights. Then, despite the fact that these contracts grow out of social inequality they are debated within the courts in terms of equality and rights. In order to explain why surrogacy arrangements are exploitative, I analyze the case of Baby M and its journey through the legal system of the state of New Jersey.[1]

The *Matter of Baby M,* as it is called by the New Jersey Supreme Court, is the appeal that Mary Beth Whitehead made to that court to challenge the earlier superior court decision that her surrogacy contract with William Stern was valid and that custody of Baby M should go to the contracting father, Stern. The original contract between Mary Beth Whitehead and William Stern was signed in February 1985. In March 1986, Baby M was born.

Whitehead refused to relinquish the baby to Stern. Early in 1987, Stern sued Whitehead for custody of Baby M and sought the enforcement of the surrogacy contract. Both were awarded to him in the superior court's opinion written by Judge Harvey Sorkow. The New Jersey Supreme Court reached a decision on Whitehead's appeal on February 3, 1988. Their opinion, written by Chief Justice Robert Wilentz, held that the surrogacy contract was invalid, but awarded custody of Baby M to Stern.

The Logic of Rights

It is necessary to consider the logic of rights that frames contract litigation. In the courts surrogacy debates are framed within the democratic liberal postulation of rights and obligations. Trial lawyers pit the rights and obligations of the surrogate against the rights and obligations of the natural father and his wife and the rights of the child.[2] Once the rights and obligations of all parties to the surrogacy contract have been arbitrated, custody disputes are decided on the basis of the "best interests" of the child.

For example, in the *Matter of Baby M*, while Whitehead's lawyers were arguing for her right to the companionship of her child, Stern's lawyers were arguing for his right to procreate. The New Jersey Supreme Court decided that Stern's right to procreate did not automatically include the right to custody. Furthermore, the court ruled that procreation through the paid surrogacy arrangement was illegal. The court was convinced that the surrogacy arrangement violated state law that prohibits paid adoptions in spite of the fact that Stern's wife Elizabeth, a pediatrician, was not a party to the initial contract. (Stern, after all, as proponents of surrogacy argue, need not adopt his own child.) In addition, state policy requires that parental rights remain with the natural parents until at least five days after the baby's birth. Thus, the court ruled that Whitehead retained her parental rights. Since parental rights and obligations are defined by law, they can be neither claimed nor relinquished without legal sanction.

Proponents of surrogacy argue that an infertile couple has the right to procreate and a woman has the right to use her body as she pleases. But, do we really have a right to procreate or merely a right to *try* to procreate? Does every person have a right to a child or as many children as one wants? And, as Gena Corea points out in *The Mother Machine*, it is the man's right to procreate that is protected: "The overriding ethic is that the man's issue be reproduced in the world" (1985, 223). The wife of the father of the child produced as a result of the surrogacy arrangement remains infertile. It is simply not true that the surrogacy arrangement primarily benefits the infertile *couple* or, as some proponents argue, the infertile wife.[3]

Surrogacy is not, as the pseudofeminist argument maintains, one woman helping another to have children. In fact, in some cases the infertile wife already has her own children, and/or she is more or less forced into the arrangement by her husband (Corea 1985, 223–224). Katha Pollitt points out the absurdity of the situation: "How can it be acceptable to pay a woman to risk her life, health and fertility so that a man can have his own biological child, yet morally heinous to pay healthy people to sacrifice 'extra' organs to achieve the incomparably greater aim of saving a life?" (1987, 684)

In the courts the right to procreate has been invoked in order to defend limiting parental rights in the case of semen donors. Almost universally, semen donors can be legally required to relinquish their parental rights. Proponents of surrogacy have argued that if it is legal to require semen donors to relinquish parental rights, then it is legal to require womb and egg donors to relinquish parental rights as well. They argue for equal protection under the law. This argument has been used successfully (and unsuccessfully) in many surrogacy trials.[4]

Andrea Dworkin points out a crucial flaw in the analogy between donating sperm and surrogacy. She argues that there is no comparison between an ejaculate of the body and the body itself. She compares collecting semen to collecting tears from the eye and surrogacy to taking the eye itself (Corea 1985, 226). The New Jersey Supreme Court realized that the time difference between producing semen and producing a child is enough to destroy the analogy (*Matter of Baby M* 1988, 1254; Raymond 1988). In spite of this conclusion, as Janice Raymond points out, the court contradicts its conclusion that sperm is not equal to egg, gestation, and birthing when it affirms Stern's "equal right to the child by virtue of his spermatic contribution alone" (1988, 178).

The liberal framework, with its emphasis on equal rights, overlooks important gender-specific differences between the parties to the surrogacy contract. The contract would not exist if the parties were *biologically* equal. The woman must give more than her egg in order to gestate a child. Whereas a man's contribution to conception is purely genetic, a woman must do more than make a genetic contribution. She must carry the child. The man's contribution might be analogous to giving blood, while the woman's is more analogous to giving an organ.

In addition to defending surrogacy arrangements for the benefit of the infertile couple, proponents defend them for the benefit of women who want to serve as surrogates. Proponents have also argued that pregnancy is therapeutic for some women (Corea 1985, 239). All admit, however, that very few women, if any, would perform surrogacy services without payment. Many more proponents defend a woman's right to use her body as she wishes, to engage freely in any contracts that she wishes, to make money in any way in which she wishes (Andrews 1989; Sistare 1988). In the end, what they argue is that we live in a capitalist society where market demands dictate propriety.

What this argument overlooks is that the market may force women into surrogacy (Corea 1985, 228–229). Economic concerns may cause women to do something that they would not otherwise do. Proponents have responded that most people do things that they would not otherwise do in order to make a living. However, most people do not perform their service 24 hours a day, unless they are slaves. And most people sell only their labor, labor performed by the body, perhaps, but distinguishable from it. Surrogates, on the other hand, perform their service 24 hours a day and sell their bodies. Every act in which the surrogate engages may come under the scrutiny of the contracting couple—what she eats, drinks, and how she plays. She is never off duty.

Proponents argue that women should have the opportunity to engage in these kinds of arrangements if they want. They argue that women are free to choose; they are not forced into surrogacy arrangements. Andrea Dworkin finds this concern with women's freedom suspicious:

> Again, the state has constructed the social, economic, and political situation in which the sale of some sexual or reproductive capacity is necessary to the survival of women; and yet the selling is seen to be an act of individual will—the only kind of assertion of individual will in women that is vigorously defended as a matter of course by most of those who pontificate on female freedom. The state denies women a host of other possibilities, from education to jobs to equal rights before the law to sexual self-determination in marriage; but it is state intrusion into her selling of sex or a sex-class-specific capacity that provokes a defense of her will, her right, her individuality, which is defined strictly in terms of the will to sell what is appropriate for females to sell (1983, 182).

Moreover, the argument that women should be able freely to choose to sell whatever the market will bear is undermined by the fact that there are many limits on what people are legally allowed to sell in the United States. For example, while people are allowed to sell blood, they are not allowed to sell their organs or body parts. And while they are allowed to sell their labor, they are not allowed to sell themselves or others into slavery. Surrogacy arrangements are more like organ selling than plasma selling. Organs cannot be sold because we have only a limited number of them available to us and they are crucial to our quality of life, if not to life itself. To allow people to sell organs would open up the possibility of poor people being exploited and virtually forced into selling their body parts away. Just as every person has a limited number of organs, a woman can have only a limited number of children. Also each successive pregnancy may lower the quality of life or even end a life. Women can die in childbirth or from ectopic pregnancies.

The surrogate is seen as the passive incubator whose purpose and obligation is to produce and relinquish a flawless product no matter what physical and/or psychological pain she may suffer. Once she has signed the contract, she is no longer free to do as she pleases. She cannot have an abortion unless the doctor agrees that she is in great danger without one. She can be forced to have a cesarean against her will.[5] The surrogate, then, is estranged from her own body and her own pregnancy. As Gena Corea observes, surrogates' estranged representations of themselves are striking in their testimonies (1985, 213–245). Many of them maintain that the child merely resided in their body and was not their child. The infertile couple was merely using the surrogate's womb. The contracting couple has control over her womb and ultimately her life. The surrogate is not even free when she eats, sleeps, or makes love.

In addition to my general argument that women do not enter into surrogacy contracts completely voluntarily is the more specific argument that women cannot give completely informed consent to relinquish parental rights to their babies before they are born. It is unreasonable to expect a woman to be bound by a preconception contract. As Pollitt points out, a woman cannot be expected to know in advance of conception, pregnancy, and birth whether or not she will want to give up her child. And, she argues that even though most people do not plan their pregnancies, they still come to love their babies even before they are born (Pollitt 1990, 844). No state enforces predelivery adoption agreements, so why accept preconception surrogacy agreements?

In response to the Sterns' claim that Whitehead freely gave her consent to relinquish her child under the terms of the contract, Chief Justice Wilentz notes the illusion of consent inherent in surrogacy contracts:

> Under the contract, the natural mother is irrevocably committed before she knows the strength of her bond with her child. She never makes a totally voluntary, informed decision, for quite clearly any decision prior to the baby's birth is, in the most important sense, uninformed, and any decision after that, compelled by a pre-existing contractual commitment, the threat of a lawsuit, and the inducement of a $10,000 payment, is less than totally voluntary (*Matter of Baby M* 1988, 1248).

The surrogate's equality in the contract is illusory. The illusion is created through the presuppositions of the liberal framework operating within a capitalist society. Within the liberal framework all people are considered equal with equal rights. They all operate autonomously and have the freedom to exercise their rights as long as they do not interfere with the rights of others. In this framework the surrogacy contract is seen as an agreement between two or more equal parties. There is an equal exchange, money paid for services rendered.

The lower court's opinion in the Baby M case provides a striking example of this attitude. According to Judge Sorkow, this contract is a contract for services between two equal parties who freely enter the agreement. There is no question of possible financial coercion or an uninformed decision: "The male gave his sperm; the female gave her egg in their pre-planned effort to create a child—thus a contract" (*Stern v. Whitehead* 1987, 74). "Once conception has occurred the parties [sic] rights are fixed, the terms of the contract are firm . . . " (75). "A price for the service each was to perform was struck and a bargain reached" (74).[6]

Even within the law's language of equal rights some contracts can be broken and illegal contracts are unenforceable. For example, marriage is a contract, but it can end in divorce. Academics are rarely expected to keep a contract with one university if they get a better offer at another. So, just because there is a contract does not mean that it cannot be legally broken. And illegal contracts are never enforceable; an illegal bargain is not a binding bargain.

The liberal framework that arbitrates surrogacy on the basis of rights allows judges to justify enforcing surrogacy contracts.[7] It protects the contracting couple's right to procreate while limiting the surrogate's parental rights. As Pollitt says, "Judge Sorkow paid tribute to Mr. Stern's drive to procreate; it was only Mrs. Whitehead's longing to nurture that he scorned" (1987, 686).

A 1990 surrogacy case in California shows not only the classism but also the racism that the structure of surrogacy arrangements can exploit. In this case, Anna Johnson, a black woman, was the gestational surrogate through in vitro fertilization and an embryo implant for an Asian-American woman and her white husband. The Calverts hired Johnson to gestate their embryo. Johnson fought in court to keep the baby boy to whom she had given birth. Superior Court Judge Richard Parslow ruled that Johnson was not the boy's mother because motherhood is determined by a genetic relation (Pollitt 1990). As Pollitt notes, this view of motherhood discounts all of the mothering activities that we normally associate with motherhood. Given this definition, what are we to make of adoptive mothers? Pollitt argues that there is more to the physical act of motherhood than contributing an egg, even if fatherhood is merely contributing sperm (1990, 842).

With the technological advances that make in vitro fertilization and embryo implantation possible comes the real danger of the further exploitation and oppression of black women. A white couple can have a child who is genetically related to both of them without going through the trauma of pregnancy and childbirth. They can hire a poor black woman to do that for them. According to Pollitt, in a custody dispute a judge will never give a black woman any parental rights over a white child. Pollitt goes so far as to suggest that this may be a reason why white couples will seek out black surrogates. The case of Baby M shows that a surrogacy dispute may be easily reduced to a custody dispute: in custody disputes the race difference combined with racism will insure that a white couple always wins in court.

Surrogacy as Custody

Even when the surrogacy contract is not enforced, the surrogate is destined to lose her child. In the *Matter of Baby M*, the New Jersey Supreme Court ruled that surrogacy contracts are not enforceable.[8] The opinion of the court was delivered by Chief Justice Wilentz, who states:

> We invalidate the surrogacy contract because it conflicts with the law and public policy of this State. While we recognize the depth of the yearning of infertile couples to have their own children, we find payment of money to a surrogate mother illegal, perhaps criminal, and potentially degrading to women (*Matter of Baby M* 1988).

While this decision seems like a victory for those opposed to surrogate motherhood, in practice it does very little to change the exploitation of women who serve as surrogates because they nevertheless lose their children. In spite of the New Jersey Supreme Court's invalidation of surrogacy *contracts*, the precedent set by recent cases, including the *Matter of Baby M*, insures that surrogates will lose in court. In the *Matter of Baby M*, supposedly, the rights of both mother and father were considered equally and custody was based on the best interests of the child.

Whether or not surrogacy contracts are legal in a state, the precedent in the courts insures that surrogacy disputes will be decided on the child's best interest. Even in the 1986 case of *Surrogate Parenting Associates v. Commonwealth of Kentucky*, where the Supreme Court of Kentucky ruled that surrogacy contracts are not in violation of either paid adoption laws or state requirements for relinquishing parental rights, the court also ruled that custody disputes would be decided on the basis of the child's best interests. In other words, even in jurisdictions where surrogacy contracts are legal, they may be voidable (*Surrogate Parenting Associates Inc. v. Commonwealth of Kentucky* 1986, 209).

The way in which the best interests of the child is decided in these situations, however, obfuscates the socioeconomic situation that gave rise to the initial contract. The contract would not exist if the parties to it were socially equal. Given the way in which both New Jersey courts defined best interests as financial security, the surrogacy contract would not exist if the child's best interests were not already owned by the father since the surrogate engages in the contract precisely because she is not financially secure.[9]

For example, in the case of Baby M, the lower court judge, Judge Sorkow, noted that the Whiteheads' house was too small and that Whitehead's concern for her daughter's education was suspect in light of Whitehead's lack of education. In contrast, the Sterns had a new house and could provide the child with "music lessons," "athletics," and a certain college education (*Stern v. Whitehead* 1987, 74–75). Although the New Jersey Supreme Court made it clear that its primary task was not to insure the growth of a new member of the intelligentsia, it decided custody on the same grounds as the lower court (*Matter of Baby M* 1988, 1260). Chief Justice Wilentz noted that whereas the Whiteheads' "finances were in serious trouble," the Sterns' "finances are more than adequate, their circle of friends supportive, and their marriage happy" (*Matter of Baby M* 1988, 1258–1259).

An additional way in which best interests are decided in court practically insures that surrogates will lose custody disputes. The very *structure* of the surrogacy arrangement *guarantees* that the contracting couple is more likely to gain custody. Within the courts' logic, the fact that the surrogate enters into a contractual agreement to give up her child makes her an unfit mother. How could a good mother agree to give up her child? The lower court in the case of Baby M used this sort of reasoning in order to grant custody to William Stern. The trial court concluded that while the Sterns "wanted" the baby, Whitehead's motivation to have a child was not because she wanted to be a parent. In part, the best interests of the child were determined by who wanted her before she was conceived (Johnson 1987, 1345–1346).

The New Jersey Supreme Court noted that whereas Whitehead demonstrated contempt for professional psychological counseling, the Sterns endorsed it. Whitehead's contempt for professional psychological counseling, however, may well be a class issue. While academics and upper-middle-class Americans have become accustomed to the "benefits" of psychological counseling, most poor and lower-middle-class Americans simply cannot afford it. Even when financial assistance is available for such therapy, most Americans do not use it. Many people are suspicious of the benefits of psychological counseling or believe that only insane people need professional help. Also, the fact that psychological counseling is not prevalent among certain classes probably leads to the attitude toward professional psychology that the court identified as "contempt."

Chief Justice Wilentz also noted Whitehead's "omniscient" attitude toward her daughter. This attitude was evidenced by her claim that "she alone knew what the child's cries meant." Due to her attitude, the court maintained that "Baby M's life with the Whiteheads promised to be too closely controlled by Mrs. Whitehead" whereas the Sterns would encourage the child's "independence" (*Matter of Baby M* 1988, 1259). This omniscient attitude, however, is another product of the surrogacy arrangement. Whitehead's parental rights were threatened by the surrogacy arrangement, and she had to defend those rights. She was forced to demonstrate that there was a natural bond between herself and her baby. She had to argue that she was the natural mother and not merely the surrogate mother of Baby M. In this position, of course, she appeared possessive and controlling.

The issue of independence and Whitehead's control of Baby M may also be a result of the surrogacy arrangement. First, in some sense, Whitehead's control of Baby M was threatened by the surrogacy contract. So perhaps she was defensive about her control. Second, perhaps independence is a class issue. The child's independence may be a middle-class priority. Whereas middle to upper classes are socialized to be independent, poor to lower classes are socialized to be interdependent and take care of each other. In poor to lower-class households, interdependence is more appropriate for financial security. It may be that only as a group can they survive financially.

Whereas the court doubted Whitehead's "ability to explain honestly and sensitively to Baby M—at the right time—the nature of her origin," the Sterns, the court decided, "are honest; they can recognize error, deal with it, and learn from it. When the time comes to tell her about her origins, they will probably have found a means of doing so that accords with the best interests of Baby M" (*Matter of Baby M* 1988, 1258–1259). The issue of honesty "when it comes time to tell Baby M about her origins," however, seems impossible to predict. The court based its evaluation of Whitehead's honesty on her refusal to give up Baby M and her omniscient attitude toward her. Yet both Whitehead's actions and her attitudes were, in large part, caused by the severity of the situation in which the police took her child away from her. It is certainly no wonder that Whitehead felt possessive about her daughter and claimed that only she knew what the child's cries meant. On what grounds did the court prove her wrong in this claim? They did not even consider the possibility that she was right.

Moreover, why was not the Sterns' honesty challenged? They had broken the law and William Stern had intentionally signed a contract designed to circumvent the law. In fact, in New Jersey, the Sterns may be guilty of a criminal offense (*Matter of Baby M* 1988, 1227). In addition, the surrogacy arrangement provides a new birth certificate that, upon completion of adoption procedures, identifies the father's wife as the mother of the child. This arrangement, whereby the birth certificate is actually falsified, does not suggest the honesty necessary to tell the child about her origins "when the time comes."

Furthermore, Elizabeth Stern diagnosed herself as having multiple sclerosis and therefore concluded that she was unable to bear children without threatening her health. She did not have her own diagnosis confirmed until after the case was in court. Although she could have borne her husband's child, she chose not to due to health risks. Pollitt raises a legitimate concern, that the same condition which prevented Elizabeth Stern from giving birth might eventually prevent her from fulfilling her function as mother (1987, 682).

The two overriding reasons,then, for granting the Sterns custody in the *Matter of Baby M* were the Whiteheads' finances and Mary Beth Whitehead's attitude toward her daughter—both her attitude toward the unwanted fetus that she was willing to give up and her attitude toward her daughter after birth. The court held that Baby M's best interests were served by the Sterns' secure financial situation and larger house, and not by Whitehead's omniscent attitude toward her daughter, contempt for therapy, and potential dishonesty. Whitehead was never judged an unfit mother. In fact, all agreed that she was a good and loving mother to her children (*Matter of Baby M* 1988, 1239). So, it was not her qualifications as a mother, but as a member of the bourgeoisie, that were challenged.

Other factors come to play in any custody decision. First, an obvious result of the class difference between surrogates and contractors is that contractors can afford more expensive and influential custody lawyers. A second related issue is what person will have custody during the surrogacy trial. In Whitehead's case the law sided with the existing contract, granted the Sterns custody, and forcibly took the baby away before Whitehead could respond with any legal action herself. Of course, Whitehead did not have her own personal attorney. The Sterns, on the other hand, had access to legal help that could get them what they wanted immediately. In spite of the illegal contract that gave rise to the initial custody decision, the fact that the Sterns had had custody of the child longer than Whitehead became a factor in the final custody decision. Given the classism and sexism evidenced by both New Jersey courts, it seems unlikely that we can assume that pretrial judges will grant temporary custody to surrogates.

Unfortunately, the New Jersey Supreme Court's statement that its ruling alone would discourage surrogacy contracts is overly optimistic. There was no mention of prosecuting the Sterns for breaking the law, even though the court maintained that theirs was a serious crime, punishable by three to five years in prison (*Matter of Baby M* 1988, 1241). By gaining custody of Baby M, the Sterns were *rewarded* for breaking the law. The court cited precedent that the use of illegal adoption does not mean the denial of adoption (*Matter of Baby M* 1988, 1257). With this precedent and the court's present action, it is difficult to see how the court's decision will discourage surrogacy arrangements. Until state legislators take some action to regulate surrogacy contracts, women will continue to be exploited.

Notes

1. For additional accounts of the *Matter of Baby M* see Johnson 1987; Pollitt 1987; and Raymond 1988.
2. In most cases the courts assume, and some commercial agencies insist, that the contracting agent be a heterosexual married man. Often the contracting agent is referred to as the "infertile couple." And the desire for a child is referred to as the "infertile couple's desire to have *their own* children" (*Matter of Baby M* 1988, 1234) even though the father's wife is not biologically related to the child. The surrogate's services are said to alleviate infertility (Eaton 1986, 717), even though the father's wife remains infertile.
3. Katha Pollitt points out that artificial insemination is practiced to avoid infidelity not infertility (1987, 683).
4. This argument was used successfully in *Surrogate Parenting Associates v. Commonwealth of Kentucky,* 1986; *Stern v. Whitehead,* New Jersey Superior Court 1987; *Syrkowski v. Appleyard,* Michigan Supreme Court 1985. It was unsuccessful in the appeal of *Stern v. Whitehead, The Matter of Baby M,* New Jersey Supreme Court, 1988.
5. Unfortunately, forced cesareans are not unique to surrogacy arrangements. Court orders can be obtained within an hour or two to force women, against their will, to undergo a cesarean (Ladd 1989).
6. As Sandra Johnson points out, "Services are something you *do*; pregnant is something you *are*. Pregnancy changes a woman's entire body—she is not merely renting her womb—and has significant impact on her psyche as well" (1987, 1345).
7. This logic was used by the Kentucky Supreme Court and the New Jersey Superior Court (*Surrogate Parenting Associates Inc. v. Commonwealth of Kentucky* 1986; *Stern v. Whitehead* 1987).
8. Although the New Jersey Supreme Court ruled that surrogacy contracts are unenforceable and perhaps criminal, its justifications for that ruling moved them out of the liberal framework. In fact, their opinion points up contradictions in what might be called an "enlightened liberal" framework. Insofar as it is enlightened, however, it is not really liberal. As soon as the liberal position begins to consider the ways in which individuals are constructed by their class and gender, it has moved away from presumptions about human nature that are central to the liberal position. Central to the liberal framework is the presumption that the individual is prior to society and that all individuals are equal and free. This is Alison Jaggar's

critique of what she calls "liberal feminism" in her monumental *Feminist Politics and Human Nature* (1983, 27–48, 174–203). See also Raymond 1988.

9. If the surrogacy contract is not enforced and the surrogate's parental rights are not relinquished, then the father's wife may not be able officially to adopt the child. However, in New Jersey, at least, as the state supreme court points out, illegal adoption does not mean denial of adoption. In other words, even if the adoption is illegal it may hold. In addition, the court need not grant the surrogate visitation rights if it is not in the best interests of the child. Furthermore, even the enlightened liberal position of many philosophers, specifically George Annas, endorses the custody process of the status quo, thereby covering over the socioeconomic issues that give rise to the surrogacy contract in the first place (Annas 1986, 1987, 1988).

References

Andrews, Lori. 1989. Alternative modes of reproduction. In *Reproductive laws for the 1990s*, ed. Sherrill Cohen and Nadine Taub, 361–403. Clifton, N.J.: Humana Press.

Annas, George J., 1986. The baby broker boom. *Hastings Center Report* 16 (3): 30-31.

Annas, George J., 1987. Baby M: Babies (and justice) for sale. *Hastings Center Report* 17 (3): 13–15.

Annas, George J., 1988. Death without dignity for commercial surrogacy: The case of Baby M. *Hastings Center Report* 18 (2): 21–24.

Corea, Gena. 1985. *The mother machine: Reproductive technologies from artificial insemination to artificial wombs.* New York: Harper & Row.

Dworkin, Andrea. 1983. *Right-wing women.* New York: Perigee Books.

Eaton, Thomas. 1986. Comparative responses to surrogate motherhood. *Nebraska Law Review* 65:686–727.

Jaggar, Alison. 1983. *Feminist politics and human nature*. Totowa, N.J.: Rowman & Allanheld.

Johnson, Sandra. 1987. The Baby "M" decision: Specific performance of a contract for specially manufactured goods. *Southern Illinois University Law Journal* 11: 1339–1348.

Ladd, Rosalind. 1989. Women in labor: Some issues about informed consent. *Hypatia* 4 (3): 37–45.

Matter of Baby M. 1988. N.J., 537, *Atlantic Reporter*, 2nd Series, 1234.

Pollitt, Katha. 1987. The strange case of Baby M. *Nation* 23 May: 667, 682–686, 688.

Pollitt, Katha. 1990. When is a mother not a mother? *Nation* 3 Dec.: 825, 840-844.

Raymond, Janice G. 1988. In the Matter of Baby M: Rejudged. *Reproductive and Genetic Engineering* 1 (2): 175–181.

Sistare, Christine T. 1988. Reproductive freedom and women's freedom: Surrogacy and autonomy. *Philosophical Forum* 19 (4): 227–240.

Stern v. Whitehead. 1987. 217, N.J., Super., 313, 525, A.2d 1128.

Surrogate Parenting Associates Inc. v. Commonwealth of Kentucky. 1986. Ky., 704, South West Reporter, 2nd Series, 209.

Syrkowski v. Appleyard. Mich. Supr. Crt 1985. 362 N.W. 2d 211.

Chapter 24

HERITAGE, SURROGACY, AND THE ETHICS OF COMMUNITY: CHOICE AND AVOIDANCE IN AFRICAN AND AFRICAN-AMERICAN PARENTING TRADITIONS

Ruth M. Lucier, Cheryl D. Childs, Shawnda M. Parks, and Rosalie A. Yemba.

Introduction

As a recently introduced option of reproduction, "surrogacy" utilizes a woman's body as a conceptual receptacle, gestator, and bearer of offspring while requiring the woman who agrees to be utilized in these ways to relinquish in advance of conception all legal claim to parental rights.[1] Surrogacy has been regarded by a number of feminist writers to be morally wrong because of the allegedly deleterious effects surrogacy has on women's place and power (see, for example, Anderson 1990; Raymond 1990; Ryan 1990).

In this chapter, questions about the rightness or wrongness of surrogacy will be raised that specifically take into account the contexts of tradition, gender, and class within which surrogacy decisions are made. Of central interest will be attitudes drawn from the African and African-American traditions and legacies[2] that (1) bolster feminist stands against surrogacy and yet (2) differ from many modern feminist views with respect to rejecting the strong notions of procreative autonomy drawn from theories of the West. Our aim is to derive from African and African-American legacies ethical concepts that will be helpful in an overarching, cross-cultural way in determining what is morally problematic in the surrogacy transaction.

We shall consider in turn each type of individual involved in the surrogacy arrangement, namely, the man whose sperm is to be used and who will assume parenting rights, the surrogate who will bear the child and give up parenting rights, the potential adoptive mother, and the child who is produced. For each type we shall ask how that individual's situation might be different from the one he or she would have in communal settings like those of traditional Africa (or its American extension). We shall then seek principles in the African and derivative outlooks that suggest a communalistic stance that illuminates the possible wrongs to that type of individual (viz., wrongs that are inherent in his or her individual situation) and ask whether there are goods that compensate for the wrongs. We shall show that from a communalistic stance compensations (particularly for women and children) are in normal cases inadequate and that surrogacy in normal cases is therefore not a morally justified option.

Tradition, Communalism, and the Masculine Impetus Toward Surrogacy

The African communal tradition places a very high value on a man's ability to father offspring within the context of community, and this value continues to be affirmed in the African-American tradition.

In the traditional thought of Africa the importance of having children has spiritual dimensions. For both men and women having progeny defines one's place in a hierarchically arranged series of ongoing, mutually sensitive, and interrelated roles. The roles taken together comprise a supportive web that fosters (1) orderings within extended matriarchal or patriarchal family systems, (2) orderings within women's groups and men's groups where gender-specific roles are assumed, and (3) orderings within generally hierarchically arranged systems of community management with assigned roles that cause one to be revered and remembered. Through such remembrance one receives the communal nurturing that makes possible the continuation of one's life force even after death and hence one's immortality (Lucier 1989, 34).

In African traditional systems (and derivatives from such systems), having children also bestows present advantages. These include enhancement of social place and power, and hence an enlargement of options (Erny 1973, 99; Lijembe 1967, 23). Thus, as John Mbiti points out, to be without children and a home is seen, in African traditional life, as an evil that is very hard to bear.

Mbiti recounts a prayer traditionally offered by the childless that concludes that without children and a home, "Where shall I go? I am in distress: Where is there room for me?" (1975, 20).

With so much at stake a man seeks arrangements that will yield biological heirs. But whether the arrangements are for wife or concubine, the heirs are not to be his autonomously—they are to be a continuation of the man's and the woman's extended family and of the community. For this reason the so-called "bride price" (or dowry) a man gives for a connection to a designated woman "is better understood as a 'progeny price'" (Kilbride & Kilbride 1990b, 14). Not simply a symbol of agreement between the two families, it is also a transaction in which a family exchanges material goods for rights to children. Writing in the 1930s, Gunter Wagner noted that among, for example, the Abaluyia of Kenya fertility was so strongly emphasized "that a young girl could increase her chances of marriage by becoming pregnant" (Kilbride & Kilbride 1990b, 14). Wagner also notes that even among people such as the Logoli, who place a very high value on virginity prior to marriage, a girl who becomes pregnant by her fiancé is accepted in marriage if she bears a healthy child (Wagner 1949, 438).

In the transference of this masculine procreative value to the American South, the importance of children took on added significance, for while African and African-American men in bondage in the United States were initially trapped in the slave system by government policy, there was always the hope that their children would eventually be free. The link to children became an aspirational link to liberation.

Within the institution of slavery an enslaved man's relationship to his offspring was perilous; his children could be taken from him and perhaps sold to strangers, and he had no effective way of blocking such action. Under a social system that threatened traditional family values in such a dramatic way, the linkages to African heritage provided an extended notion of family and community, the common elements of which were (1) the common continent of origin, (2) shared motifs of the heritage, (3) the common shared tragedy of being systemically deprived of basic human rights, and (4) the shared circumstance of being regularly subjected to difficult, dangerous, inhumane, and potentially life-threatening circumstances. Survival of the community through mutually supportive acts and the heroism of shared offspring opened the way for generalized conceptions of "nurturing one's own," where "one's own" became any of the children of one's community who were in need of care. Hence, the African-American man in the context of his community eventually became a mentor, adviser, nurturer (a practicing parent) to an extended group of children who suffered from the same legally enforced constraints.[3]

This parenting relationship was valued whether or not the children were genetically his own.[4]

Ideas that might seem in this communal tradition to be somewhat analogous to surrogacy are (1) (from the African tradition) the endorsement of the "progeny price" paid for liaisons that produce children, and (2) (from the African-American tradition) the notion that it is appropriate for a man to act as father to children of his community who are not by his designated mate and who are not, in the immediate sense, genetically his own. But the difference between the traditional arrangements and what occurs in modern surrogacy is marked, for the "bride price," while being in a sense a "progeny price," is also a gift to a bride's family. It is not paid, as modern surrogacy fees are paid, for children only. Moreover, this gift, given to obtain parenting rights to children, is not given to divest the biological mother of legal claim to her offspring. The transaction itself is not entered into for the purpose of allowing the payers to remove a child from its extended family connections. The woman who produces the offspring is to become part of the extended family of the man who is seeking to acquire offspring by her. Once the relationship is confirmed, moreover, it is expected that the man's family would be part of the extended family of the woman who is selected as well as for any children produced.

The principles that seem implicit in the African traditional context are ones that endorse the propriety of seeking a woman by whom to have offspring (even a woman in addition to a first or primary spouse) on the supposition that this will foster an ongoing connection with her as a part of one's family and community. The principles at work in the African-American derivative of this "probonding" view are ones that endorse the rightness of considering children of one's community to be one's own to nurture simply because they are part of one's own community and bearers of its legacy. The first sort of principle places emphasis on genetic lineage, but not in the absence of association with the mother of the child. The second sort, while not excluding the positive value of nurturing children of one's direct genetic line, widens this value to include nurturing of shared offspring. The first principle suggests a permanent, socially recognized liaison plus procreation. The second suggests *adoption.* These are appropriate traditional ways in which a man might acquire a direct and permanent parenting connection to a child.

Suppose a man accepts these principles as "ideals" but opts for surrogacy as a way of obtaining offspring. Will he forfeit any good that is crucial to his ability to live strongly and well—to flourish as a person? And will he be wronged in a way that will cause him to suffer moral harm?

One good that is obviously forfeited in rejecting principles of the first sort is the experience of forming a family with the birth mother of a "spouse-produced" genetic heir and thus the forfeiture of a personal, historic good. The harm that would result from not acting in accordance with principles of the second sort would be loss of an important sense of community—a sense that itself provides a source of strength, comfort, and psychological power.

Failure to act in accordance with the ideal expressed in the initial principle, might be unavoidable given physical limitations and acceptance of monogamy. But failure to act on the second principle (thus, in effect, opting for surrogacy *in preference to adoption*) signals, from a communalistic point of view, a rejection of community responsibility and therefore possible forfeiture of entitlement to community support. This would be especially true where there are children from one's community available to be adopted and desperately in need of care and where the surrogate does not have, and will not have, any community connection.

A man who resorts to surrogacy in preference to adoption may, therefore, suffer not only loss of ongoing historic connection to a community-associated birth mother of his genetic child, but also loss of community support due to his apparent defection. While he seems not to be subject to any treatment by others that could be regarded as morally wrong, he does wrong to himself by divesting himself of these goods.

But, suppose what "motivates" the man is the good of having, as his child, a child of his own immediate genetic lineage. Would this good outweigh the harm? From a communalistic perspective it would not, for the man would be giving up something quite positive (an opportunity for bonding with and taking responsibility for a family formed within his community) and would be giving this up for an irrelevant value, namely, an "outsider-produced," historically isolated, genetic heir.

The harm done by the man to himself does constitute a moral harm, but it is a self-inflicted one. Since the harm is self-inflicted and not socially disruptive in any ongoing way, the man need not be protected, especially when such protection goes against his will.

Biological Mother/Surrogate Mother: Communalistic Considerations

Unlike the man who elects surrogacy over adoption, the woman who serves as surrogate normally relinquishes *both* parental power *and* communal connection to the child she has produced. Comparisons between the surrogate's role and analogues in the African and African-American traditions are useful for suggesting a perspective from which the surrogate's situation can be assessed.

In the surrogate case a woman previously unassociated with the prospective father is sought to bear a child, presumably because the present spouse of the prospective father is unable or unwilling to do so. In the African tradition a variant of this is certainly allowed through the institution of polygamy. While permitting men to have biological offspring by acquiring additional wives or concubines, polygamy also imposes requirements that protect women. Usually, a woman brought into the family is given her own compound and enjoys a rights-entailing place in the total system of communal farming on communally held land (Kilbride & Kilbride 1990a, 58). Moreover, the woman retains her nurturing connection to the children she bears. In contrast, in surrogacy with the complete, post-fee/post-birth, economic and family disassociation, a woman is assured of neither ongoing support nor ongoing social connection to her child.

In the traditional African context the closest approximation to the surrogate situation where a mother is separated from her child would occur only as a consequence of servitude or war. A woman might be given as a concubine to a foreigner of high status and taken to a territory far from her community. If she becomes a mother of a child, however, she would still be honored. Since the biological mother's status in the family where the child is to be an inheritor of wealth and power might be increased by the birth regardless of whether the biological mother became the man's wife, such a woman might pose a definite threat to the status and power of the first wife—but only in an extreme case would the biological mother be excluded from the home.

In war women and children were taken as "property," as valuable resources for the perpetuation of the work force. Captives in war were separated from other family members and placed where useful, but no one was expected to choose to be a captive. To be a captive, to be enslaved, was a great tragedy—not a voluntary choice.

The African and African-American perspectives suggest that as a matter of principle a woman who bears a child (1) should be allowed ongoing family and social connection to the child, (2) should receive, and has a right to receive, ongoing support for herself and for the child, (3) should have a firm basis for economic security within family and community, and (4) should receive ongoing respect for her contribution as the gestator and birth mother of the child. Deviation from principles 1 through 4 in the African context would indicate that the woman had undergone a socially tragic situation, one that led her to be divested of the normal entitlements associated with her role.

In using these principles to judge the surrogate case, one wrong identified in most instances would be the failure to give the surrogate fair and ongoing compensation; another wrong would be the denial of ongoing social recognition for motherhood that is traditionally due.

Is the harm done greater than the self-inflicted harm done to the father of the surrogate's child? Clearly, it is. While the father may suffer social stigma and partial connectional loss (viz., some loss of community connection and also loss of family connection as spouse to the birth mother of his genetic child), he may gain ongoing custody of the child and generally enjoys both gender and class-based advantages that in some measure offset the loss. The surrogate, in contrast, loses custody of the child and generally enjoys no comparable contravening gender or class-based advantages. Indeed, it may be argued that, in contrast to the prospective father, the prospective surrogate/birth mother is likely to agree to surrogacy only because of socially induced gender and class *handicaps*—handicaps imposed by traditions that encourage women's sacrifice to masculine interests (Raymond 1990) and that place limits on women's economic options (Anderson 1990). These handicaps might well compound the harm. For example, a woman conditioned to feel that femininity is affirmed through producing and giving up a child or a woman who is in dire economic straits might be attracted to the rewards of being a surrogate with an intensity that prevents her from objectively assessing (and protecting herself from) the negative consequences of the surrogacy choice.

The possible advantages of income seem at this time rather minimal from a middle-class perspective. But even the rather moderate fee of, say $10,000, might appear quite substantial to women from working-class households, especially those economically hard pressed by the expense of raising other children. So the fact that a woman is offered money over and above the hospital expenses certainly would provide an incentive that traditional adoption would not. Traditional adoption is costly, but the money goes to agencies and lawyers—not to the woman who produced the baby. Thus the birth mother's reason for bearing the child would not, in the traditional case, be motivated by monetary gain.

What goods are there that might outweigh the harm? The goods might be these: (1) the income to be acquired as surrogate, (2) the contribution the birthing experience might make to the variety of experiences in the surrogate's life due to the interest value of the experience of having given birth, and (3) the opportunity the surrogacy agreement might give for making others happy —and thus the personal satisfaction that might be obtained from knowing one had given a parenting opportunity to others who want very much to be parents and the personal satisfaction of giving life itself to the child.

Do these advantages outweigh (or further compensate for) the harm? Evidence that they do not may be seen in the fact that some surrogates have made attempts (indeed desperate and passionate attempts) to invalidate the arrangement once the child is born, even though they apparently freely agreed to the arrangement prior to conception. What being a surrogate asks of women may entail pain and loss for some too extensive to be outweighed or offset either by material rewards or by the anticipated psychological benefits of being perceived as a generous and altruistic person. Altruism is laudable only if it is a response to authentic needs by a contributor who is fully aware of the cost.

If the emotional damage to the surrogate is as great as cases such as that of Baby M suggest (Kantrowitz 1987), surrogacy may be judged morally wrong simply because (1) it interferes with a woman's ability to make a reasonable choice (the choice *after* the birth of the child to *keep* that child) and (2) it excludes her without adequate compensation from enjoying the status and rewards that that instance of childbearing would otherwise give her in the social setting within which she must live.

The Adoptive Mother and the "Surrogate-produced" Child

Unlike the situation of either the surrogate or the potential father, the situation of the potential adoptive mother appears on the surface to involve only a net *gain*, namely, the addition of an offspring to her home. Her position resembles that of a traditional adoptive mother's in many respects. However, there are important differences. Again, cross-cultural reflection will be helpful for making significant features clear.

Mothering children is a social good. In African tradition it is crucial. The woman without children loses status in a dramatic way. The pregnant woman is praised and admired: she contributes to the economic security of her family by providing the workers needed for food production and the offspring needed to form valuable social and political connections (Erny 1973, 102–103; Kilbride & Kilbride 1990a, 58; Lijembe 1967, 22; Wagner 1949, 275).

Since the husband of a woman with no children, according to African tradition, can have multiple wives, a woman's lack of children does not mean a lack of children in the family. Since "having one's own" is viewed as a positive good, social convention permits analogues of adoption. One striking analogue among East African people is the possibility of a childless woman adopting the child of another and becoming a "female husband" (Kilbride & Kilbride 1990b, 14). Here the tradition of inclusiveness and standard adoption blend, for the mother as well as the child is taken into the female husband's home.

In the African-American extension of this tradition such inclusiveness is reflected in the willingness of a very large extended family network to take in and raise children of their kin while keeping the kinship relations intact. Hence, the adopted child might find that her birth mother was, in fact, someone she had known as her aunt or cousin—but at the appropriate age the child would know her birth mother as mother and be reconciled to her in deference to her past.

Principles to be drawn from these traditions include the ideas that (1) the adoption of children by a woman—so she can have the benefits of being parent to specific offspring—is a positive good, particularly when the woman has been biologically unable to have children of her own, (2) the children adopted should be under the parental authority of the adopter, and yet (3) the adopted children need not, and should not, be estranged from their biological roots.

In the surrogate case, the adoptive mother does receive the good of principles 1 and 2 but resists principle 3, for the *point* of the surrogacy is to receive the child unencumbered by any ongoing relationship with the woman who produced the child.

In reference to these principles, no apparent harm appears done to the adoptive mother as long as the claim she has to the child remains firm. But some possible harms may be hidden at the time the surrogacy decision is made. The adoptive mother is not, in Western practice, a "female husband"; her entitlement may be subordinate to that of the biological father (her husband) and hence subordinate to that of "her man."

This asymmetry of claims is an especially strong threat to the woman's acquired parenting power if her egg is not used and her parenting power is gained only through adoption, for in a society that systematically pays higher wages to men, allows no fault divorce, favors a biological parent's claims to children and tends to give children to the parent who can best afford to pay the expenses of child-rearing, the chance of the man receiving custody of the surrogate-produced offspring is very great indeed. Therefore, in the case of the dissolution of the marriage (and there is a 50 percent probability of this), the adoptive mother in the surrogate case is more likely than the traditional adoptive mother to lose not only her spouse but also her child.

When a woman is put at risk of losing her entire family if the marriage ends, her power within the marriage is clearly reduced. Therefore, while the genetically unrelated adoptive mother by agreeing to the surrogacy situation gains by having a child to be a parent to, she may also lose by being made the most vulnerable and hence disimpowered parent; she may lose, in effect, traditional adoption's more favorable male/female parenting equilibrium.

Even if the adoptive mother in the surrogate case is also the genetic mother of the child, she will still lose the bonding implicit in the birth-mother experience and will also face the threat of the birth mother's (the surrogate's) possible attempt to reacquire the child. The latter threat may be more pronounced in surrogacy cases than in traditional adoption.

In the case of traditional adoption of a nonrelated child, each adoptive parent would have to base his or her claim to the child on the ability to provide good parenting "services." Although the adoptive mother might still be at an economic disadvantage, at least she would not have a less well-based genetic claim.

Children in the Web

If there are wrongs to both the surrogate and the adoptive mother, as our analysis suggests, then, insofar as one cares about strengthening the position of women in society (and preventing situations that could cause women unnecessary pain), a stance favoring the adoption of already existing children over the use of surrogacy would appear to be the more reasonable and sound. This same conclusion can be reached by considering the possible wrongs to the child.

To be without parents or to lose one parent (father or mother) has been regarded in African tradition as a major handicap for the child, even if the child is too young to be conscious of the loss. The lack of knowledge of parent deprives the child of knowledge of its social roots and of possible economic support as well. In traditional Africa, among the Kele, the tragedy of being an orphan is significant enough to be permanently affixed to a person's spoken name and to be preserved in the person's drum name as well (Carrington 1969, 43). Among the Dogon, a boy "born without a father" has "neither house nor fields, nor protective spirits" (Erny 1973, 102), and among the Kavirondo, if the mother dies in childbirth, the infant is left to die as well, probably because its position in the community is unclear (Wagner 1949, 302).

In the African-American context where group care is offered, the pain connected with the knowledge that there is a missing parent has often prompted a child to search for the parent it has lost.

In both African and African-American traditions univocal strands suggest these principles: (1) one should prevent, if possible, the loss of, or separation of, children from their biological parents because the loss is a social evil for the child, and (2) one should avoid placing the child in a socially ambiguous situation—for this too is a harm.

If being without one or both biological parents (either because they no longer exist or because the child cannot find and know them) *is* a handicap and a source of pain to the child in the modern context, then the surrogacy arrangement might be regarded as premeditatively wronging the child because it involves, in advance, the planned divestiture of the child's associations with, and personal knowledge of, its biological mother. The handicap may encompass the loss of the adoptive mother as well due to a more tenuous genetic claim, as explained above.

To bring about any situation where a child is more vulnerable than necessary is surely morally questionable strategy, for children are already extremely vulnerable (Cohen 1980; Vardin & Brody 1979). Surely, justice has as one of its many aims the protection of the vulnerable (Goodin 1985). While surrogacy arrangements in an immediate sense do not make a child more vulnerable to loss, since at the time of the arrangement (at the time the agreement is first struck) no child exists, such arrangements do institutionalize a future child's vulnerability to profound, ongoing, and legally mandated loss.

One kind of understanding of birth involved in African traditional views that might be thought to give some supporting rationale for surrogacy over adoption, is that in African traditional views the new birth of a child in one's genetic line may present the possibility of a relived life of an ancestor. Similarly, the possibility of the new birth from surrogacy may offer to the person whose sperm or egg is used a sense of the continuation of his or her ancestry. The genetic child of one's body, after all, carries the physical heritage of one's own biological family and is likely to resemble forebears in one's ancestral line. Hence, the child links one's personal present to one's family's past.

Whether this value of genetic family resemblance is a value for the child might depend on the degree to which a parent's genetic strain is uniquely good for the child. One unique good might be that a physical resemblance to the parent, manifested in the child, can provide a concrete basis for family bonding that reinforces the child's position and claim to physical support and other social goods. This would be especially so in a family with few members or one that has little sense of belonging to any wider community. Therefore, seeking a child through surrogacy to secure for the child genetic resemblance to oneself or one's spouse could be a benefit to the child and cannot be rejected out of hand as either irrational or prejudicial to children whom one might otherwise adopt. However, the sense of community achieved for the child in such a case is very minimalist, and the minimalism (the lack of a wider view) might itself be injurious to the child.

The Adoption Dilemma

To this point we have argued that in the modern context the principles we have elicited strongly favor adoption over surrogacy. A dilemma concerning adoption, however, emerges from the concept of community in its ethnic connection and complicates attempts to apply the traditional African notion of community in advocating adoption. If, on the one hand, potential adopters are from, say, the European-American mixed stock and the children available for adoption are, say, from the African-American or other non-European yet American heritages and potential adopters decline to adopt a child *because* the children available for adoption are of such heritages, their stance would appear morally wrong. To decline such adoption is to deny a child the opportunity to be one's child *simply* because of heritage or race. In addition, to make heritage or race the determining factor in excluding a child from the possibility of being one's child is to take into account a factor that should not be considered in deciding which children's basic needs for love, nurturing, and a secure home are met.

If the child is born of parents of a distinctive ethnic or racial heritage, an equally pressing concern emerges if individuals adopt in spite of ethnic heritage or racial difference. The problem here becomes one of loss of legacy. Could adoptive parents with no ethnic attachments themselves communicate to the child the distinctive legacy of the child's own natural community? Or will they, by adopting a child in order to provide it with a home, break the child's connection to its natural community—the community from which in later times the child may need to seek comfort and support? In a society where prejudice and discrimination run deep and where ethnicity is often "color-coded," such a loss of community associations could be very detrimental to the well-being of the child.

When, then, the African and African-American principles of nurturing all in need are applied in contexts where the notion of community is stretched to include groups of persons who do not share a heritage that enables the group to function as a community in the deep and supportive sense, the principle flounders. In such cases the child rather than gaining the more enduring community connections, instead loses them. The child loses through extraethnic adoption an important attachment to an ethnic community to which it will be assigned by the dominant groups and to which it may need to look for support. If in a given case adoption would entail such a loss, then in spite of the availability of adoptable children there could be (even for decidedly moral persons) hard cases where there was no appropriate child to adopt.

A Note on the Outsider: General Moral Constraints

If one accepts and ascribes to the values of community and care-giving to all, found in African and African-American traditional thought, and universalizes these values to very loosely connected communities, one might still develop a perspective that would allow surrogacy arrangements in hard cases such as those indicated above. While accepting the view against surrogacy that has thus far been advocated, one might still firmly believe that what it means to be a virtuous member of an ethnically diverse society is that one is tolerant in a positive way—a way that allows one to participate in diverse heritages by celebrating whatever in each is life enhancing, interesting, and good. Such tolerance involves allowing others to do some things that one's own values and/or one's own community's values would disallow. Hence, positive tolerance could reasonably give the basis for supporting options for outsiders that one would never approve of for oneself and would never utilize. Among these might be an option for "outsiders" to seek and obtain a surrogate-produced child if they can not obtain an appropriate child through adoption. In our view, however, surrogacy in even the hard cases should be tolerated only if (1) the surrogacy situation *does not* involve the violation of moral rules (such as the rule that one should not deceive another person to get what one wants), (2) *does promote* human flourishing, and (3) *does achieve* a good that substantially outweighs any harm and avoids, or minimizes, the doing of wrong.

One wrong to be avoided is the wrong of tempting any person to engage in surrogacy when it is likely that the person will be deeply hurt by it. Since there are so many possible harms, impartial monitoring of specific contractual processes is required. Only through such monitoring can one know in what instances the good is likely to outweigh the harm. Such monitoring is politically appropriate, for whenever engagement in potentially harmful activities is allowed, a responsible society must institute monitoring so that there are protections for those put at risk. Options are important, but no options should allow some to ride roughshod over the interests of others.[5]

Persons who might profit by promoting surrogacy should not monitor the process or grant legal permission for these arrangements. Rather, the monitoring process should provide, in effect, a support system oriented to prevent the surrogate from being wrongfully persuaded to give up the child, to strengthen the adoptive mother's connection to the child, and, especially, to safeguard the interests of the child. Attention should be given to compensating for missing networks of kinship and community—the social web—that in traditional systems would have provided a context within which a child's well-being could be promoted and secured (Bellah et al. 1985, 134–138; Kilbride & Kilbride 1990a, 237–238).

Conclusion

Drawing from the African and African-American traditions, we have advocated a principle-based analysis that suggests that normally surrogacy should not be used. Exceptions might be envisioned only for hard cases in which some goods (e.g., family bonding or tolerance) would outweigh the harms.

Reflections on the African and African-American traditions have brought forward principles that are protective of women and children. As social and legal systems are being reshaped, concerned persons need to participate actively in defending traditional principles (or enlightened modifications thereof) that will maintain and augment the needed protections. These principles should not be abandoned in the rush to obtain parenting opportunities or any other goods.

Notes

1. We shall follow convention in using the term "surrogacy" for the option and surrogate for the birth mother involved in such an option, even though the surrogate birth mother is the actual (not the substitute) birth mother of the child.
2. By African traditions and legacies the authors mean, in the context of this article, primarily those of agricultural village peoples of Sub-Saharan Africa whose languages generally fall within the Bantu language families (see Galake 1978, 11; see Kagame 1976, 328). The extension of these traditions and legacies found in the United States stems both from assimilation of cultural motifs brought by African people under slavery (McPherson 1971, 32–35; Miller & Smith 1988, 10–31) and by the later rediscovery of cultural patterns by American citizens returning to Africa and bringing knowledge of the culture back to the United States (Asante & Asante 1985).

   Of the people from Africa brought in bondage to the United States between 1690 and 1807, 24.5 percent were from Bantu territories (Angola/Congo), and 27.6% were from the Bights of Benin and Biafra, which are adjacent to such territories (Miller & Smith 1988, 12).
3. Africans and African-Americans enslaved in the United States could not tell their own story or exhibit cultural awareness or concern for one another publicly without risking reprisals by European-Americans who attempted to control them. For this reason it is not surprising that stories of nurturing by enslaved men (noticeably absent in European-American accounts of the slave period) surface publicly only after the fact in memoirs and autobiographies of ex-slaves or in novels based on family oral traditions (see Haley 1976; Walker 1966; Washington 1896).

   Such nurturing when noticed by slave owners could be brutally suppressed. One memorable example that is widely known (because of its discovery and because of the achievements of the nurturer) is the account of Frederick Douglass's founding of a Sunday school for young slaves on a Maryland plantation. For doing this, Douglass was "beaten and for his effrontery threatened with the same punishment given Nat Turner" (Miller & Smith 1988, 448).

4. Booker T. Washington's autobiography, *Up From Slavery*, provides a clear example of this. Washington's stepfather, owned by a master other than the master of his mother, seldom saw his family while enslaved in Virginia. But, immediately after emancipation, the stepfather sent for his family, composed of Washington's mother and her three children, to come and live with him in West Virginia. Washington's stepfather apparently did this without raising any questions about the directness of his lineage to his wife's children and certainly without rejecting Washington and his brother (who were reportedly fathered by a white man from a nearby plantation—a man who presumably never visited Washington or his brother and never contributed to the family's support in any way) (Washington 1896, 8, 16).
5. For an interesting *noncommunalistic* argument to this effect, see Machan 1982, 123–142.

Acknowledgments

For support for basic research on the cross-cultural ethical views in this essay we thank the Women's Studies Program of Bennett College (directed by Teresa Jo Styles) and the Faculty Research, Development, and Support Program of Bennett College (directed by Gloria Wentowski).

We are also indebted to members of the 1989 Humanities Symposia at Bennett College, especially to Kimberly Grant, Terrilynne Jenkins, Shavaughn Neal, Tina Nelson, Lorraine Patton, Sara Williams, Melissa Rivers, and Taundra Woodard. In addition special thanks is owed to Barbara Woods, Doris Strange, Mary Stewart, Juanita Lewis, and Krishna Kasibhatla for technical assistance with the manuscript.

References

Anderson, Elizabeth S. 1990. Is women's labor a commodity? *Philosophy and Public Affairs* 19 (1): 71–92.

Asante, Molefi Kete, and Kariamu Welsh Asante. 1985. *African culture: The rhythms of unity*. Westport, Ct.: Greenwood Press.

Bellah, Robert, Richard Madsen, William M. Sullivan, et al. 1985. *Habits of the heart: Individualism and commitment in American life*. Berkeley: University of California Press.

Carrington, J. F. 1969. *Talking drums of Africa*. New York: Negro University Press.

Cohen, Howard. 1980. *Equal rights for children*. Totowa, N.J.: Rowman & Littlefield.

Erny, P. 1973. *Childhood and the cosmos: The social psychology of the black African child.* Washington, D. C.: Black Orpheus Press.

Garlake, Peter S. 1978. *Kingdoms of Africa*. Oxford, Eng.: Elsevier-Phaidon.

Goodin, Robert E. 1985. *Protecting the vulnerable: Reanalysis of our social responsibilities*. Chicago: University of Chicago Press.

Haley, Alex. 1976. *Roots*. New York: Dell.

Kagame, Alexis. 1976. *La philosophie Bantu comparie*. Paris: Presence African.

Kantrowitz, Barbara. 1987. Who keeps 'Baby M'? *Newsweek* 19 Jan.: 44–49.

Kilbride, Philip, and Janet Capriotti Kilbride. 1990a. *Changing family life in East Africa: Women and children at risk*. University Park and London: Pennsylvania State University Press.

Kilbride, Philip, and Janet Capriotti Kilbride. 1990b. Moralnets. *Bryn Mawr Bulletin* 72 (1): 12–17.

Lijembe, Joseph. 1967. *East African childhood: Three versions*. Oxford, Eng.: Oxford University Press.

Lucier, Ruth M. 1989. Dynamics of hierarchy in African thought. *Listening: Journal of Religion and Culture* 24 (1): 29–40.

Machan, Tibor. 1982. Property rights and the decent society. In *Ideology in American experience: Essays on theory and practice in the United States,* ed. John K. Roth and Robert C. Whittemore. Washington, D. C.: Washington Institute for Values and Public Policy Press.

McPherson, James M. 1971. *Blacks in America: Bibliographical essays*. Garden City, N.Y.: Doubleday.

Mbiti, John S. 1975. *The prayers of African religion*. New York: Orbus Books.

Miller, Randall M., and John David Smith. 1988. *Dictionary of Afro-American slavery*. Westport, Ct.: Greenwood Press.

Raymond, Janice G. 1990. Reproductive gifts and gift-giving: The altruistic woman. *Hastings Center Report* 20 (6): 7–11.

Ryan, Maura A. 1990. The argument for unlimited procreative liberty: A feminist critique. *Hastings Center Report* 24 (4): 6–12.

Vardin, Patricia A., and Ilene N. Brody. 1979. *Children's rights: Contemporary perspectives*. New York: Teacher's College Press, Columbia University.

Wagner, G. 1949. *The Bantu of North Kavirondo*. London: Oxford University Press for International African Institute.

Walker, Margaret. 1966. *Jubilee*. Boston: Houghton Mifflin.

Washington, Booker T. 1896. *Up from Slavery*. Mattituck, N.Y.: Amereon House. Reprint 1990.

Chapter 25

SLAVERY AND CONTRACT MOTHERHOOD: A "RACIALIZED" OBJECTION TO THE AUTONOMY ARGUMENTS

Sarah S. Boone

Introduction

In the last decade much controversy has centered around the issue of commercialized contract or so-called "surrogate" motherhood. In exchange for payment a woman who is capable of gestation and childbirth—the contract mother—agrees at the onset to surrender all parental claims to the child to the party who has contracted for her reproductive services. This party is typically an "infertile couple," consisting of a the biological father and his spouse (who may or may not be a genetic mother of the issue), who later will become the adoptive mother. The stormy legal battles that have often resulted over custody and recognition of parental ties to "contract babies" (see Oliver, this volume) have done much to publicize the legal, prudent, and moral difficulties created by commercialized contract motherhood (henceforth CCM).

CCM has gained supporters from a variety of political camps. Its feminist supporters argue that women have a right to enter into such contracts as do infertile couples who seek their reproductive services. Such rights are viewed as subsumable under the exercise of personal freedom in pursuit of one's perceived interests (and even in pursuit of further more explicit rights to procreate). For women, we are told, the right to become contracted mothers (i.e., gestators and childbearers) is a part or natural extension of their personal autonomy or self-determination, both bodily and economic. To prohibit, generally restrict, or invalidate CCM contracts would violate fundamental rights for autonomy of women, thereby undermining them. Prohibition would also tend to reinforce the negative stereotype of women as incapable of full rational agency.

Pro-CCM arguments usually rely centrally upon a deontological defense of expressions of personal autonomy and the successful casting of CCM as such. It is clear why the autonomy arguments draw substantial support from mainstream feminists. CCM appears to allow women to "sell services they once did for free," as defenders have put it (Sistare 1988). They can now capitalize their important bodily capacities for personal gain. However, the autonomy arguments share a conceptual weakness of most traditional (rights-based) contract-modeled moral theory. Because they assume the common status of CCM's participants as "free," "equal," and naturally vested with autonomy (which the state should not contravene), they ignore important issues of *actual status*. The socially constructed statuses conferred by gender, race, and class have profound impact upon the degree to which any actual social/legal practice functions as a vehicle of autonomy or of continued repression.

Other proponents of autonomy arguments shy away from a strict deontological defense of women's rights to engage in CCM. Those less committed to the absolute sanctity of individual (autonomy) rights buttress their arguments with a utilitarian style consequentialism: they argue that the benefits (or good consequences) of society's allowing CCM outweigh its potential harms. Central among the benefits is, of course, the increased personal freedom and economic opportunity that women will enjoy and the satisfaction of infertile couples' desire for genetic offspring. Regardless of how much of an absolutist one is about rights, there are at least two lines of defense for CCM that are based upon the notion of enhanced autonomy: (1) CCM is an exercise of women's fundamental right of self-direction and is prima facie defensible as such, and (2) CCM is likely to enhance the actual power of self-determination among women by expanding their economic control over their reproductive powers.

In this chapter I intend to cast serious doubt upon both autonomy claims. I shall do so from the vantage point that treats women of color (i.e., the conceptually and socially marginalized category of women not of European descent) as a primary object of analysis. The experience of enslaved African-American women, in particular, helps historically to enrich and put the CCM debate into a broader context. The slave women's experience of sexual and reproductive exploitation uniquely informs us about patriarchy's particular denigration of racially and economically marginalized women. I shall attempt to show how the popular acceptance of CCM (like the exploitation of slave women) results from the hybrid interplay of sexism and racism. In the end, CCM is morally objectionable because it reinforces the multi-tiered oppression of all women and devalues both women and people of color.

Why Look at Slavery?

Issues of exploitation and commodification of mother and child are at the forefront of the CCM debates, yet virtually no consideration is given to the looming historical example we have, as a society, of women (and men) along with their children being wholesalely exploited and commodified.[1] The presumption seems to be that whatever the experience of women slaves, it can be ignored because slavery is too fundamentally dissimilar to CCM to be relevant. If we flesh it out, the claim seems be that the socioeconomic institutions, and even the ideologies, that supported slavery and shaped the oppressive life circumstances of the slave woman are too fundamentally different from those that shape the experiences of the contract mother *as such*. Therefore, the two sets of experiences cannot be compared. Such a claim is far from self-evident, however. In fact, its ready acceptance should be disturbing, given this society's propensity for effacing all historical experiences of its non-European members. The extreme reluctance of European Americans to look to the self-conceived experiences of African Americans to inform any of its intellectual inquiries is an oblique aspect of racism which continues to distort mainstream perceptions of African-American life and worth.

The assumption that the slave woman's experience is irrelevant is unsupported, and we have good reason to be suspicious of its motivations. Only a fuller examination of those experiences could allow an informed determination of relevancy. The aim here is not to draw simplistic analogies showing that CCM is a form of slavery. Rather, it is to suggest that (the circumstances of) African-American female enslavement and CCM are two very different social expressions of the same underlying ideological forms.

An Overview of the "Peculiar Institution"

To understand the exploitation of slave women one must have some understanding of the peculiar social dynamics of slavery as a whole. The European/American slave trade differed in at least two important ways from previous forms of slavery, in particular from the pre-European Islamic slave trade that it transformed and supplanted (Lovejoy 1983). Various forms of involuntary servitude dotted the African continent as they did much of the premodern world. However, the form of slavery that emerged in the Americas was striking (1) in the extensive economic reliance upon slave labor for mass (agricultural) production and (2) in the increasing systematic reliance upon concepts of racial superiority for its justification.

Under European domination, slavery coalesced with the advent of modern capitalism and colonial expansion to place slaves in a new global socioeconomic role. Africa became incorporated into the capitalist world economy as the mass supplier of agricultural producers for the "New World" (Wallerstein 1976). The numbers of exported Africans increased from thousands to millions and later tens of millions, and their coerced labor became a central economic and political institution.

European/American slavery itself was not rationalized by claims of religious or cultural superiority (or even simply by the assertion of brute power, which would have been very much against the spirit of the "Enlightenment"). It was rationalized by claims of racial superiority. This departure is significant, for while religious and cultural standing could be acquired (more or less) by individuals, racial "standing" could not. Phenotypically denoted categories of race were constructed and were treated as the biologically fixed determinant of all important human attributes, from intelligence to moral propensities. "Black" Africans were viewed as necessarily inferior to "White" Europeans. As a result, the American slave community was a physically identifiable and socially fixed rather than fluid population. Preexisting Islamic slave systems justified slavery in terms of religious/cultural superiority; it was supposed to represent a proselytizing station. As a result, despite their very real exploitation, slaves and particularly the children of slaves could be "assimilated" through formal mechanisms into many African societies, gaining full status as free persons.[2] For example, under Islamic law the children of concubines were free upon birth (Lovejoy 1983, 7–8). In contrast for African-American slaves, in particular, the stigma defining slave status was racial status, determined by one's African features and/or one's African descent. As constructed, "race" became an indelible accompaniment to the person and marking her and her offspring for generations to come.[3]

The point is not to laud other slave systems but to show that the European slave system was unique in the power and "universality" of the negative stereotypes of Africana peoples that it ingrained. The social realities of slavery and the racist ideology that supported it became mutually reinforcing. Together they once made the assumption of African-American natural suitability to servitude seem as unquestionable as the assumption of women's natural suitability to motherhood.

Property . . . Being

There is a tendency to view American slavery and its brutalizations as anomalies that stood very much apart and in contrast to prevailing American social ideals. But, in fact, slavery reflected various ideologies that were prominent underpinnings of the collective American self-image. The exploitation and abuse of slaves (particularly women) is consistent and continuous with the abuse and exploitation associated with the doctrines of laissez-faire capitalism and Manifest Destiny. All reflect various (European-American male) agendas of sexual, ethnic, economic, and environmental domination carried out against "others."

The African-American slave represents the quintessential colonized person. He or she is stripped of all recognized rights (the hallmarks of human identity), radically displaced in the cultural/historical continuum of (self-directed) human activity, and redefined as the property of others.

The slaves' thorough subjugation was legally articulated by the state-validated bill of sale. This bill of sale also became an unequivocal assertion of the superior worth of European Americans, as southern society increasingly articulated the view that "whites" could not be bought/sold as property (i.e., either as slave or indentured servant). But by presumption all "blacks" could. (African Americans who were not slaves had to be able to prove their nonslave status by producing "freedom papers.") Yet however infatuated southern slave-holding society was with the idea that slaves were merely chattel, they had compelling reasons at least partially to recognize their humanity. The slave had to possess free will, or be inherently self-directing, in order to be held morally (and legally) accountable for her actions. But recognition of a being's natural free will or sophisticated (i.e. humanlike) powers of self-direction are exactly the grounds upon which the individual is said to be endowed with natural rights (Genovese 1974, 29).

Slavery thus emerged as a "partializing" social/legal construction. It clearly divided this society into two polar ranks, those who were true Americans, citizens, and full persons and those "others" who could be the objects of bills of sale. The latter group, consisting mostly of African Americans,[4] was forever suspended in a state of partially recognized humanity. Patricia Williams (1988) first suggested some conceptual link between the enslavement of African-American women and CCM. She coined the very useful term "partializing social constructions" to denote social and conceptual schema that cause us to recognize only those human capacities in a subordinate group that, in the end, facilitate their exploitation. One's attention becomes systematically focused away from the full range of human attributes when regarding these "others."

The dual oppression of the slave woman (and indeed the contemporary woman of color) can be described as twice "partializing" her, by the distorting ideologies of racism and sexism.

The Partialized Woman: Slave, "Mistress," Mother

Until very recently, virtually all studies of slavery have centered upon the experiences of African-American men. Even the rape of slave women was analyzed in terms of its impact upon African-American men, as a mechanism of their further "emasculation" (Davis 1983). The slave woman remains among the most obscured figures of American history. It is difficult to give a generalization of her experiences for another reason. Since there was no real regulation or monitoring of the treatment of slaves, very much of their experience depended upon the mental health and moral leanings of particular slaveholders.

One abuse that virtually all slaves endured was the intervention by slaveholders into their sexual and reproductive lives. Such intervention ranged from the relatively benign practice of granting material rewards to slave women for producing children to the (less common) castrating of "undesirable" males. There is a good deal of controversy over the extent to which slaveholders forced and controlled sexual contact among slaves in order to promote high reproductive rates. There is also some debate about the extent to which slave women were coerced into unwanted sexual contact with masters and overseers. But most contemporary scholars would agree (and the narratives attest) that such practices were widespread, more the unspoken rule rather than the exception of the slaveholders' conduct (see Gutman & Sutch 1978).

The reproductive exploitation of African-American women may have been rooted entirely in economic motives. However, their sexual exploitation resulted from far more complex motivations.

The slaveholding society's gender double standard, divided into a quadruple standard for European-American male slaveholders, not only embraced a different code of conduct toward women than the one they embraced toward men, but also obviously embraced a different code of conduct toward white women than toward black.[5] As Angela Davis notes, in a society that idealized female delicacy and modesty, African-American women were routinely stripped and brutally beaten. These darker members of the "weaker sex" were required to perform the same back-breaking field labor as male slaves in addition to the work of gestation, childbearing, and early child care. And even as they honored asexualized ideals of European-American women, slave owners humiliated and raped African-American women (Davis 1983, 8–10).

Perhaps slaveholders sexually exploited African-American women simply because they could with full impunity, since they and other European-American males controlled southern society. However, at another level of analysis, it can be argued that white male access to black female bodies was (ipso facto) endorsed because it served several important social functions:

> It would be a mistake to regard the institutionalized pattern of rape during slavery as an expression of white men's sexual urges, otherwise stifled by the specter of white womanhood's chastity. That would be far too simplistic an explanation. *Rape* was a weapon of domination, a weapon whose covert role was to extinguish slave women's will to resist, and in the process to demoralize their men (Davis 1983, 24).

African-American women resisted slavery as vigorously as the male slaves. They ran away, "stole" their children, plotted against overseers, and bodily resisted sexual advances, beatings, and assaults upon themselves and loved ones.[6] Rape served then, as it does now, as a way of "putting women in their place," especially women whose assertions of autonomy are particularly offensive to the dominant group. What better way to remind her that her female embodiment is precisely what suits her for subordination? . . . or so the pathologies of sexism prescribe.

For slaveholders, sexual coercion of slave women was a natural extension both of male rights over female bodies and of white property rights over black bodies. While it is a mistake to view the sexual coercion of slave women primarily for its impact on African-American men, it is important to see how it was twice motivated by the view that access to female bodies is a matter of *hierarchical* male rights. As "top men" in the social/political order European-American men categorically claimed the right of sexual access to all women below. And, at the same time, they insisted that sexual access to their "top women" be reserved for themselves. Of course, factors of class intervened making actual spheres of sexual exclusivity relativistic and the category of top subdivisional. For example, a hired (European-American) overseer could openly have sexual contact with a slave woman but not with the plantation owner's daughter.

The social acceptance/tolerance of slavery and the sexual exploitation of slave women further partialized all women by creating a social structure that mirrored patriarchy's proverbial schizophrenic image of woman as "good girl" and "bad girl." The mirror, however, was really a "racialized" lens, clearly delineating which was which. The white woman as top woman became the physically delicate asexual mother/wife, subordinate helpmate, deserving of all the privileges white men, as top men, could bestow upon her. The black woman, on the other hand, as bottom woman became seen as the physically sturdy, lusting and promiscuous, emasculating drudge, deserving of all the exploitations and abuses that white men, as top men, had a right to heap upon her. These particularly negative stereotypes were grafted onto the African-American woman as she was brutally forced into the social role of bottom woman, and they have haunted her ever since. The bottom slave women also provided a buffer zone between European-American women and men. Their powerlessness to retaliate made them ideal for adsorbing much sexual hostility.

Perhaps the beginning of the partializing of mothers and the role of mothering (in Western society) lay in the experience of African-American slave women. The slave mother stood in a very peculiar relationship to her biological children, namely, that of having in no legally recognized relation. Although she was acknowledged to be the biological mother, that relationship carried for her no custodial rights or claims to her children. Since southern law infamously decreed that the child "follow in the condition of the mother," from conception to birth, she carried children that were not legally hers. They were the property of the slaveholder who held her bill of sale. By their own assertion, for African-American women, this was one of the most personally devastating realities of slavery (whether or not pregnancy was the result of a chosen sexual liaison).

Other unpleasant intricacies of the slave mother's position are worth noting. If a slave woman could gain freedom by the time of her child's birth, the child was also free. Freedom achieved at a later date, however, could not undo her child's slave status. This meant that the maternal claims of the biological mother, free or slave, could never contravene "valid" property claims to her child. The subjugation of the African-American woman was the fundamental economic basis of the slaveholder's world. Her enslavement guaranteed the reproduction of the desired product, an enslaved population, since property status passed directly from daughter to daughter. For this reason, a slaveholder often tolerated a slave marrying a free husband, but never a free wife.

The slave woman's life was a grim panorama of dehumanization as she was forced into various partializing roles: slave mother/breeder, bottom woman/mistress, person/property. Fortunately for her sanity, she was not socially defined exclusively by the slaveholders. Slave women by and large functioned within mutually supportive communities of fellow slaves. And here alone her full humanity was acknowledged.

The slaves regarded marital and parental ties, often adoptive, as of the utmost importance. Accepting and fulfilling familial/communal roles was fundamental to their collective redefinition of self as human. As Nathan Huggins (1972) notes, the crucial tutelage of slave children in the "common school in survival without power" had many participants besides biological parents. He also speculates that the fact that slave men had no property (and thus no "problem of legitimacy in inheritance") factored in making them more willing than other men to accept parental responsibility for children of whom they were not biological fathers (Huggins 1977, 169, 172).

The integrity of the bonds forged among women and men within slave communities was probably the single most important factor in slave women's cross-generational survival.[7]

CCM: A "Racialized" Overview

The experience of African-American women in slavery suggests that rather than function as a vehicle for greater autonomy for all woman (through greater economic opportunity), CCM is likely to generate greater repression along gender, race, and class lines. It reinforces the partializing of women into top and bottom women, encourages the continued subjugation of those relegated to the status of bottom women, and negates the full human standing of all women. If this is true, then both the deontological and consequentialist autonomy claims about CCM fail.

The likely impact of CCM upon women of color in particular and people of color in general has been marginalized from the mainstream debate. However, the great irony is that the advancement of CCM, as a social institution widely sanctioned by public opinion and law, only makes sense once we "racialize" our analysis. We must pay attention to the constructed categories of race and class, and the tremendous importance society places on them, before we can even understand the terms of reference used by its proponents (e.g., the shortage of "adoptable" children and "the gift of motherhood"). Better to strip away the euphemisms and critically examine all the ideologies that CCM embodies. Without a complementary interplay of both racism and sexism, it is unlikely that CCM, as such, would have emerged.

"Bottom Woman," Contract Mother

In our discussion of the sexual coercion of slave women we noted the role that sexual access played in defining both female and male hierarchical social positions. Top women (southern European-American women in the case of slavery) were reserved for top men, but top men claimed unspoken rights of sexual dominion over all women below. This particular facet of (European) male domination is not unique to slavery. Indeed, it finds expression in a variety of societal contexts around the world today.[8] In Western societies (and many others) men have long gained status in the gendered hierarchy by having, or being presumed to have, sexual access to more women. Women, conversely, tend to drop in status by becoming (or being presumed to be) more sexually accessible. Now CCM may allow not only sexual access but also reproductive access to become a patriarchal measure of women.

For all the same reasons that the bulk of prostitutes have come from the rank of those socially defined as bottom women, the bulk of contract mothers are likely to come from the same socioeconomic rank. The experiences of African-American women under slavery give stark and grim testament to the degree to which European-American male power-brokers have been able to partialize women and "women's work," along race and class lines. Rather than reflecting an agenda of full emancipation for all women, CCM seems to align far more closely with older schemes of domination.

CCM allows men and privileged women to purchase or rent the gestational capacities of other women in order to produce a genetic heir. These other women are told that their sale of gestational services, unlike the sale of sexual services, is a good thing. Unlike the prostitute, the end the contract mother serves is a pure one. She is bestowing the gift of parenthood, in particular the gift of motherhood, and this is in itself a good thing, or so society tells her. But in fact, the form of motherhood that is good for a particular woman depends upon the (gendered) social status patriarchy assigns her. In CCM bottom women are rewarded for the role of gestating and bearing a child for someone else with more social standing. If motherhood in all that it ordinarily entails were really valued, then social praxis would encourage and reward all women for carrying, giving birth to, and successfully rearing biological and (to the degree possible) adoptive children (Gibson 1988).[9]

With the growth of CCM even the work of mothering may be partialized into roles appropriate for top and bottom women, reinforcing the historically entrenched dichotomy. Indeed, all we need do is add a few modernizations to our old familiar female stereotypes. Top woman remains helpmate/wife (unsuited for taxing physical labor). Now a career woman in her own right but naturally drawn to motherhood, she is fully appropriate for the more refined roles of genetic contributor and rearer of children, real motherhood after all. She is the "superwoman," society's highly visible proof that women need not give up traditional roles in order to succeed in a male world. And what of her invisible counterpart the bottom woman: mistress, menial laborer, and now reproductive drudge? Already viewed as appropriate for the more demanding forms of physical labor, few will oppose her being assigned the "unrefined" work of gestation and childbearing for men and more privileged women who are incapable of or unwilling to do this work.

The top woman's advance through patriarchy (and the maintenance of her new superwoman ideal) will be possible largely because of the society's oppressive reliance upon bottom women. They will continue at the necessary and demanding but devalued "woman's work" of housekeeping, childbearing, wet nursing, physically caring for the infirm, the very young and very old, etc., for society at large. In addition, because they are least insulated (by resources and privileges), these women will continue to bear the brunt of male sexual hostilities.

Most of those who argue for CCM on the grounds of increased practical autonomy for women, in general, fail to pay enough attention to who the contract mothers will be. Historical patterns and underlying ideology virtually assure that they will be those cast as bottom women. These women represent an unacknowledged class that has and continues to be much maligned and much exploited. Whatever the negative consequences of CCM, they will be most directly and thoroughly felt by those most subject to past injustices and least in a position to defend themselves.

Because they suffer the adverse effects of both gender and racial domination, CCM may seem like relatively appealing work, given the options, for many women of color around the world. So, unless other factors intervene, they may end up comprising a significant proportion of the contract mothers.

Let me stave off an initial objection to the likelihood of women of color becoming contract mothers (in significant numbers). This is the objection that racism will make it highly unlikely that wealthy white couples seeking the services of a contract mother will employ a "nonwhite"—particularly a black—woman. There are several responses to such a claim. First, it should be noted that the new reproductive technologies now make it possible for the contract mother to be implanted with an "in vitro" fertilized ovum, taken from another woman. This means she need not make any genetic contribution to the fetus she carries. This option is likely to be preferred, whenever possible (and affordable). It allows the contracting couple, man and woman, to both be progenitors (genetic parents) of the child. At the same time it weakens any claims the contract mother might wish to press upon the child she produces. And, from her point of view, it may seem less emotionally costly to sever parental ties to a child with whom she has only a gestational relationship rather than a genetic one also. Thus technology makes it possible for women of color to produce phenotypically European infants with whom they have no genetic link.

Yet one might still suppose that European and European-American antiblack and antibrown sentiments would be strong enough to prevent widespread acceptance of African-American or Third-World (mostly women of color) contract mothers. Although this may well be the case, we should not assume it nor be reassured by it.

Partializing ideologies of racism and sexism have always held the woman of color/bottom woman as ipso facto unworthy and defiled. Nevertheless, utilization of her physical labor in the more odious and demanding tasks of "women's work" has always been perfectly acceptable, despite the intimacy of contact with those deemed more worthy.

European-American slaveholders did not react in horror as white infants suckled black breasts or as black hands bathed and cared for aging and infirm white bodies. In fact, most probably viewed these things as reflections of the natural order, with blacks performing menial tasks, fulfilling their basic needs, and whites being freed for the high pursuits of life. (Those who dared reflect upon the sexual exploitation of slave women probably came to similar conclusions.)

The services of a contract mother of color might be less objectionable (to European and European-American couples) than imaged, especially if the price is right. In her powerful polemic, *The Mother Machine*, Corea quotes early social architects of CCM who envision making it available to more infertile couples by driving the contract mother's fee down. Their plans entailed the successful exploitation of Third-World women, who could be paid substantially less than their American (and European) counterparts (Corea 1985, 230–231, 276).

The degree to which women of color may be utilized globally as contract mothers is an open question. It depends in part upon the dynamics of racism in various societies, and with respect to various nonwhite groups, with economic considerations undoubtedly playing an important role (given historical patterns of disenfranchisement). It will also depend greatly on the extent to which various populations of women of color are willing to be contracted gestational mothers. Clearly many social/cultural variables will go into that determination (e.g., religious prohibitions, awareness of one's oppression, etc.).

Whatever their numbers, contract mothers who are also women of color will be in a position of extreme vulnerability, despite popular rhetoric about women's autonomy and rights. European-American feminism has a disturbing history of collusion with racism. Its early support of and continuing complacency over the widespread coerced sterilization of African, Hispanic, and Native American women belie any commitment to these women's reproductive interests (Davis 1983, 208–221). Given the historical track record, it would be unwise for contract mothers of color to imagine that mainstream feminism's defense of "women's reproductive autonomy" is likely to defend them against potential exploiters and abusers.

CCM is likely to reinforce existing cross cultural patterns of racial and gender oppression by giving new "reproductive" forms to the same old partialized conceptions of women.

Property . . . Again

Should CCM be viewed as an expression of women's autonomy? To answer this question we need to return to its basic premises. Ostensibly, CCM is a social construction centered around a legal one, the motherhood contract. Valid contracts paradigmatically generate special rights by creating or transferring them. A valid bill of sale for an automobile, for example, gives the buyer "exclusive use" or property rights to the item. Similarly, a valid rental agreement creates for the renter a more limited set of "appropriate use" rights to an item owned by another for a set duration of time. Contracts involving the exchange of specific forms of labor for money become even more complex.

For CCM it is appropriate to ask what special rights valid and binding motherhood contracts would produce. The most conceptually clear answer is blunt in terms of its ideological implications. Minimally, CCM guarantees male rights (i.e., the contract father's) to the reproductive use of female bodies, a reality reflected by the popularized description of CCM as womb renting. While conceptually on target on one level, the description is less than complete, for until and unless society produces artificial ones, wombs necessarily come attached to female persons. There are, moreover, good moral grounds for objecting to social policy that allows and encourages the rental of person-attached wombs.

One might propose that what is being rented is not the person, in any sense, but only the use of a womb, and this really amounts to the sale of a specific form of labor.[10] But the distinction between marketing persons' bodies and the intimate use of persons' bodies cannot be coherently maintained. (The distinction between renting the item verses renting the "use" of the item falters immediately. Consider the example of the car.) As Sara Ann Ketchum argues, allowing parts and capacities of women's bodies to be sold on the open market violates our most fundamental societal presumptions about the proper regard for "full humans" (viz., persons):

> An identity or intimate relationship between persons and their bodies . . . is essential to a minimal moral conceptual scheme. . . . [W]e cannot make sense out of the concept of assault [for example] unless an assault on S's body is ipso facto an assault on S. By the same token treating another person's body as a part of my domain—and among the things that I have a rightful claim to—is, if anything is, a denial that there is a person there (Ketchum 1984, 34–35).

It seems inconsistent to regard another as a person, an autonomous moral equal (i.e., one whose best interests are prima facie as important as mine or any other's) and at the same time regard them as the legal object of another's use. The same Kantian arguments that weigh against allowing slavery (even "voluntary") or a market in body parts weigh against CCM: sale of bodily parts and intimate capacities violates the full human standing of those who in part are being vended. Rather than express basic human autonomy, CCM contradicts it.

In addition, a compelling "slippery-slope" argument can be made. Allowing some to acquire recognized property/use rights over others encourages social practices that fundamentally partialize human beings. However, we define them, in actuality there will be some people whom it is "okay" to treat as objects, as the physical means to satisfy the needs and ends of others, and those whose needs and ends are treated as paramount or good in themselves. Given Western historical propensities for evoking (by word and deed) this dangerous social dichotomy, CCM is one precarious step in an alarming direction that we can ill afford.[11]

Patriarchy has always created ways for men to acquire property claims (or use-rights) over women. Indeed, if there is one experiential commonality of gender oppression that cuts across race/class lines, it may be the threat of being claimed as the property of some man or group of men.

The contract mother like the slave mother stands in a very peculiar relationship to her child. A motherhood contract like a slave bill of sale strips the birth mother's tie to her offspring of any legal meaning. It completely devalues her unique experiences of gestation and childbearing. Unfortunately, in an effort to prove themselves as coolly rational as men, many feminists have joined in effacing the moral and epistemic importance of the gestational mother's bodily experience.

Whatever the particular experience of carrying this child has meant to this woman and her family, she has a moral and legal obligation to keep the CCM contract (see Ketchum 1989, 124). She cannot justify changing her mind by appeal to the fact that she has undergone a personally and metaphysically profound experience that no one could guarantee the effects of beforehand. Rather, she has simply been weak willed, fickle, and overcome by sentimentality, indeed, "just like a woman."

Western philosophy has long claimed that women are not capable of full rationality and therefore full moral agency, because of their female embodiment. The great pity is that by responding to this charge by denying any significance, moral or epistemic, to bodily states—particularly those that men do not share—women devalue themselves. They also participate in the conceptual narrowing of the definition of *human* experience to all and only those experiences that are typical of white males. Fortunately, some feminist theorists, such as Annette Baier (1985) and Sandra Harding (1987), have recognized and challenged biases in the basic premises of traditional moral/social theory that reflect their emphasis upon European male life experiences and cognitive styles.

Presumably, the greatest virtue of the contract mother's work lay in the value of its end, the production of a genetic offspring for others. Unlike the production of a slave, we are told, this is a good thing, despite involving us in some moral "technical" difficulties. To be sure, reproducing children for others is better than reproducing slaves for others. But it may be less laudable than it at first seems.

The experience of African-American women and their children in slavery belies the importance of a genetic link alone, for many slaveholders were genetic fathers of the children they sold as property. So, to some extent, does the abundance of "imperfect" (e.g., handicapped and chronically ill) children who have often been placed in institutional care by their genetic parents. (Of course, many factors come to bear here.) Although the social climate of this country is not the same as it was a century and a half ago, many of its racialized values prevail. CCM undoubtedly serves to counteract the shortage of healthy phenotypically white infants (so-called "adoptable" children). Clearly, the societal desire for them is quite strong. As such, CCM reinforces the ideology that places a higher premium on such individuals and their reproduction.

CCM is a social/legal device that insures that infertile couples who can afford it may obtain a genetic *and racial* heir. The readiness with which our society has swept aside obvious and profound ethical concerns and complex legal difficulties in order to clear its way expresses the underlying ideological commitments all too well. No price is too high for providing the world and those worthy souls who desire them with premium offspring, whose progenitors can be assured to be successful and similarly worthy souls. When one places CCM alongside the rush to adopt Eastern-European children and the U.S. immigration regulations that categorically favor those of European descent, on the one hand, and the deplorable increases in infant mortality rates among African Americans, which is at best the result of gross societal neglect, on the other, a circumspect cynic would conclude that the ultimate operative value is not motherhood, parenthood, or respect for personal autonomy—it is simply the guarantee of the re-production of a ruling caste, as such.

Conclusion

Rather than deal conclusively with the ideological and social links between the slave woman's experience and CCM (and the importance of the legacy of the former for the latter), I have endeavored to provide insights and provoke a greater awareness of the powerful ongoing interplay between forms of racial and sexual domination. The historical experiences and living voices of African-American women and women of color around the world must actively inform the feminist agenda for increased female autonomy and, indeed, any agenda for a more humane social order.

Notes

1. One rare exception is Means (1987), who discusses the reproductive exploitation of slave women in arguing that CCM "imposes a form of bondage upon mother and child" that is prohibited under the Thirteenth Amendment. However, his side assumption that it was probably a common practice of free (African-American) husbands to rent slave women as "surrogates" seems unwarranted.
2. For a closer look at the various circumstances of slave women within the African context see Robertson and Klein (1983).
3. Notice that while the physical and genealogical attributes delineating race are "indelible," the categories themselves ("races") and the social meanings we assign to them are arbitrary. Stephen Jay Gould (1981) offers a highly instructive overview of failed "scientific" attempts to establish physical evidence for European racial distinction/superiority. Also of value is Cornell West's (1985) radical critique of Enlightenment manipulation of the notion of human races.
4. For example, some Chinese-American women and Native Americans were subject to formal enslavement.
5. Hurtado (1989) also discusses the male European "deconstruction" of women along racial lines, from slavery to the present.
6. Hine and Wittenstein (1981) discuss the slave women's forms of sexual and reproductive resistance (e.g., sexual "abstinence," abortion, and infanticide).
7. Slave women's narratives provide a cornucopia of accounts of extraordinary efforts made by individuals and small communities to resist overtly and covertly forced separation and defend loved ones from slaveholder abuse. See, for example, Brent (1973); also from Andrews (1989), especially "The History of Mary Prince, a West Indian Slave" (1831), "The Story of Mattie J. Jackson" (1866), and "From Darkness Cometh the Light, Or Struggles for Freedom" (1891).
8. Women of color seem to be widely relegated to the sociosexual role of mistress/prostitute within Western societies. My experience has been that to be an ostensibly nonwealthy woman of color traveling without male accompaniment is to be presumed to be selling sexual favors in most major European cities.
9. See also Stanworth (1987) for further discussion of social meanings and manipulation of the notion of motherhood.
10. Notice that the contract mother is paid both to perform the work of bodily producing a child *and* to surrender her parental claims to the child, in effect, to the

contracting progenitor(s). Thus analogies with ordinary labor contracts fail, and the baby-selling objection is ushered in.

11. The slippery-slope argument is available even if our Kantian constraint against using the bodies of true persons is seen as arising from social consensus rather than logical or nomological necessity.

Acknowledgments

I would like to thank Mary Gibson for her initial interest, encouragement, and inspiring pedagogy; also Howard McGary, Stephanie Woods, and Gina Bailey for their support of this endeavor and Ruth Lucier for her comments on an earlier version of this paper. Special thanks to Maryellen Tria, Uma Narayan, and Anjana Mebane-Cruz, with whom I shared many "kitchen-table" discussions that helped inspire and sustain this effort.

References

Andrews, William A. 1989. *Six women's slave narratives*. New York: Oxford University Press.

Baier, Annette. 1985. What do women want in a moral theory? *Nous* 29:53–63.

Corea, Gena. 1985. *The mother machine*. New York: Harper & Row.

Davis, Angela. 1983. *Women, race and class*. New York: Vintage Books.

Genovese, Eugene. 1974. *Roll, Jordan, roll: The world the slaves made*. New York: Pantheon Books.

Gibson, Mary. 1992. Contract motherhood: Social practice in social context. *Women & Criminal Justice* 3(1): 55–99.

Gould, Stephen Jay. 1981. *The Mismeasure of man*. New York: Norton.

Gutman, Herbert, and Richard Sutch. 1976. Victorians all? The sexual mores and conduct of slaves and their masters. In *Reckoning with slavery: A critical study in the quantitative history of the American Negro slave*, ed. Paul A. David et al. New York: Oxford University Press.

Harding, Sandra. 1987. The curious coincidence of feminine and African moralities: Challenges for feminist theory. In *Women and moral theory*, ed. Eva Feder Kittay and Diana T. Meyers. Totowa, N.J.: Rowman and Littlefield.

Hine, Darlene and Kate Wittenstein. 1981. Female slave resistance: The economics of sex. In *The black woman cross-culturally*, ed. Filomina Steady. Cambridge, Mass.: Schenkman.

Huggins, Nathan Irvin. 1977. *Black odyssey*. New York: Vintage Books.

Hurtado, Aida. 1989. Relating to privilege: Seduction and rejection in the subordination of white women and women of color. *Signs* 14(4):833–855.

Jacobs, Harriot (Linda Brent). 1973. *Incidents in the life of a slave girl*, ed. L. Maria Child. New York: Harcourt Brace Jovanovich.

Ketchum, Sara Ann. 1984. The moral status of the bodies of persons. *Social Theory and Practice* 10:34–35.

Ketchum, Sara Ann. 1989. Selling babies and selling bodies. *Hypatia 4(3):116–127.*

Lovejoy, Paul E. 1983. *Transformations in slavery*. New York: Cambridge University Press.

Means, Cyril C. 1987. Surrogacy v. The Thirteenth Amendment. *New York Law School Human Rights Annual* 4 (Part 2):445–478.

Robertson, Claire, and Martin Klein. 1983. *Women and slavery in Africa*. Madison: University of Wisconsin Press.

Sistare, Christine. 1988. Reproductive freedom and women's autonomy. *Philosophical Forum* 19(4):227–240.

Stanworth, Michelle. 1987. Reproductive technologies and the deconstruction of motherhood. In *Reproductive technologies: Gender, motherhood and medicine*, ed. Michelle Stanworth. Minneapolis: University of Minnesota Press.

Steady, Filomina Chioma. 1981. The black woman cross-culturally: An overview. *The black woman cross-culturally*, ed. Filomina Chioma Steady. Cambridge, Mass.: Schenkman.

Wallerstein, Immanuel. 1976. The three stages of African involvement in the world-economy. In *The political economy of contemporary Africa*, ed. P.C.W. Gutkind and Immanuel Wallerstein. Beverly Hills, Calif.: Sage.

West, Cornell. 1984. A genealogy of racism: On the underside of modern discourse. *Journal of Black Philosophy* 1(1):18–25.

Williams, Patricia. 1988. On being the object of property. *Signs* 14(1):5–24.

Chapter 26

SOCIAL CONTROL OF SURROGACY IN AUSTRALIA: A FEMINIST PERSPECTIVE

Heather Dietrich

Introduction

In August 1988 the newly established Australian National Bioethics Consultative Committee (NBCC) met for the first time. An advisory committee to the government on "bioethical and associated legal and social issues," it received its references[1] jointly from the welfare and health ministers of the six Australian states and reported directly to the Australian Health Ministers Conference. Its existence was the outcome of public demand for a national body to be set up to consider the social implications of the new reproductive technologies and genetic engineering. In fact, women's formal and informal networks had been central to the mobilization of this demand.

In April 1990 the NBCC released Report 1 on surrogacy. It recommended that surrogacy arrangements be legally permitted and that a formal institutional arrangement, such as a surrogacy licensing board, be created in each of the six states of Australia. Two members (including the author) dissented and argued for prohibition of surrogacy, issuing our minority reports as Appendices A and B.

One year later (March 1991) a joint meeting of the state ministers of welfare and health in Adelaide recommended against our majority report on surrogacy. The ministers recommended, instead, uniform national legislation to make surrogacy arrangements unenforceable by law and to apply criminal sanctions to any third party to a surrogacy agreement. That meeting also endorsed the recommendation of Brian Howe, the federal minister for community service and health, to disband the committee. Thus the surrogacy report was pivotal in the demise of the NBCC.

This chapter analyzes the story of the creation and destruction of the NBCC as a valuable case study for progressive public policy action and for feminist thinking. I describe the polarized ideological positions on surrogacy that developed among the committee members. Principles of liberal individualism, proposed by the dominant male members of the committee, were countered in the dissenting arguments by the principles of social responsibility and equity.

Creation of the NBCC

The NBCC had been set up as a response to growth in public concern over social outcomes that might arise from the new reproductive technologies (NRTs). This concern stemmed from eight years of in vitro fertilization (IVF), from proposals for scientific experimentation on human embryos, and from media coverage of controversial legal cases of surrogacy arrangements.

Issues of family formation and the definition of human life were already on the public policy agenda by 1986 when the Australian chapter of the feminist organization FINRRAGE (Feminist International Network of Resistance to Reproductive and Genetic Engineering) convened the conference Liberation or Loss, Women Act on the New Reproductive Technologies. That conference, in a wide-ranging agenda of critique and proposals for social action, called for a national body to control the NRTs.

Only the previous year (1985), the Family Law Council of Australia had reported on its inquiry into the welfare issues arising from artificial reproduction. Named after the inquiry's chair, this Asche Report had called for a National Council on Reproductive Technology that would

> develop and foster a national approach to reproductive technology and the creation of children and families and to the questions of public policy thus raised (Family Law Council 1985, ix).

This proposal was consistent with the individual inquiries in most states, which also had called for a multidisciplinary body to regulate and control reproductive technology.

Australia has a formal network of public policy advice on women's issues at the state and federal levels. Each state has a women's bureau, an adviser to the government, and an independent council on women's issues. These maintain liaison with the federal Office on the Status of Women (in the prime minister's cabinet) and with the National Women's Consultative Council. Thus there is a highly effective public policy input for women's issues. This lobby was crucial in presenting a formal demand to the government for a national body on reproductive technology.

In 1986, moreover, the New South Wales Women's Advisory Council (NSW-WAC) and Women's Co-ordination formed a working party on the NRTs and in July hosted a National Consultation on reproductive technology. This forum brought together a group with high status and experience from the fields of law, medicine, social science, welfare, ethics, and health. In an intensive workshop this consultation produced a proposal for a national commission on reproductive technology to coordinate and monitor a national reproductive technology program that would include research practice, community education, and information. The proposal was sent to the prime minister and to all state premiers and relevant ministers.

It was also sent to a round-table conference of the National Health and Medical Research Council (NH&MRC), which just at that time was considering reproductive technology among a range of issues. These deliberations by NH&MRC were seen as an attempt to address the concerns being raised about medicine but yet to keep any control body within the medical arena. At that time there was a debate over whether the control and scrutiny of medical research and practice in the NRTs should be exercised by an independent body or left to the medical profession, i.e., to traditional professional practice and ethics measures as they were carried out by the NH&MRC.

The feminist movement and women's bureaus, on the other hand, were clear and active in articulating the necessity, instead, for social control of the NRTs—control to be outside the medical community.

The final component of the public demand for a national body was the Federal Parliament's Senate Inquiry into Human Embryo Experimentation. This inquiry followed a 1985 bill, introduced by Senator Brian Harradine, which had called for a ban on such experimentation. Its charge was to inquire into the necessity and desirability of human embryo experimentation in Australia. Chaired by Senator Michael Tate, the inquiry reported in 1986.

The majority report of the inquiry called for a ban on destructive, nontherapeutic experimentation on human embryos and for establishment of a licensing body to oversee any permitted experimentation. Two women senators dissented from this report and argued for decision-making mechanisms that empowered the mother of any embryo in question. The report also called for a national body to be set up to examine research protocols for compliance with those guidelines.

Thus, by the end of 1987 there was a broad-based but well-focused demand for social control measures with respect to IVF, embryo experimentation, and other NRTs.

The Labor government (socialist) responded by creating the NBCC in 1988. This committee's charge was broader than reproductive technology, but the terminology used and the membership were close to the Asche and NSW-WAC proposals. "It seemed to offer a solid framework for a national consensus" (West 1991).

One word in this new committee's title—bioethics—summarized the social control of technology function. This particular representation turned out to be highly significant in the way in which the committee would interpret its brief to pursue the legal, social welfare, and bioethical issues arising from new developments in reproductive technology and biotechnology.

The NBCC received its references jointly from the six states' welfare and health ministers. It reported directly to the Australian Health Ministers Conference (AHMC), the top health policy body in Australia, composed of all the states' ministers of health plus the federal minister of health. The members of the NBCC had been selected from a list provided by each state health minister; the secretariat recommended from this list to the federal health minister who made the appointments. For the names and affiliations of the members, see Table 26–1.

1990 Report on Surrogacy

The surrogacy report fundamentally split the NBCC on principles and led to widespread criticism of the committee's internal processes, its lack of community consultation, and the poor quality of its decision making. In its surrogacy deliberations the implications of "bioethics" in its title were made clear.

The majority report relied on three main principles: personal autonomy, justice, and common good. These principles, as applied to surrogacy, led to the conclusion that surrogacy arrangements should indeed be allowed and should be legally regulated by some form of state agency. The core ideas expressed were:

- That in a liberal democratic society the individual's right to make autonomous decisions is paramount.
- That state intervention should be minimized in those decisions.
- That the individual's right to make such decisions should be limited only in situations where harm could ensue for others from that individual's actions.

TABLE 26–1

Membership of the National Bioethics Consultative Committee

Member	Occupation & relevant previous experience
Chair: Robyn Layton*	Barrister, South Australia Commissioner, Health Insurance Commission
Rebecca Albury	Lecturer, Sociology, Univ. Wollongong; Member, New South Wales Women's Advisory Council Working Party on Reproductive Technologies
Hilda Bastian	Chair, Consumers Rights Task Force, Consumer Health Forum; Coordinator, Maternity Alliance and Homebirth Australia
Don Chalmers*	Professor & Head, Law Dept., Univ. Tasmania; 1984/1985 Chair, Tasmanian Committee of Inquiry into Artificial Conception & Related Matters
Max Charlesworth*	Professor, Philosophy, Deakin Univ.; Member, Victorian Government's Standing Review & Advisory Committee on Infertility
Sheryl de Lacey	Lecturer, School of Nursing Studies, Sturt College of Advanced Education, S. Australia; Representative of infertile people, S. Aus. Reproductive Technology Council
Heather Dietrich	Lecturer, Science & Technology Policy, Univ. of Technology, Sydney
Regis Mary Dunne*	Sister & Director, Provincial Bioethics Centre, Queensland Catholic Dioceses; Member, Queensland special committee of inquiry re AI & IVF
John Funder*	Deputy Director, Medical Research Centre, Prince Henry's Hospital, Victoria; Endocrinologist
Sandra Gifford*	Lecturer, Dept. Social & Preventive Medicine, Monash Medical School; formerly a senior policy adviser, Victorian Health Department
Charles Gurd	Retired Secretary, Northern Territory Department of Health; President, St. John Ambulance
Colin Honey	Master, Kingswood College, Univ. W. Australia; Member, Ethics Committee, King Edward Memorial Hospital for Women; Member, interim Western Australia Reproductive Technology Council
Con Michael	Professor, Obstetrics & Gynaecology, Univ. W. Australia; Chair, interim Western Australia Reproductive Technology Council

* Appointed in 1991 to serve on the new committee within the National Health and Medical Research Council (NH & MRC).

Justice applied to surrogacy would require that all parties be treated fairly and equally, and that care be taken to ensure that:

> the best interests of the surrogate mother are safeguarded (and also the best interests of her family if there are any) and also that the best interests of the child born as a result of a surrogacy arrangement [and] that any potential for the exploitation of the surrogate mother, the child, or in fact any of the parties, is minimalized (NBCC 1990, 14).

The principle of common good was interpreted as requiring that:

> parent-child relationships be established in an orderly way, that information about parentage be valid and accessible, and that institution of the family should not be subverted (NBCC 1990, 14).

The application of these principles, as interpreted by the majority report, means that regulation and facilitation by a state-run agency would prevent any harm by weeding out persons or situations deemed undesirable. The agency would also ensure fair (but enforceable) contracts of agreement between the parties and would provide a formal mechanism of complaint.

The report concluded that there was no intrinsic harm to individuals, or to society as a whole, in surrogacy arrangements. The risks involved, it considered, are within limits comparable to those in other areas of family formation. The state's duty, therefore, would be to formalize and legitimize surrogacy arrangements through an agency and to ensure the best practice to minimize possible harm.

Much also was made of the abortion debate. The argument was presented that if a woman has the right to choose abortion and to do what she wants with her body, then she must have the right of choice to be a surrogate mother as well.

In summary, the majority report proposed that individuals have the right to form a family in any way they want, unless there be harm to others. The adoption analogy was considered invalid, and the view was expressed that little evidence from existing surrogacy arrangements "proves" that they are intrinsically harmful. Consequently, surrogacy arrangements should be allowed but be regulated by the state.

These conclusions rest heavily on Mill's principle of personal autonomy with its championing of the "rights" of individuals to pursue their own "happiness" with minimal interference. The comparison made with the adoption experience (as evidence of harm to the relinquishing mother or to the child who is born) was dismissed as insufficient to demonstrate risk of harm.

In bioethics, as in economics, an emphasis on liberal individual rights is a conservative ideology. It neither recognizes nor includes the differentials of power between people in the society to which it is applied. The poor and the rich stand equal in the analysis. Bioethics as a discipline is currently dominated by this liberal, individualistic analysis. This framework, however, proved to be inadequate in the NBCC discussions, since issues of social equity clearly affect the outcomes of surrogate acts.

I suggest that bioethics in this form is inadequate as a discipline to apply to social control agencies looking at the NRTs. In the final section of this essay

I shall show that the alternative perspective of a feminist ethics may be a richer framework.

Although the application of the three principles in the NBCC majority report was fairly straightforward in its discussion and conclusions, the arguments on the social desirability of surrogacy were more confused. Both within the committee and in the final report, there was extensive and incoherent discussion of the "morality" and the "desirability" of surrogacy and of the necessity of formalizing and controlling it rather than letting it go underground. Some members who thought that surrogacy was both immoral and undesirable still thought it should be legalized in order to control it. Others thought it not immoral but undesirable. No majority report member considered it totally desirable, but some advocated a neutral position: "It is not my place or business to decide on the desirability of surrogacy arrangements undertaken by other people." All concluded that control was necessary. The committee members envisioned that the state agency, which would include a component of counseling for participants, would minimize harm and maximize justice.

There is a clear separation here between abstract intellectual principles and moral, emotional desires or liking. That is to say, the head and the heart are divided. This polarization was crucial in the conclusions reached on surrogacy. Significantly, in the gender-equal membership, arguments that began "surrogacy does not seem or feel right" could not hold their own against propositions based on intellectual principles attributed to prominent philosophers and steeped in historical references.

Such historical, philosophical, and legal arguments were put forward predominantly by high-status male members of the committee. Many of the women—all except the chair were of lower status than the male members—struggled noticeably to articulate the "heart" perspective, but they ultimately bowed to the "principles" in reaching agreement on prosurrogacy legislation.

What was lost between the head and the heart poles was the notion of the "social"—the social context and social construction of the surrogacy arrangements being considered. Without this perspective it was impossible to consider factors of power and equity that would affect the outcomes of surrogate births. The social-construction arguments came to be championed by the two dissenters, Sister Regis Dunne and myself, and finally were annexed, in the committee discussion, to dissenting reports.

Sister Regis Dunne's Dissenting Opinion

The two dissenting opinions raised notions of the power, status, and welfare imbalances between men and women as factors to be considered in predicting surrogacy outcomes. These opinions projected a strong possibility of harm to the individuals involved and to society at large. They also cited evidence from adoption (which, in fact, is analogous) and from current surrogacy arrangements, which pointed to the likelihood of harm. The dissenters proposed that principles of social responsibility, based on visions of collectivity, are the best ones to apply to the complex issues of family formation. These principles are the most applicable because they are based on the view of our social order as a dynamic collective structure of interacting lives making a whole, rather than a sum, of individuals with individual interests.

Sister Dunne viewed the principle of personal autonomy, as it was applied in the majority report, as unconvincing:

> . . . this principle pays small regard to the common interest, is unevenly applied to the woman who bears the child, and mainly supports the interests of the commissioning couple (NBCC 1990, Appendix A, 47).

Sister Dunne regarded surrogate motherhood as an act of alienation requiring the woman to distance herself in the deeply intimate act of bearing a child and to deny her own maternity. Thus the experience of pregnancy is denied, and motherhood is defined only in terms of biological/genetic determinants and of possession in law. The child is treated in many respects as a commodity, especially in the cases of commercial surrogacy. Sister Dunne drew attention to the fact that surrogacy was being discussed as a medical treatment, and she rejected the validity of this representation. Following from this reasoning, she rejected the application of a strict and individualistic ethic of health care without regard to pertinent common interest concerns, and thus she questioned the rightness of surrogacy. She questioned also the interpretation of justice and freedom, as those words were used in the majority report:

> The ultimate irony of surrogacy is that, while it may provide some women with their heart's desire, it can only do this by reducing others to their biological function, and putting them socially at risk in their families and places of living. The practice of surrogacy contains the seeds of injustice for women and children. If justice is diminished in a democratic society, so also is freedom (NBCC, 1990, Appendix A, 54).

A Feminist Analysis[2]

In my dissenting view I placed surrogacy in its social context and asked what would be the likely outcomes for most women, given the social structure of inequality between men and women:

> We live in an unequal society, where there is unequal access to resources, information, and life opportunities. Women as a group still occupy the

> lower rungs of income statistics and skill status. Those who are especially disadvantaged may be susceptible to use any capacity they have to survive materially. This could mean bearing a child in a surrogacy arrangement in order to receive some material or social advantage. Even if a direct exchange of money is disallowed by law, if surrogacy arrangements are made legal there is every likelihood that ways will be found to 'repay' the act of relinquishing a child (NBCC, Appendix B, 57).

I placed surrogacy in its medical and technological context and therefore viewed it as a further medicalization of reproduction. In this process it may be seen as an extension of IVF, in that it denies:

> . . . the vital role played by the mother in the psychological and social structuring of new human life as well as in the physical creation of it (NBCC 1990, Appendix B, 58).

I cited the adoption experience as demonstrating that we form a secure sense of personal and social identity through knowledge of, and continuity with, our birth into a family. A family is a social construct of time, place, and culture. The mother places us in this family and gives us this "place" in the world. Denial of origins and of the truth of this important social construct has led to confusion and alienation in adoption. I suggested that the current discussion on surrogacy is making the same mistakes as (or worse ones than) the early adoption practice. Surrogacy defines family and motherhood in terms of ownership law and ignores the important emotional and social linkages. The social and the biological thus are separated, whereupon it is all too easy to lose the social by narrowly defining the borders of the argument. In my dissent I viewed the justifications for surrogacy as deeply exploitative of women and as consistent with the use of motherhood ideology as a disempowering act:

> The ideology of motherhood has served to justify the exploitation of the real work and gift of mothering to the world. Women have come to be praised and not rewarded for their mothering. They have been expected to fulfill the complex tasks of mothering at the cost of economic dependency on a husband, social isolation, and low status. Deeply ingrained in our society is the notion of the self-sacrificing and all-giving mother. Sacrifice in this case of even the fulfilment and pleasure of the child in relationship to the mother (NBCC 1990, Appendix B, 58).

In considering the appropriate principles to apply to surrogacy arrangements, I suggested in my dissent that the biological and the social be considered together. Bearing a child needs to be seen as a social, as well as an individual, act. In fact, the issue needs to be seen as one of family formation, not of biological reproduction. We are discussing the creation of lives and social relationships that go beyond the gestational time of nine months and the physical boundaries of birth.

I proposed that the appropriate analysis from which to draw was one which "recognizes the political, economic, and social reality that we exist in a system of interconnecting lives, responsibilities, and actions" (NBCC 1990, Appendix B, 60).

I rejected individualistic analysis:

> The concept of society as made up of autonomous, freely acting individual units which add up to a whole is no longer a useful one. Society is a system of individuals. We cannot polish and protect the rights and controls of individuals to act thereby keeping the whole society working well and in the best interests of all. Firstly, every individual affects others in the exercising of these rights. Secondly, individuals are not equal in power, status and material position in society. This differently affects their ability to act (NBCC 1990, Appendix B, 60).

I urged policy recommendations that are progressive and based on notions of social responsibility:

> [This] means consideration must be given to analysing which parties have most and least power. Public policy can then determine where the duty of maximum care lies .... [Then] surrogacy is not viewed from the perspective of competing interests. The question is, with respect to families, where does the maximum duty of care reside? ... The duty of care at the individual level must be to the person born ... they have least power ... and are at most risk of harm. At the social level, the duty of care lies with maximising humane and equitable family and social relations (NBCC 1990, Appendix B, 61).

The contrast between principles of personal autonomy and social responsibility is most sharply drawn in discussions on abortion and its comparison with surrogacy. The majority report defined abortion as an issue of choice and of individual control of a woman's body: the "right to choose." This, of course, is the language of the feminist abortion campaign. In my report I offered a contrasting view:

> [T]his emphasis on rights and control is a partial picture of abortion. A woman deciding on an abortion is taking an individual and socially responsible act in the light of information she has about the likely personal and social future of herself and the child if born. It is a responsible act with respect to her individual life and her role and function as a mother ... least harm is done in abortion by not creating a stressed family, a damaged child, or an unwanted life.... Abortion is a decision taken about family formation which includes elements of social responsibility and least harm done (NBCC 1990, Appendix B, 62).

The surrogacy issue as discussed by the NBCC highlights the urgent need for a thorough alternative to individualistic notions of social structure and therefore for alternative principles appropriate for the radical developments occurring in the NRTs and genetic engineering. I suggest that the arguments taken from Mill and other liberal theorists are also "masculinist," since they assume that social relations consist of equally powerful individuals who are inherently in competition for needs to be met. This competition is somehow supposed to be balanced by the social or economic market. (Remember, Mill was a founding father of laissez-faire capitalist economic theory.) The role of law and government, then, is supposed to be to remove barriers to the market or to balance injustice. This picture is masculinist because it assumes an existential relationship of human life, with separation as the bottom line of the human state. I propose that women's experience and feminist theory both view our relationship to each other and to the environment in terms of connection—not of separation.

In a powerful analysis, feminist legal theorist Robin West has characterized the difference of perspective between the masculinist and the feminist world views as the separation thesis versus the connection thesis. The separation thesis claims:

> A human being, whatever else he is, is physically separate from all other human beings. I am one human being and you are another and that distinction between you and me is central to the phrase "human being." Individuals are . . . distinct and not essentially connected with one another (West 1988, 1).

West describes how this assumption underlies both liberal and radical theory. By contrast, feminist theory proposes the following:

> [T]he claim that we are individuals "first" and the claim that what separates us is epistemologically and morally prior to what connects us—while "trivially true" of men are patently untrue of women. Women are not essentially, necessarily, inevitably, invariably, always, and forever separate from other human beings: women are . . . "connected" to another human life when pregnant. . . . [W]omen are in some sense "connected" to life and to other human beings during [several] recurrent and critical material experiences: heterosexual penetration, which may lead to pregnancy; . . . menstruation, which represents the potential for pregnancy; and the post-pregnancy experience of breast feeding. Indeed, perhaps the central insight of feminist theory of the last decade has been that women are "essentially connected," not "essentially separate," from the rest of human life . . . (West 1988, 2–3).

In considering the issues arising from the NRTs, we must develop an alternative vision and an alternative set of principles to the liberal-masculinist ones. The connection thesis offers a progressive notion of what it is to be human. The economic, social, and ecological crises that we face at the end of the twentieth century make it clear that the old notions of competition, win-lose, power over, etc., have run their course of usefulness. A model is needed of human life—biological and social—that is based on systemic understanding and connectedness. This seems most obvious when we try to develop public policy and law in response to these radical ways of reproducing ourselves. How can the "right" of the child in the womb be separated from the "right" of its mother?

> Feminists have . . . seen the shortcomings of abstract individualism in that the abstract individual looked so little like a woman or a child. There is something distinctly hairy-chested about Hobbes's state of nature, about the social contract, about revealed preference theory, about the conception of equality that accords to every rational individual equal rights regardless of gender, economic class, race or age. As Virginia Held remarks, "It stretches credulity even further than most philosophers can tolerate to imagine babies as little rational calculators contracting with their mothers for care (Held 1987,120)" (Nelson & Nelson 1989, 89).

With rights come responsibilities. If one has the right to life or procreation, there is a concomitant responsibility for conditions of living and procreation. Feminist ethics is creating principled arguments that can support such new "connection thesis" attitudes to developing public policy.

Carol Gilligan, in her empirical study comparing moral development and decision making between men and women, describes women as having a "care perspective." This contrasts with the men's moral language being based on "autonomy, rights, and justice." There are, of course, dangers of emphasizing care and the perspectives gained from childbearing and nurturing because this may perpetuate the social ghetto of women and buy into the essentialist arguments on women's inherently passive and self-sacrificing nature. Vigilance is needed. However, I believe the feminist alternative vision is more powerful and challenging than this. Feminist ethics is also concerned with the social and historical context in which events are happening. As interpreted by Anne Donchin, Hilary Rose (1987, 158) proposes an integration between essentialist and social constructivist arguments:

> [S]he [Hilary Rose] urges the development of an alternative feminist epistemology that takes into account both the material reality of social relations and the material reality of nature (of which our bodily selves are a part). She argues that only this kind of epistemology has the capacity to embrace both the commonality and diversity of women's experiences and provide the standpoint needed to deal effectively with the issues raised for women by the new reproductive technologies (Donchin 1989, 148).

Lessons from the NBCC

Although feminist ethics would see no separation between the "health" and "welfare" aspects of the surrogacy issue, the NBCC majority report in applying classical bioethics did just this. The ethical considerations, which the report took to be its main concern, excluded any consideration of class, gender, or race. Equity was not interpreted in the current socioeconomic context, but it was taken to mean individual rights and how to promote them. The fact that the surrogacy issue caused the demise of the NBCC clearly demonstrated its failure to integrate the social with the ethical. The committee will be merged with the medical ethics committee of the NH&MRC and the welfare ministers will be given back their references from the NBCC portfolio (West 1991). Only a few of the existing members, however, will be transferred to the new committee. The directive from the minister for welfare and health was for the welfare issues to be "withdrawn and the (welfare ministers) consider alternative methods of progressing these issues." The "social" proved too difficult for the NBCC, and so the social control of reproductive technology has been lost.

This failure makes it all the more imperative that feminist thinking and social action continue and that feminists expand their development of alternative social visions, ethical structures, and public policy programs. The next time that a gender-balanced committee considers an issue such as surrogacy or embryo experimentation it would be good to have thorough, documented, clear sets of feminist and progressive arguments. These would include developed notions of social responsibility, social equity, and the ethic of care. Elite and removed professional committees may be able to separate medical and health science from the welfare and the social, but the human population and the planet clearly cannot afford this luxury.

The frontier in modern science lies in the biological sciences: most prominent are the programs of the NRTs, genetic engineering, and the mapping of the human genome. "Big" science is pushing for money and human effort to be directed into these endeavors. All these efforts are occurring in the context of increased globalization of human societies and their social and environmental problems. These radical developments in the control of human reproduction pose challenges for the notion of what is acceptable to do with human life, in fact, what *is* human life. Clearly, an integrated science and social welfare perspective is needed. I am hopeful that positive creative thinking from feminism can provide such a policy framework. The critique is important but so is the vision.

Notes

1. "References" is the term used in Australia for the duties assigned to the committee, the issues they were to discuss.
2. For additional Australian feminist critiques of the NBCC surrogacy report, especially on use of language, see Ewing 1990 and Rowland 1990.

References

Donchin, Anne. 1989. The growing feminist debate over the new reproductive technologies. *Hypatia* 4(3):136–149.

Ewing, Christine. 1990. Draft report on surrogacy issued by the Australian National Bioethics Consultative Committee—The debate on surrogacy in Australia continues. *Issues in Reproductive and Genetic Engineering: Journal of International Feminist Analysis* 3(2):143–146.

Family Law Council. 1985. *Creating children—A uniform approach to the law and practice of reproductive technology in Australia.* Canberra: Australian Government Publishing Service.

Held, Virginia. 1987. Non-contractual society: A feminist view. *Canadian Journal of Philosophy* 13(Suppl.):111–137.

National Bioethics Consultative Committee (NBCC). 1990. *Surrogacy: Report 1.* April. Canberra: Australian Government Publishing Service.

Nelson, Hilde Lindemann, and James Lindemann Nelson. 1989. Cutting motherhood in two: Some suspicions concerning surrogacy. *Hypatia* 4(3):85–94.

Rose, Hilary. 1987. Victorian values in the test-tube: The politics of reproductive science and technology. In *Reproductive technologies: Gender, motherhood and medicine*, ed. Michelle Stanworth. Minneapolis: University of Minnesota Press.

Rowland, Robyn. 1990. Response to the draft report of the National Bioethics Consultative Committee (NBCC), *Surrogacy*. *Issues in Reproductive and Genetic Engineering: Journal of International Feminist Analysis* 3(2):147–157.

West, Robin. 1988. Jurisprudence and gender. *University of Chicago Law Review* 55(1):1–72.

West, Rosemary. 1991. IVF birth: A question of ethics. *Age* 11 April:13.

Chapter 27

CONTRACT PREGNANCY: AN ANNOTATED BIBLIOGRAPHY

Helen Bequaert Holmes

In the last decade hundreds of articles have appeared on "surrogate" motherhood, the bulk of them in newspapers, news magazines, and especially law review journals, many written before the "hard" cases of Stiver, Baby M, Muñoz, and *Calvert v. Johnson.* This bibliography includes only a few selected entries from those three sources. Rather it concentrates on English-language books and articles that discuss ethical, social, and feminist issues. Not intended to be inclusive, it focuses primarily on pieces written after 1986.

The present bibliography comprises five sections: I, authored books; II, edited books; III, special issues of journals or sections in journals; IV, papers, essays, and articles; and V, bibliographies and resource guides. The largest section, IV, gives exact citations to articles in the anthologies listed in II and III. To find citations to the popular press and legal literature, use the bibliographies in Section V and the papers by Radin and Rothenburg in Section IV.

I. Authored Books

This section lists books written by one author or by a team of authors. Two committee reports are included. Some books give personal accounts of a surrogate's experience; most of the others include topics other than surrogacy.

Books with only brief discussions of surrogacy have not been listed. Several of these books have been reviewed a number of times. To find these reviews, look under Surrogacy in *Book Reviews Index, Social Science Citations Index,* or *Women Studies Abstracts.*

Adair, Patricia. 1987. *A surrogate mother's story.* Tallahassee, Fla.: Loiry Publishing House. 140 pp.

Surrogate Adair describes her experience in detail with a positive glow, including how she defied the broker in order to meet the commissioning couple and the dishonest overcharges to that couple.

Andrews, Lori B. 1985. *New conceptions: A consumer's guide to the newest infertility treatments, including in vitro fertilization, artificial insemination, and surrogate motherhood.* New York: Ballantine. 230 pp.

The section on surrogacy comprises 40 pages of "how to" and "should you" advice, with specific examples from real cases.

Andrews, Lori B. 1989. *Between strangers: Surrogate mothers, expectant fathers & brave new babies.* New York: Harper & Row. 288 pp.

In a personal journalistic style, Andrews describes the development of commercial surrogacy and the drama of the Muñoz and Baby M cases and then discusses proposed legislation. Upbeat, she claims true feminists are pro-IVF.

Birke, Lynda, Susan Himmelweit, and Gail Vines. 1990. *Tomorrow's child: Reproductive technologies in the 90s.* London: Virago. 340 pp.

In the little space on surrogacy, this book describes generally hostile "official attitudes" toward the practice; argues that this distaste arises from surrogacy's overstepping of boundaries between public and private; proposes that a responsible public agency make surrogacy arrangements, *without* any contracts.

Blank, Robert H. 1990. *Regulating reproduction.* New York: Columbia University Press. 280 pp.

This brief, scattered, discussion of surrogacy describes controversies, especially over payment; anticipates that the practice may lead to pressure for responsible behavior during any pregnancy; and describes legal statutes.

Chesler, Phyllis. 1988. *Sacred bond: The legacy of Baby M.* New York: Times Books. 212 pp. To find excerpts, see Chesler in Section IV.

Polemic and lively, strongly against surrogacy.

Corea, Gena. 1985. *The mother machine: Reproductive technologies from artificial insemination to artificial wombs.* New York: Harper & Row. 374 pp. Chap. 11: "Happy breeder woman," on surrogacy.

Strongly antisurrogacy. Corea includes analysis of surrogate firms, fragments of case studies. The free-will argument is debunked. A classic.

Cotton, Kim, and Denise Winn. 1985. *Baby Cotton: For love and money.* London: Dorling Kindersley. 189 pp.

This is Kim's personal narrative as first British surrogate with the American Surrogate Parenting Agency, including the media attention forced on her, the split in her family, and protective custody of the baby girl before her release to the commissioning parents.

Field, Martha. 1988. *Surrogate motherhood: The legal and human issues.* Cambridge: Harvard University Press. 224 pp. (2nd ed. 1990).

This even-handed, competent explication of legal issues for the lay reader presents arguments for a spectrum of positions; it advocates unenforceable surrogacy contracts, with mothers retaining custody. Excellent bibliography.

Freedman, Warren. 1991. *Legal issues in biotechnology and human reproduction: Artificial conception and modern genetics.* Westport, Conn.: Quorum Books. 229 pp. Chap. 5: "Baby selling and surrogate motherhood."

There are excerpts from state court decisions and discussion of contract provisions and litigation. The volume is valuable for its extensive citations to the legal literature. Chapter 10 has the text of the proposed Uniform Surrogate Parenthood Act.

Humphrey, Michael and Heather. 1988. *Families with a difference—Varieties of surrogate parenthood.* London and New York: Routledge, Chapman and Hall. 225 pp.

Defining a surrogate family as one without a complete genetic linkage between parents and children, the authors propose eliminating pitfalls by preventive action. Five pages on contract pregnancy.

Kane, Elizabeth. 1988. *Birth mother: America's first legal surrogate mother tells the story of her change of heart.* San Diego: Harcourt Brace Jovanovich. 320 pp.

This is the day-to-day story of an early advocate's insistence on being a surrogate, her pregnancy, her experiences with the media, her change of mind, and some consequences for her other children.

Keane, Noel P., and Dennis L. Breo. 1981. *The surrogate mother*. New York: Everest House.

A pioneer entrepreneur of surrogacy describes many cases, some quite bizarre. The issues involved are analyzed. A classic.

Kirkman, Maggie and Linda. 1988. *My sister's child: Maggie and Linda Kirkman—Their own story*. Ringwood, Australia: Penguin Books. 351 pp.

In diary form, with alternating chapters by the two sisters, this tale's position is that their good experience with surrogacy should provide an example for others—yet it depicts Linda's misery while undergoing IVF and in the pregnancy and Maggie's frantic search for ways to adopt baby Alice.

Landau, Elaine. 1988. *Surrogate Mothers*. New York: Franklin Watts. 144 pp.

For grades 7 and up, there are the usual pro and con arguments. Uninspired.

Lasker, Judith N., and Susan Borg. 1987. *In Search of Parenthood*. Boston: Beacon Press. 232 pp. Chap. 5: "Surrogate motherhood."

The authors give a detailed case study of the positive experience of Sarah with Alex and Lisa (pseudonyms); analyze policy differences in screening couples and surrogates at three programs.

National Bioethics Consultative Committee (NBCC). 1990. *Surrogacy: Report 1*. Commonwealth of Australia.

The report examines principles and options; recommends to Australian health ministers that surrogacy be legally permitted and controlled by government bodies.

New York State Task Force on Life and the Law. 1988. *Surrogate parenting: Analysis and recommendations for public policy*. Albany, N.Y. Reprinted in Appendix E of Gostin, Section II.

Society should discourage surrogate parenting; legislation should declare contracts void and bar surrogate brokers from operating in New York State.

Overall, Christine. 1987. *Ethics and human reproduction: A feminist analysis*. Boston: Allen Unwin. 245 pp. Chap. 6: "Surrogate motherhood."

Overall compares free-market and prostitution models of surrogacy; she comments on various policy recommendations. "Surrogate motherhood [should not] be fostered or benignly tolerated."

Overvold, Amy Z. 1988. *Surrogate parenting*. New York: Pharos. 223 pp.

Basically prosurrogacy. Overvold presents a detailed narrative of the McRobbie family's experiences hiring a surrogate; how-to-do it information; lists of clinics.

Robbins, Sara. 1990. *Baby M case. A collection of the complete trial transcripts*. Buffalo: William S. Hein.

This set of six volumes costs $450.

Rothman, Barbara Katz. 1989. *Recreating motherhood: Ideology and technology in a patriarchal society*. New York: Norton. 282 pp.

The story of Baby M is told two myths: feminism and patriarchy. One chapter gives antisurrogacy arguments regarding policy and values.

Schwartz, Lita Linzer. 1991. *Alternatives to infertility: Is surrogacy the answer?* Frontiers in Couples and Family Therapy Series No. 4. New York: Brunner/Mazel. 200 pp.

This book aims to alert mental health professionals to problems in surrogacy situations. Topics covered include mental health issues in the Baby M case, surrogacy "pro" and "con" arguments, psychosocial and legal issues, and the draft ABA Model Surrogacy Act. The answer to the title's question is "not yet."

Shalev, Carmel. 1989. *Birth power: The case for surrogacy*. New Haven: Yale University Press. 201 pp.

More space is devoted to adoption and IVF than to surrogacy. Shalev is against IVF, yet prosurrogacy, arguing for women's choice and the duty to keep contractual obligations.

Shannon, Thomas A. 1988. *Surrogate motherhood: The ethics of using human beings*. New York: Crossroads. 212 pp.

This is a strong con argument without polemics that is well done. Recommended.

Sloan, Irving. J. 1988. *The law of adoption and surrogate parenting*. Legal Almanac Series: No. 3. Dobbs Ferry, N.Y.: Oceana Publications. 148 pp.

Chapter 6 discusses the (probably slight) impact of the Baby M case on developing law of surrogate parenting; Appendix B is a surrogate contract agreement.

U.S. Congress, Office of Technology Assessment. 1988. *Infertility: Medical and social choices*. Washington, D.C.: U.S. Government Printing Office. 403 pp. Chap. 14: "Legal considerations: Surrogate motherhood." Appendix G: "OTA survey of surrogate mother matching services."

Results of the survey are given, e.g., who hires, characteristics of surrogates, involvement of physicians and attorneys, typical contract provisions. Five different models of state policy are identified.

Whitehead, Mary Beth [with Loretta Schwartz-Nobel]. 1989. *A mother's story. The truth about the Baby M case*. New York: St. Martin's. 224 pp.

Detailed narrative: "... if [Baby M] grows up and finds out that you *sold* her, she will hate you." "I learned in the most painful way that the rental of a women's body ... is wrong."

II. Edited Collections

This section lists anthologies that deal exclusively with surrogacy as well as ones that include related topics but contain at least three articles on surrogacy. For citations and annotations of each paper included, see Section IV.

Bartels, Dianne M., Reinhard Priester, Dorothy E. Vawter, and Arthur L. Caplan, eds. 1990. *Beyond Baby M: Ethical issues in new reproductive techniques*. Clifton, N.J.: Humana Press. 288 pp.

These essays on moral assessments of assisted reproduction include seven on surrogacy and an appendix with the Baby M contract and excerpts from the Vatican "Instruction on respect for human life."

Baruch, Elaine Hoffman, Amadeo F. D'Adamo, Jr., and Joni Seager, eds. 1988. *Embryos, ethics and women's rights: Exploring the new reproductive technologies*. New York: Harrington Park Press. 259 pp. From a special issue of *Women & Health* 13(1/2), 1987.

Amidst contributions on IVF and prenatal diagnosis, surrogacy is discussed in competent pieces by Schuker, Lifton, and Charo.

Cohen, Sherrill, and Nadine Taub, eds. 1989. *Reproductive laws for the 1990s*. Clifton, N.J.: Humana Press. 472 pp.

The outcome of a project from Rutgers University Law School and its Institute for Research on Women, this book deals mostly with topics such as time limits on abortion, prenatal screening, and hazards in the workplace. Surrogacy is covered in a strong position paper by Andrews, a rebuttal by Chavkin et al., and a commentary by Davis.

Gostin, Larry, ed. 1990. *Surrogate motherhood: Politics and privacy*. Bloomington: Indiana University Press. 366 pp. From a special issue of *Law, Medicine, and Health Care* 16(1/2), 1988.

This anthology, entirely on surrogacy, contains 16 essays with positions running the gamut from strong pro to strong anti.

Holmes, Helen Bequaert, and Laura M. Purdy, eds. 1992. *Feminist perspectives in medical ethics*. Bloomington: Indiana University Press. 308 pp. From two special issues of *Hypatia: A Journal of Feminist Philosophy* 4(2) and 4(3), 1989.

The section on surrogacy has antisurrogacy essays by the Nelsons, Oliver, and Ketchum and a prosurrogacy one by Malm.

Klein, Renate, ed. 1989. *Infertility: Women speak out about their experiences of reproductive medicine*. London: Pandora Press. 328 pp. Part Three: "Exploiting fertile women in the name of infertility."

Statements from five surrogate mothers describe their extremely negative experiences.

McCuen, Gary E., ed. 1990. *Hi-tech babies: Alternative reproductive technologies*. Hudson, Wis.: McCuen. 160 pp. Chap. 4: "Surrogate mothers."

From the "Ideas in Conflict" series of readings for schools on political, social, and moral issues. This volume includes readings on surrogacy by Andrews, Reimer, Corea, and Balboni, as well as points to consider and questions to stimulate classroom discussions.

Quebec Council on the Status of Women, ed. 1988. *Sortir la maternité du laboratoire* (Departure of motherhood from the laboratory). Montreal: Government of Quebec. 423 pp.

In these proceedings of a 1987 bilingual conference on the new reproductive technologies, about two-fifths of the papers are in English. On the topic of surrogacy are pieces by Corea (opening session) and Raymond (closing session) and two from the surrogacy workshop (Utérus recherché) by Dickens and Eichler.

Richardson, Herbert, ed. 1987. *On the problem of surrogate parenthood: Analyzing the Baby "M" case*. Lewiston, N.Y.: Mellen. 135 pp.

These 10 essays were assembled within a month after the initial decision by Judge Sorkow in the Baby M case.

Whiteford, Linda M., and Marilyn L. Poland, eds. 1989. *New approaches to human reproduction: Social and ethical dimensions*. Boulder, Col.: Westview Press. 224 pp.

Part Three, "Ethical implications of family formation by surrogacy," contains six papers, four of which (Whiteford, Wolfram, and two by Garcia) discuss surrogacy.

III. Special Issues or Sections of Journals

Listed here alphabetically by journal name, these collections are either entire special issues or clusters of at least three papers. Papers dated after 1986 are cited completely and annotated in Section IV, except for those in legal journals.

Against the Current. Vol. 2, September-October issue (1987). Essays by Reagan, Swerdlow, and Wrigley.

Bioethics. Vol. 3 No. 1 (1989). Essays by Dodds and Jones and by Purdy; then responses of these authors to each other.

Biomedical Ethics Reviews—1983. Includes discussions of surrogacy by Benditti and by Newton. Not annotated in Section IV.

Family Law Quarterly. Vol. 22, No. 119 (1988). "Special issue on surrogacy." Draft American Bar Association Model Surrogacy Act; five articles or comments, plus a bibliography. See Peritore in Section V.

Georgetown Law Journal. Vol. 76, No. 5 (June 1986). "Colloquy: *In re Baby M*." Seven essays. Not annotated in Section IV.

Harvard Journal of Law and Public Policy. Vol. 13 (Winter 1990). "Property: The founding, the welfare state and beyond." The Eighth National Federalist Society Symposium on Law and Public Policy. Four essays.

Hypatia: A Journal of Feminist Philosophy. Vol. 4, No. 3 (1989). Four essays. Published also in the book *Feminist perspectives on medical ethics*. See Holmes and Purdy in Section II.

Law, Medicine & Health Care. Vol. 12, No. 3 (June 1984). Papers by Furrow, Gersz, and Holder. Not annotated in Section IV.

Law, Medicine & Health Care. Vol. 18, No. 1/2 (Spring/Summer 1988). Forum on "Surrogate motherhood: Politics and privacy." Also published as a book, same title. See Gostin in Section II.

Ms. Vol. 1, No. 6 (May/June 1991). Special Report "Women as wombs." Articles by Raymond, Snitow, Rowland, Williams, and Buttenwieser. Not cited in Section IV because all pieces devote more space to other reproductive technologies and other forms of traffic in women.

New York Law School Human Rights Annual. Vol. IV Part 2 (Spring 1987). "Symposium: Surrogate mothering." Five essays by Field, Means, Shifman, Taylor, and Wolf. Not annotated in Section IV.

Nova Law Review. Vol. 13 (Spring 1989). Four articles, including ones by Rothman and Keane. Not annotated in Section IV.

Politics and the Life Sciences. Vol. 8, No. 2 (February 1990). "The politics of surrogacy contracts." Four papers by Hill, Merrick, Shevory, and Woliver with five commentaries on them by Bonnicksen, Field, Okin, Richard, and Shanley.

Seton Hall Law Review. Vol. 18 (Fall 1988). "Baby M and its aftermath." Nine papers, not annotated in Section IV.

Society. Vol. 25, No. 3 (March/April 1988). Section: "Controversies: Surrogate motherhood." A position paper by Neuhaus plus reactions by Heyl, Morris, Rothman, and Zelizer.

Women & Health. Vol. 13, , No. 1/2 (1987). Also published as the book *Embryos, ethics, and women's rights*. See Baruch et al. in Section II.

IV. Articles

This section lists single papers in academic journals, anthologies, and a few popular magazines. Not included are book reviews and articles that discuss various reproductive issues, but surrogacy only in passing.

Aaron, J. 1987. High tech births: Jewish laws based on view of the world. *Jewish Exponent* 4:63.

Aaron reports his interview with Moses Tendler, Yeshiva University professor of Jewish medical ethics. Use of third-party sperm leads to concern that children might ultimately intermarry.

American College of Obstetricians and Gynecologists, Executive Board. 1983. Ethical issues in surrogate motherhood. Statement of policy. Washington, D.C.: ACOG. 2 pp.

The ACOG gives cautious approval of physician participation in surrogate motherhood; lists issues; makes recommendations to physicians.

American Fertility Society, Ethics Committee. 1990. Ethical considerations of the new reproductive technologies. *Fertility and Sterility* 53(6)(suppl. 2):1S-109S.

Chapters 21 and 22 are on surrogate gestational mothers and surrogate mothers, respectively. Surrogacy is approved with reservations, to be pursued only as a clinical experiment. These chapters are identical to chapters 24 and 25 in their 1986 ethics statement [*Fertility and Sterility* 46(3)(suppl. 1):1S-94S].

Anderson, Elizabeth S. 1990. Is women's labor a commodity? *Philosophy & Public Affairs* 19(1):71–92.

Antisurrogacy. Anderson urges reader to "resist the encroachment of the market upon the sphere of reproductive labor."

Andolsen, Barbara. 1987. Why a surrogate mother should have the right to change her mind: *A feminist analysis of changes in motherhood today.* In Richardson, Section II.

Questions are raised about human dignity, "disembodied" rational judgment as well as how to minimize the "need" to resort to surrogacy.

Andrews, Lori B. 1987. The aftermath of Baby M: Proposed state laws on surrogate motherhood. *Hastings Center Report* 17(5):31–40.

This is an excellent analysis of bills in the various U.S. states, proposed to forbid or regulate surrogacy or to set up study commissions; and whether matters such as informed consent, screening, parental rights, and decision making during pregnancy are included.

Andrews, Lori B. 1989. Position paper: Alternative modes of reproduction. In Cohen and Taub, Section II.

Andrews's detailed, well-referenced presentation of a strong feminist case for surrogacy is necessary reading for feminists.

Andrews, Lori B. 1990. Prohibiting new reproductive technologies: The counterpoint. In McCuen, Section II. Excerpted from her testimony before the House Select Committee on Children, Youth, and Families, 21 May 1987.

The author argues that "families created through alternative reproduction are particularly strong ones" and that desire for a biological child is morally appropriate and protected by our constitutional principles.

Andrews, Lori B. 1990. Surrogate motherhood: The challenge for feminists. In Gostin, Section II.

Prosurrogacy. Andrews "claims that anti-surrogacy sentiments [may turn] *all* women into reproductive vessels." "By breathing life into arguments that feminists have put to rest. . , the current rationales opposing surrogacy could undermine a larger feminist agenda."

Anleu, Sharyn L. Roach. 1990. Reinforcing gender norms: Commercial and altruistic surrogacy. *Acta Sociologica* 33(1):63–74.

Anleu summarizes arguments that condemn commercial contracts and support altruistic agreements. Examining the cases of Baby M and the Kirkman sisters, she claims that the distinction "is based on gender norms . . . that love . . . not self-determination . . . should underlie women's motivation to have children."

Annas, George J. Many papers. See bibliography in Gostin. In *Hastings Center Report* before 1987: (1981) 11(2):23–24; (1986) 16(3):30–31.

Annas, George J. 1987. Baby M: Babies (and justice) for sale. *Hastings Center Report* 17(3):13–15.

Annas claims that "paying women to have children for other people is a bad idea," that we should not "permit the power of the state. . . to be used to seize children from their mothers on the basis of preconception contracts."

Annas, George J. 1988. Death without dignity for commercial surrogacy: The case of Baby M. *Hastings Center Report* 18(2):21–24.

Here the author asserts that the decision of the New Jersey Supreme Court in *Baby M* (which determined surrogate contracts invalid) is "well-reasoned" and "will set the legal agenda for future discussion of surrogate motherhood."

Annas, George J. 1989. Surrogacy revisited. *Hastings Center Report* 19(3):45

In this reply to a letter from Tomlinson, who objects to his views (Annas 1988 above), Annas says the *real* policy issues are dehumanizing of the mother and commodification of children. See Tomlinson, this section.

Annas, George J. 1990. Fairy tales surrogate mothers tell. In Gostin, Section II.

Strong antisurrogacy arguments. One fairy tale is that babies are consumer products and that by permitting their sale "we will all live happily ever after." He recommends a statute that the child's gestational mother be the child's legal mother.

Annas, George J. 1991. Crazy making: Embryos and gestational mothers. *Hastings Center Report* 21(1):35–38.

The decision in the Johnson/Calvert case is criticized as is the view that genetics is more important than gestational experience.

Arditti, Rita. 1987. "Surrogate mothering" exploits women. *Science for the People* 19(3):22–23.

An antisurrogacy position is argued in describing the Muñoz case.

Arditti, Rita. 1987. The surrogacy business. *Social Policy* 9(1):42–46.

The antisurrogacy arguments, using the Baby M and Muñoz cases as examples, are similar to those in the preceding article.

Arditti, Rita. 1987. Wombs for rent, babies for sale. *Sojourner* (March):10–11.

Arditti, as above, considers Baby M and Muñoz cases and raises commercial and patriarchal issues in her antisurrogacy arguments.

Arditti, Rita. 1988. A summary of some recent developments on surrogacy in the United States. *Reproductive and Genetic Engineering: Journal of International Feminist Analysis* 1(1):51–64.

This analysis of the Baby M case quotes extensively from the contract, Judge Sorkow's decision, the legal briefs submitted, and women's antisurrogacy activities.

Arditti, Rita. 1990. Surrogacy in Argentina. *Issues in Reproductive and Genetic Engineering* 3(1):35–43.

Translation of a 1987 interview with the first surrogate mother in Argentina, from the women's magazine *Emmanuelle*.

Arditti, Rita. 1990. Who's the mother? Ask the infertility industry! *Sojourner* (December):10–11.

Arditti analyzes the Johnson/Calvert case and the primacy of genetics; criticizes the profit motivation in surrogacy.

Argus, Arlene. 1988. Surrogacy in Jewish law. *Lilith* No. 19 (Spring):20, 31.

Orthodox to Reform Jewish thinkers use four principles to object to surrogacy: family integrity, human dignity, rights of the the child, contract legitimacy.

Asch, Adrienne. 1990. Surrogacy and the family: Social and value considerations. In Bartels, Section II.

Asch takes no position but urges consideration of the value of the family, consequences for children and society and the analogy with adoption.

Baber, H.E. 1987. FOR the legitimacy of surrogate contracts. In Richardson, Section II.

Baber argues that surrogacy is typically highly beneficial to all concerned; presents logical arguments against such objections as right to relinquish parental rights, baby selling, and exploiting women.

Balbioni, Michael. 1990. The right of procreative choice. In McCuen, Section II. Excerpted from his testimony before the House Subcommittee on Transportation, Tourism, and Hazardous Materials, 15 October 1987.

Balbioni asserts that prohibition of surrogacy is the wrong response, that regulation is "the avenue best suited to protect all parties."

Barrass, Nancy. 1989. Women who experienced surrogacy speak out (USA). In Klein, Section II.

Barrass recounts her miserable experiences during and after pregnancy as a surrogate for the Center for Reproductive Alternatives in California.

Bartels, Dianne M. 1990. Surrogacy arrangements: An overview. In Bartels et al., Section II.

This is a brief essay on definitions, demographics, reasons for participation, public policy alternatives.

Berer, Marge. 1987. surrogacy≡adoption. Letter. *off our backs* (October):27.

Berer urges that surrogacy contracts not be made legal—legal status would undermine all women in relation to claims over children.

Berquist, Richard. 1990. The Vatican *Instruction* and surrogate motherhood. In Bartels et al., Section II.

Berquist suggests approaching the *Instruction* in a spirit of dialogue; discusses ethical principles, the American Fertility Society's ethics statement, and many aspects of assisted reproduction. Little space to surrogacy.

Bettenhausen, Elizabeth. 1987. Hagar revisited: Surrogacy, alienation and motherhood. *Christianity & Crisis* 47:157–159.

Antisurrogacy. The author discusses financial aspects, analogies, contracts, social forces, and more.

Bezanson, Randall P. 1990. Solomon would weep: A comment on *In the Matter of Baby M* and the limits of judicial authority. In Gostin, Section II.

Bezanson objects that the New Jersey Supreme Court should not have addressed the surrogacy problems but merely resolved the dispute in the best interests of Baby M.

Bhimji, Shabir 1987. Womb for rent: Ethical aspects of surrogate motherhood. *Canadian Medical Association Journal* 137:1132–1135.

(Winner of the Dr. William Logie medical ethics essay contest for students at Canadian medical schools.) The author suggests a dual-mother solution: surrogate to share child as a co-parent.

Bonnicksen, Andrea. 1990. A commentary on four papers on surrogate motherhood. *Politics and the Life Sciences* 8(2):195–198.

After summarizing main themes and differences in the four papers, the author attempts to find "intuitively acceptable resolutions" in their conclusions, claims understanding the roots of value differences is important.

Bopp, James, Jr. 1990. Surrogate motherhood agreements: The risk to innocent human life. In Bartels et al., Section II.

Appropriate legislation can eliminate such risks as mandated abortion, prenatal tests, and devaluation of pregnancy and the unborn child.

Brahams, Diana. 1987. The hasty British ban on commercial surrogacy. *Hastings Center Report* 17(1):16–19.

Brahams claims that the 1985 British Surrogacy Arrangement Act making it a criminal offense for third parties to benefit from surrogacy is neither logical nor fair; better to license stringently and control agencies.

Brahams, Diana. 1987. Surrogacy, adoption, and custody. *Lancet* i:817.

Two cases in Britain are detailed: one in which the surrogate gave up the child but did not take all the payment because she made money from a book; another in which the surrogate was awarded custody of twins, unwisely, according to Brahams.

Brenner, Johanna, and Bill Resnick. 1987. Baby M, family love & the market in women. *Against the Current* 2 (May/June):3–6.

The authors are critical of Mary Beth Whitehead's behavior, argue that the Sterns should get the baby because they were expectant parents; otherwise it is biological essentialism. Surrogacy ought to decline, not through regulation but through a fundamental restructuring of society.

Brodribb, Somer. 1989. Delivering babies: Contracts and contradictions. In *The future of human reproduction*, ed. Christine Overall. Pp. 139–158. Toronto: The Women's Press.

Brodribb analyzes the reasoning in the 1985 Ontario Law Reform Commission report—the only government report before 1990 to recommend legalizing surrogacy; she urges women to "resist . . . the patriarchal assertion of rights to children."

Brody, Eugene B. 1987. Reproduction without sex—but with the doctor. *Law, Medicine & Health Care* 15:152–155.

Brody questions to whom, in surrogacy, do physicians owe primary allegiance. He urges doctors to consider their roles as unwilling agents of social control and moral arbiters in the reproductive arena.

Butzel, Henry M. 1987. The essential facts of the Baby M case. In Richardson, Section II.

Butzel presents a chronology, an assessment of genetic issues, and some legal aspects of the case. Judge Sorkow's decision is considered a landmark and possible model for future cases.

Cahill, Lisa Sowle. 1990. The ethics of surrogate motherhood: Biology, freedom, and moral obligation. In Gostin, Section II.

Surrogacy should not be given legal protection. One objection is that it denies moral obligation.

Callahan, Sidney. 1987. Lovemaking & babymaking: Ethics & the new reproductive technology. *Commonweal* 114(8)(24 April):233–239.

Antisurrogacy. With third parties there are too many risks to dignity and well-being.

Calling King Solomon. 1987. *New Republic* (23 February):9–10.

This editorial argues for giving Baby M to Stern.

Capron, Alexander M. 1991. Whose child is this? *Hastings Center Report* 21(6):37–38.

Capron describes the 1991 Johnson/Calvert decision, claims that it was a flagrant, lamentable misreading of the Uniform Parentage Act, and worries that it makes gestational surrogacy legally attractive.

Capron, Alexander M., and Margaret J. Radin. 1990. Choosing family law over contract law as a paradigm for surrogate motherhood. In Gostin, Section II.

Procreative liberty does not support enforcing surrogate arrangements, which should be handled from the perspective of adoption.

Charo, R. Alta. 1988. Problems in commercialized surrogate mothering. In Baruch et al., Section II.

Laws to regulate commercial surrogacy could set a dangerous precedent for regulating all women during pregnancy.

Charo, R. Alta. 1990. Legislative approaches to surrogate motherhood. In Gostin, Section II.

Charo gives data from demographic surveys of surrogate mothers; discusses matters for legislative regulation; groups approaches into categories: static, private ordering, inducement, regulatory, and punitive. Extensive, useful references. Very worthwhile reading.

Chavkin, Wendy, Barbara Katz Rothman, and Rayna Rapp. 1989. Position paper: Alternative modes of reproduction: Other views and questions. In Cohen and Taub, Section II.

The authors rebut succinctly and powerfully six feminist prosurrogacy arguments. Recommended.

Chesler, Phyllis. 1988. Baby M; NJ outlaws surrogacy. *off our backs* (March):20.

The author applauds the New Jersey Supreme Court decision, even though it "custodially sacrifices" Mary Beth Whitehead; she invents "Miranda Warnings" to read to women before they are "reproductively arrested."

Chesler, Phyllis. 1988. What is a mother? *Ms.* (May):36–39.

Adapted from Chesler's *Sacred bond.* See Section I.

Chesler, Phyllis. 1990. Pound of flesh. *New Statesman & Society* (9 March):29–31.

Extract from Chesler's *Sacred bond.* See Section I.

Chollar, Susan. 1989. Two views of surrogate motherhood. *Psychology Today* June:76.

From their books, Chollar summarizes and contrasts the views of Andrews and Whitehead. See Section I.

Cohen, Barbara, and Teresa Lynn Friend. 1987. Legal and ethical implications of surrogate mother contracts. *Clinics in Perinatology* 14:281–292.

For health professionals, this is an overview of legal issues and ethical considerations for deciding about their involvement in surrogate arrangements and for counseling patients; urges serious consideration of ramifications before choosing this method.

Corea, Gena. 1989. Introduction [to the congress's proceedings]. In Quebec Council, Section II.

The author describes the industrialization of most steps of reproduction, with about one-third of the text on surrogacy; she summarizes the stories of seven surrogates and lists numerous public policy questions, such as policies about police enforcement and on catalogues for choosing surrogates.

Corea, Gena. 1989. Surrogacy: Making the links. In Klein, Section II.

Corea claims that the American Fertility Society's ethics report medicalizes the sale of women's bodies; she introduces the stories of eight surrogates, five of whom then give longer narrations.

Corea, Gena. 1990. Human slavery. In McCuen, Section II. Excerpted from her testimony before the House Subcommittee on Transportation, Tourism, and Hazardous Materials, 15 October 1987.

The excerpt includes brief case studies of seven surrogates; asks "Is reproductive slavery good for women?"

Corea, Gena. 1990. Junk liberty. In Gostin, Section II. From testimony before the California Assembly Judiciary Committee, April 1988.

Corea quotes from surrogates, gives bits of case stories. She emphasizes surrogacy's violation of human dignity.

Craig, Sue. 1990. Infertility counselling: Should surrogacy be an option? *HealthRight* 9:29–39.

"Doctors and counsellors should be able to provide information and support to clients who are considering surrogacy" but "involvement by medical staff [may] become illegal" in New South Wales.

Dahlem, Michael. 1992. Contract motherhood and the morality of care. *Women & Criminal Justice* 3(1):101–126.

Dahlem examines judicial and legislative responses and public policy implications of surrogate parenting contracts from the perspective of a (Gilligan-inspired) morality of care; provides arguments against granting of specific performance.

Daniels, Ken, and Karyn Taylor. 1991. Surrogacy: The private troubles and public issues. *Community Mental Health in New Zealand* 6(2):28–50.

The authors describe in detail a New Zealand case in which a surrogate reported to the news media her distress in relinguishing her baby. The authors urge mental health professionals to play a key role in assisting all involved parties in surrogacy and also the policymakers.

Davies, Iwan. 1985. Contracts to bear children. *Journal of Medical Ethics* 11:61–64.

Davies favors the minority view in the Warnock Report: careful regulation of surrogacy rather than outright prohibition.

Davis, Peggy C. 1989. Commentary: Alternative modes of reproduction: The locus and determinants of choice. In Cohen and Taub, Section II.

Prosurrogacy. Surrogacy should be permitted and wisely regulated in order to liberate us from role stereotypes based on sex.

Deegan, Mary Jo. 1987. The gift mother: *A proposed ritual for the integration of surrogacy into society*. In Richardson, Section II.

Deegan proposes a scenario of celebration, a rite of passage for a gift relationship between surrogate families and parents-to-be.

Despreaux, Michele Ann. 1989. Surrogate motherhood: A feminist perspective. *Research in the Sociology of Health Care* 8:99–133.

This detailed analysis of several feminists' ethical theories and principles is followed by application to surrogacy.

Dickens, Bernard. 1988. Introduction [to workshop on surrogacy]. In Quebec Council, Section III.

With general yet low-key approval, Dickens discusses recognition of surrogacy contracts, commercialization, benefits to women, and whether to amend common law.

Doane, Janice, and Devon Hodges. 1989. Risky business: Familial ideology and the case of Baby M. *differences* 1(1):67–81.

Doane and Hodges point out that in the Baby M case all participants defend the centrality of the family; Whitehead's double bind is analyzed; a decision of an imaginary feminist judge is proposed.

Dodds, Susan, and Karen Jones. 1989. Surrogacy and autonomy. *Bioethics* 3(1):1–17.

The authors argue that surrogacy contracts pose serious risks to personal autonomy and pay insufficient regard for the resultant child; they should be not only unenforceable but also illegal.

Dodds, Susan, and Karen Jones. 1989. A response to Purdy. *Bioethics* 3(1):35–39.

Dodds and Jones rebut Purdy's arguments on transferring risks, paternalism, separating sex and reproduction, and selling babies.

Eichler, Margrit. 1988. Preconception contracts for the production of children—What are the proper legal responses? In Quebec Council, Section II.

Eichler considers how to identify desirable legal responses, first clarifying the relationship of the contractual parties to each other, parenthood relations to the child, involvement of middle persons, and commercial aspects. Guided by the Ontario Law Reform Commission Report, she discusses the Baby M case.

Ewing, Christine. 1990. Draft report on surrogacy issued by the Australian National Bioethics Consultative Committee—The debate on surrogacy in Australia continues. *Issues in Reproductive and Genetic Engineering: Journal of International Feminist Analysis* 3(2):143–146.

Ewing summarizes the objections to the draft report from Australian FINRRAGE groups (Feminist International Network of Resistance to Reproductive and Genetic Engineering), especially to the recommendation for legislative control of surrogacy. See Chapter 26, this volume.

Faulkner, Ellen. 1989. The case of "Baby M." *Canadian Journal of Women and the Law* 3(1):239–245.

This essay is a feminist critique of the two legal proceedings: the decisions by Judge Sorkow and by Chief Justice Wilentz.

Feldman, David M. The Jewish response to surrogate motherhood. *Women's League Outlook* 57(4):9–10.

"Issues raised by surrogate motherhood pose a clash between two desirable goals: procreation and family. The first should be pursued through alternatives that do not destroy the second."

Field, Martha A. 1990. The case against enforcement of surrogacy contracts. *Politics and the Life Sciences* 8(2):199–204.

Commenting on four papers, Field is strongly critical of Hill's views. "Allowing surrogacy contracts and using police and courts to enforce them undermine a strongly felt attitude that some things in life should escape the market economy."

Fischer, Susan, and Irene Gillman. 1991. Surrogate motherhood: Attachment, attitudes and social support. *Psychiatry* 54:13–20.

Standardized questionnaires administered to 21 surrogates and 21 controls found significant differences in attachment to the fetus, social support, and familial support.

Ford, Marcus P., and Sandra B. Lubarsky. 1987. An ecological evaluation of surrogacy: *A wrong idea for our time*. In Richardson, Section II.

Since an organism is linked to its environment by a web of connections, surrogacy is wrong for this world.

Foster, Patricia. 1989. Women who experienced surrogacy speak out (USA). In Klein, Section II.

This surrogate mother describes her pain in relinquishing her son in "doing this wonderful thing for humankind."

Franks, Darrell D. 1981. Psychiatric evaluation of women in a surrogate mother program. *American Journal of Psychiatry* 138:1378–1379.

For the ten women in the evaluation there were high levels of femininity; increased energy; social extroversion. Their reasons for entering the program were altruistic and financial.

Frederick, Winston R., Robert Delapenha, Graciela Gray, et al. 1987. HIV testing of surrogate mothers. Letter. *New England Journal of Medicine* 317:1351–1352.

The authors describe the case of a surrogate who did not reveal past drug abuse. The child was seropositive for HIV; both parties refused custody.

Freeman, Michael. 1989. Is surrogacy exploitative?. In *Legal issues in human reproduction*, ed. Sheila McLean. Brookfield, Vt.: Aldershot.

The principle objection to surrogacy—that it exploits or dehumanizes women—does not stand up to critical examination. Freeman argues away other objections but admits the possible danger of making children into a consumer durable.

Gavin, Kathleen. 1987. Surrogate issue demands resolution. *New Directions for Women* March/April:9.

Taking no strong stance, Gavin reports contrasting feminist views. She urges "social, medical and corporate responsibility" to prevent infertility.

Gallagher, Maggie. 1987. Womb to let. *National Review* 39(24 April):27–30.

After describing her interviews with two happy surrogates, Carol Pavek and Jan Sutton, and with prosurrogacy New York Senator Mary Goodhue, Gallagher argues a strong case against surrogacy. Well written and lively.

Garcia, Sandra Anderson. 1989. The Baby M case: A class struggle over undefined rights, unenforceable responsibilities, and inadequate remedies. In Whiteford and Poland, Section II.

Garcia gives the chronology of the Baby M case; raises questions about specifics throughout the procedure; quotes from the Sorkow decision; outlines the Whiteheads' claims; summarizes arguments of attorneys on both sides. She provides some very useful excerpts.

Garcia, Sandra Anderson. 1989. Surrogacy in the marketplace: Will sales law act as surrogate for surrogacy law? In Whiteford and Poland, Section II.

The author describes surrogacy as a transaction under Article Two of the Uniform Commercial Code: discusses preagreement, contract formation, preperformance, delivery, receipt and inspection, payment, and warranty liability; clearly shows how joy can turn into sorrow. Interesting unique analysis, recommended.

Gellman, Marc. 1988. "I'll take the head": The ethics of surrogate motherhood. *Journal of Reform Judaism* 35(2):7–11.

In applying aspects of Jewish law to the Baby M case, the author discusses barrenness, adoption, the commandment to procreate, exploited labor, polygamy, and adultery.

Gibson, Mary. 1992. Contract motherhood: Social practice in social context. *Women & Criminal Justice* 3(1): 55–99.

Using a socialist feminist approach, Gibson discusses social context and defends objections to surrogacy on grounds of exploitation, commodification, and alienation and then recommends prohibiting commercial surrogacy.

Gladwell, Malcolm, and Rochelle Sharpe. 1987. Meet the surrogacy entrepreneur: Baby M winner. *New Republic* 196(7):16–18.

This article is a detailed and harsh criticism of Noel Keane, who prospers despite the Stiver and Baby M cases.

Gordon, Linda. 1987. Reproductive rights for today. *Nation* (12 September):230–232.

Gordon covers other conflicts raised by medical technologies; recommends that surrogacy contracts have no legal force.

Gostin, Larry. 1990. A civil liberties analysis of surrogacy arrangements. In Gostin, Section II.

Civil liberty prevents prohibiting surrogacy, exchange of money, or contracts requiring the surrogate to waive her parental rights. Custody, if disputed, should be determined without regard to the surrogacy.

Guinzburg, Suzanne. 1983. Surrogate mother's rationale. *Psychology Today* 17 (April):79.

Summary of findings reported in Parker 1983.

Harris, Arlene, and Donald S. Klein. 1988. New biology poses new problems. *Trusts & Estates* (February):50, 53–54, 56, 58, 60.

The authors analyze several cases to shed light on the problem of the rights, contractual or not, of persons who have a legal interest in a surrogate birth.

Harrison, Barbara Grizzuti. 1987. Surrogate mothers: No way to treat a baby. *Mademoiselle* (January):96.

Harris avers, "Everything about this transaction is fraught with risk for the child, and nothing about it seems sane or good to me."

Harrison, Michelle. 1987. Social construction of Mary Beth Whitehead. *Gender and Society* 1:300–311.

This meticulous review (with quotes) of the mental health experts' evaluation of the participants and testimony in the Baby M case reveals their unsubstantiated conclusions, middle-class biases. A unique analysis, highly recommended.

Henry, Alice. 1985. Feminists debate surrogate motherhood. *off our backs* (April):12–13.

Henry reports the lively discussion on 8 December 1984, at the Women's Reproductive Rights Campaign Centre in London.

Heyl, Barbara Sherman. 1988. Commercial contracts and human connectedness. *Society* 25(3)(March/April):11–16.

The role of class factors in surrogacy is probed. Heyl argues that to balance the rights and risks of the key parties we should not deny their interconnectedness. Definitely worth reading.

Hill, John Lawrence. 1990. The case for enforcement of the surrogate contract. *Politics and the Life Sciences* 8(2):147–160.

Hill argues that when policy options are evaluated by benefit/harm, the enforceable contract gives the least added burden. He proposes an intentional theory of parenthood that revolves around the *intent* to have and raise a child, not around a biological contribution.

Hill, Michael R. 1987. A cross cultural analysis of several forms of parenting: *Mother, genitrix, and mater*. In Richardson, Section II.

Hill analyzes the institution of "family," multiple parenting, the ideology and praxis of parenting. Baby M's life "is worth celebrating and protecting."

Hirsch, Bernard J. 1983. Parenthood by proxy. *Journal of the American Medical Association* 249:2251–2252.

After presenting an imaginary "worst case" scenario, Hirsch recommends that physicians involved in surrogacy arrangements use extreme caution to minimize many problems, including genetic risks.

Holbrook, Sarah M. 1990. Adoption, infertility, and the new reproductive technologies: Problems and prospects for social work and welfare policy. *Social Work* 35(4):333–337.

This brief history of traditional adoption includes problems. The author provides suggestions for social workers in surrogacy situations and emphasizes the necessity for research.

Holder, Angela R. 1990. Surrogate motherhood and the best interests of children. In Gostin, Section II.

Strong antisurrogacy stance. "If the courts accept commercial surrogacy as a legitimate enterprise, . . . we have again reverted to the concept of child as chattel." The author also raises concerns about the effect on the surrogate's other children.

Hubbard, Ruth. 1987. A birthmother is a birthmother is a . . . *Sojourner* 13(1)(September):20–21.

A woman has the right to choose the conditions under which she will bear a child *and* the right to refuse to relinquish the baby. We must not "pretend that the ideal of the two-parent family can stand unchallenged."

Hynes, H. Patricia, Janice G. Raymond, and Gena Corea. 1990. Women and children used in systems of surrogacy: Position statement of the Institute on Women and Technology. In Appendix F, Gostin, Section II.

The authors describe the social, political, economic, personal, and physical exploitation of women by surrogacy; they support federal legislation making surrogate contracts void and unenforceable.

Ince, Susan. 1984. Inside the surrogate industry. In *Test-tube women*, ed. Rita Arditti, Renate Duelli Klein, and Shelley Minden. London: Pandora.

Questionable practices in surrogacy agencies are exposed when Ince pretends to want employment as a surrogate. A classic.

Isaacs, Stephen L., and Renee J. Holt. 1987. Redefining procreation: Facing the issues. *Population Bulletin* 42(3):1–37.

Eight pages herein summarize the practice of surrogacy, noteworthy cases, ethical/legal/social issues, regulation, protecting the parties.

Kane, Elizabeth. 1989. Male order babies. *Broadsheet* 167 (April):16–19.

A talk in Auckland, as excerpted by editor Pat Rosier; why Kane changed her mind, formed the National Coalition Against Surrogacy, and took the position that surrogacy is not good for our society.

Kane, Elizabeth. 1989. Surrogate parenting: A division of families, not a creation. *Reproductive and Genetic Engineering: Journal of International Feminist Analysis* 2(2):105–109. Also in Klein, Section II.

In this condensed narrative of her book (Section I) Kane describes her change from advocate to opponent of surrogacy.

Kasindorf, Martin. 1991. And baby makes four. *Los Angeles Times Magazine* 20 January:10–14, 16, 30–34.

Thorough investigation of Johnson/Calvert case. Recommended.

Ketchum, Sara Ann. 1989. Selling babies and selling bodies. *Hypatia: A Journal of Feminist Philosophy* 4(3):116–127. Also in Holmes and Purdy, Section II.

The free market in babies and women's bodies is contrary to Kantian principles of personhood and to the feminist principle that men do not have a right to the sexual or reproductive use of women's bodies

Kirby, Michael D. 1985. From Hagar to Baby Cotton—Surrogacy. *Australian and New Zealand Journal of Obstetrics and Gynaecology* 25:151–158.

Kirby describes the Baby Cotton case; lists possible undesirable parliamental reactions; urges Australians to an informed national debate.

Kopecky, Gini. 1983. Womb for hire: Life. *Omni* 5(9):18, 23, 142–144.

Comments from Richard Levin about his procedures in Surrogate Parenting Associates in Kentucky. Happy surrogates' experiences.

Krauthammer, Charles. 1987. The ethics of human manufacture. *New Republic* 4 May:17–21.

The author examines the Vatican's position regarding manipulation of embryos, artificial families, and artificial insemination; he proposes discouraging, not prohibiting, surrogacy.

Kruse, Richard A. 1987. The strange case of Baby M. *Human Life Review* 13:27–34.

Kruse discusses Judge Sorkow's lack of due process in the Baby M case, including use of hostile lawyers and "experts." Strong condemnation of surrogacy as "commercialization of humanity."

Kuo, Lenore. 1989. The morality of surrogate mothering. *Southern Journal of Philosophy* 27(3):361–380.

Kuo argues that surrogacy as currently practiced is morally unjustifiable. After describing "current practice," inveighing against "profit," and urging adoption of unadoptable children, she analyzes at length procreative rights and the desire to have (genetic) children.

La Puma, John, David L. Schiedermayer, and John L. Grover. 1989. Surrogacy and Shakespeare: The Merchant's contract revisited. *American Journal of Obstetrics and Gynecology* 160:59–62.

"Obstetricians should not be placed in the position of Portia in *The Merchant of Venice*, that of an arbiter of an unethical contract. [They] should not prescribe or acknowledge surrogacy as a medical treatment and should not knowingly participate. . . ."

La Puma, John, David L. Schiedermayer, and John L. Grover. 1990. Reply *American Journal of Obstetrics and Gynecology* 163(2):680.

Responding to Wettstein's letter (this section), the authors reaffirm, "Surrogacy is not a medical treatment" and argue "[A] fetus is not a kidney."

Laqueur, Thomas W. 1990. The facts of fatherhood. In *Conflicts in feminism*, ed. Marianne Hirsch and Evelyn Fox Keller. New York: Routledge, Chapman & Hall.

Biological "facts are but shifting sands for the construction of motherhood and fatherhood." "In parenthood emotional work should count."

Leeton, J., C. King, and J. Harman. 1988. Sister-sister in vitro fertilization surrogate pregnancy with donor sperm: The case for surrogate gestational pregnancy. *Journal of in Vitro Fertilization and Embryo Transfer* 5(5):245–248.

In this case history of gestational surrogacy in Melbourne, the authors advocate using relatives or close friends.

Lifton, Betty Jean. 1988. Brave new baby in the brave new world. In Baruch, Section II.

A plea to consider the psychological effects of surrogacy on children because of the experiences of many adopted children.

McDowell-Head, Leila. 1987. On surrogate motherhood. *Essence* (July):136.

A broadcast journalist, who interviewed Mary Beth Whitehead, warns that "where the poor. . . and people of color are routinely exploited, . . . surrogate motherhood is a dangerous approach to addressing the legitimate concerns of the childless."

McFadden, Terese. 1988. Surrogate motherhood—Refusing to relinquish a child. In *The baby machine: The commercialisation of motherhood*, ed. Jocelynne A. Scutt. Carlton, Victoria: McCulloch.

Personal story of an Australian surrogate mother who succeeded in keeping her son.

McGoldrick, K.E. 1988. Baby M: Surrogacy and the law. *Journal of the American Medical Women's Association* 43:131.

The author commends the N.J. Supreme Court's decision in the Baby M case and the opposition to surrogacy in France and Germany; hopes N.J. decision will be a "persuasive precedent affirming . . . that women's bodies or wombs can't be rented."

Macklin, Ruth. 1990. Is there anything wrong with surrogate motherhood? An ethical analysis. In Gostin, Section II.

Macklin uses a carefully argued formalist approach to demonstrate that surrogacy is not a morally flawed activity, except in its commercial features.

Macklin, Ruth. 1991. Artificial means of reproduction and our understanding of the family. *Hastings Center Report* 21(1):5–11.

The author holds that with new reproductive technologies we are forced to rethink the concept of family and to distinguish between ethical and conceptual questions.

Mahoney, Joan. 1990. An essay on surrogacy and feminist thought. In Gostin, Section II.

Mahoney poses questions and explores issues of sex equity and gender neutrality in regard to prohibiting surrogacy contracts, enforcing them, and determining custody of children.

Malm, H. 1989. Paid surrogacy: Arguments and responses. *Public Affairs Quarterly* 3(2):57–66.

Malm considers and rejects five arguments that others have raised to prohibit contracted child-bearing arrangements: selling babies, selling bodies, exploitation, transferring rights, and the needs of noninvolved persons.

Malm, H. 1989. Commodification or compensation: A reply to Ketchum. *Hypatia: A Journal of Feminist Philosophy* 4(3):128–135. Also in Holmes and Purdy, Section II.

Similar to above, this article more specifically rebuts arguments raised by Ketchum. See Ketchum, this section.

Meehan, Mary. 1987. Wombs shouldn't be for rent. *U.S. Catholic* (September):16–21.

The author sets forth six arguments for outlawing surrogacy; gives the results from a readers' opinion poll; includes letters commenting pro and con on her views.

Merrick, Janna C. 1990. The case of Baby M. In Bartels et al., Section II.

This thorough, straightforward description of the Baby M background facts, the trial court and Supreme Court decisions, and some legal implications is informative and easy to read.

Merrick, Janna C. 1990. Selling reproductive rights: Policy issues in surrogate motherhood. *Politics and the Life Sciences* 8(2):161–172.

The author argues powerfully that surrogacy *does* involve child selling, discusses the case of Elizabeth Kane, and claims that practices limiting surrogacy will not solve the inequalities surrogacy exposes.

Michelow, M.C., J. Berustein, M.J. Jacobson, et al. 1988. Mother-daughter in vitro fertilization triplet surrogate pregnancy. *Journal of in Vitro Fertilization and Embryo Transfer* 5(1):31–34.

The authors detail a South African case: daughter with hysterectomy; mother, perimenopausal; son-in-law, poor sperm motility; use of oral contraceptives to synchronize menstrual cycles.

Miller, Tracy E. 1988. A resounding NO to commercial surrogacy. *Hastings Center Report* 18(4):4.

Summary of the surrogate parenting report of the New York State Task Force on Life and the Law. See Section I.

Milne, David. 1987. Panel calls for ban on pay to surrogates. *American Medical News* 1 May:32.

Milne reports that the Symposium on Evolving Reproductive Technology held in Detroit recommended that states ban payments to surrogate mothers.

Morgan, Derek. 1990. Surrogacy: An introductory essay. In *Birthrights: Law and ethics at the beginning of life*, ed. Robert Lee and Derek Morgan. New York: Routledge, Chapman & Hall.

The author analyzes the situation in Britain in regard to definition of mother, nature of surrogacy; estimates the incidence (including results of the author's survey); gives reasons for surrogacy's contemporary visibility. An impressionistic history.

Morris, Monica B. 1988. Reproductive technology and restraints. *Society* 25:16–21.

Responding to Neuhaus, Morris says we first need research on what happens to people involved in surrogacy; recommends regulating surrogacy, considering approaches of other countries.

Muñoz, Alejandra. 1989. Women who experienced surrogacy speak out (Mexico). In Klein, Section II.

As told to Gena Corea, this is the story of an illiterate Mexican woman who was tricked into being a surrogate mother for her cousin Nattie Haro in California.

Neff, David. 1987. How not to have a baby. *Christianity Today* 3 April:14–15.

This antisurrogacy editorial lists "common sense considerations" as reasons for outlawing, not merely regulating, surrogacy.

Nelson, Hilde Lindemann, and James Lindemann Nelson. 1989. Cutting motherhood in two: Some suspicions concerning surrogacy. *Hypatia: A Journal of Feminist Philosophy* 4(3):85–94. Also in Holmes & Purdy, Section II.

"The assumptions [underlying surrogacy] hold an impoverished view of the full significance of women's freedom and an inadequate recognition of the child's moral stake."

Nelson, Sara. 1988. Making babies. *Lilith*. No. 19 (Spring):18–20.

Nelson interviewed Ada Greenberg, active proponent of surrogacy, who bore Eamon Samuel for Lynne and Jerry Schwartz-Barker in 1984; she volunteered to do it, talked them into it, and took no pay.

Neuhaus, Richard John. 1988. Renting women, buying babies and class struggles. *Society* 25(3):8–10.

In a position paper, Neuhaus declares that the "baby trade rudely rips the veil off class divisions and hostilities in American life" and that court decisions reveal that "the world of which [Mary Beth Whitehead] is part is unfit for Mr. Stern's baby."

Neuhaus, Richard John. 1988. Power, money and high-minded intentions. *Society* 25(3):28–29.

Neuhaus comments on the responses to his paper (above) by Heyl, Morris, Rothman, and Zelizer.

Okin, Susan Moller. 1990. A critique of pregnancy contracts: Comments on articles by Hill, Merrick, Shevory, and Woliver. *Politics and the Life Sciences* 8(2):205–210.

Criticizing points in all four articles, Okin argues that the freedom to sign away one's rights to a child, not only before birth but even before conception, is a "freedom not to be free." She also worries about effects on the birth mother's other children.

Oliver, Kelly. 1989. Marxism and surrogacy. *Hypatia: A Journal of Feminist Philosophy* 4(3):95–115. Also in Holmes and Purdy, Section II.

Oliver suggests that "Marx's analysis of estranged labor can reveal the class and gender issues" concealed by a liberal framework and that the inequality of the parties ensures surrogates will lose in court.

Ollenburger, Jane, and John Hamlin. 1987. "All birthing should be paid labor"—A Marxist analysis of the commodification of motherhood. In Richardson, Section II.

The authors deplore the class inequalities in the Baby M case, yet approve surrogacy because it provides "payment for labor that exists and until now has gone unpaid," if safeguards about sufficient wages and satisfactory work conditions are built into the agreement.

Overall, Christine. 1987. Surrogate motherhood. In *Science, morality & feminist theory*, ed. Marsha Hanen and Kai Nielsen. Supplementary Vol. 13, *Canadian Journal of Philosophy.*

Nearly the same argument as Chapter 6 in her book (Section I) but without her policy commentary.

Overall, Christine. 1989. The misuse of feminist values in the defence of contract motherhood: A case study. *Resources for Feminist Research (RFR/DRF)* 18(3):67–71.

Overall examines in detail Baber's (1987) paper, as "a striking example of the use of pseudo-feminist language . . . in defence of a reproductive practice, surrogacy, that oppresses women." See Baber, this section.

Overall, Christine. 1991. The case against the legalization of contract motherhood. In *Debating Canada's future: Views from the Left*, ed. Simon Rosenblum and Peter Findlay. Toronto: James Lorimer. Pp. 210–225.

Parker, Philip J. 1983. Motivation of surrogate mothers: Initial findings. *Journal of Psychiatry* 140(1):117–118.

From interviews, Parker finds motives such as guilt from previous loss of a fetus or baby and perceived need for money; women distance themselves; there are no serious consequences, only transitional grief.

Peterson, Iver. 1987. Baby M's future. *New York Times* 5 April:1, 7.

Interviews with 18 legal experts, ethicists, religious leaders, surrogate mothers, feminists, and surrogacy entrepreneurs just after Judge Sorkow's decision that the Whitehead/Stern surrogacy contract was legal. Recommended.

Pierce, Calvin. 1988. Many states enacting, studying surrogacy laws. *Ob.Gyn. News* 23(17):1:42–43.

Pierce describes legislation in several states to ban surrogacy for pay or declare the contracts void and unenforceable; comments on specific organizations that welcome or challenge these actions.

Pollitt, Katha. 1987. The strange case of Baby M. *Nation* 23 May:667, 682–686, 688.

This lively antisurrogacy polemic is peppered with good points: Baby M trial was "riddled with psychobabble, class prejudice and sheer callousness... welter of half-truths, bad analogies, logical muddles and glib catch phrases." Recommended.

Pollitt, Katha. 1990. When is a mother not a mother? *Nation* 3 December:825; 840–844.

Pollitt gives a pungent analysis of the Johnson-Calvert case; claims that Judge Parslow's decision degrades women, that gestational surrogacy invites the singling out of black women for exploitation.

Posner, Richard A. 1989. The ethics and economics of enforcing contracts of surrogate motherhood. *Journal of Contemporary Health Law and Policy* 5:21.

The popularity of surrogacy is due to scientific advances, decline in conventional attitudes toward family, shortage of babies for adoption, and desire for genetic continuity.

Purdy, Laura M. 1989. Surrogate mothering: Exploitation or empowerment? *Bioethics* 3(1):18–34.

After countering many feminist arguments against surrogacy, Purdy concludes that surrogacy "has the potential to empower women and increase their status," but also admits the "frightening potential for deepening their exploitation."

Purdy, Laura M. 1989. A response to Dodds and Jones. *Bioethics* 3(1):40–44.

Here the author describes details of her partial agreement with several of their arguments and concludes by agreeing that contract pregnancy must be strictly regulated in societies like our own.

Rachels, James. 1987. A report from America: Baby M. *Bioethics* 1(4):357–365.

Rachels describes the Baby M case, digresses by giving examples of baby situations brought to the Phil Donahue Show on TV, gives Judge Sorkow's reply to six arguments against surrogacy contracts, and concludes with "distrust created by the Baby M case seems to me most unfortunate."

Radin, Margaret Jane. 1987. Market-inalienability. *Harvard Law Review* 100(8):1847–1937.

Radin explores the significance of market-inalienability (things that may be given away but not sold) and applies the theory to contested market-inalienabilities, including surrogacy. A classic.

Ratterm, Debra. 1987. Whitehead vs. sperm. *off our backs* May:1, 12.

The author gives the background and case history of the Baby M situation with an extended commentary on Judge Sorkow's "vindictive" 121-page opinion.

Raymond, Janice G. 1988. Making international connections: Surrogacy, the traffic in women and de-mythologizing motherhood. In Quebec Council, Section II.

Raymond criticizes the liberal American argument that surrogacy is a "women's right to choose what to do with her body" and shows that the practice increases international traffic in women; she argues that women cannot have rights without first being accorded human dignity.

Raymond, Janice G. 1988. The spermatic market: Surrogate stock and liquid assets. *Reproductive and Genetic Engineering: Journal of International Feminist Analysis* 1(1):65–75.

Antisurrogacy. Raymond analyzes how the Baby M case illustrates essentialist constructs, manipulation of the maternal instinct, and baby craving.

Raymond, Janice G. 1988. At issue: In the matter of Baby M: Rejudged. *Reproductive and Genetic Engineering: Journal of International Feminist Analysis* 1(2):175–181.

Although pleased that the New Jersey Supreme Court declared surrogate contracts illegal, Raymond details many problems illustrated by the gender neutrality of that decision.

Raymond, Janice G. 1989. The international traffic in women: Women used in systems of surrogacy and reproduction. *Reproductive and Genetic Engineering: Journal of International Feminist Analysis* 2(1):51–57.

The author here describes the international traffic in babies and women; compares surrogate brokers with pimps; likens "regulating" surrogacy to regulating slavery to make it less obviously oppressive.

Raymond, Janice G. 1990. Reproductive gifts and gift giving: The altruistic woman. *Hastings Center Report* 20(6):7–11.

"Altruistic reproductive exchanges leave intact the status of women as a breeder class." In surrogacy, "altruism reinforces the role of women as *mothers for others*."

Reagan, Leslie. 1987. Surrogacy is a bad bargain. *Against the Current* 2 (Sept./Oct.):56–58.

Reagan argues vigorously against surrogacy but recommends discouraging, not forbidding, it; discusses how one can support the right of a biological mother to keep her child and still challenge biological determinism.

Reame, Nancy E. 1988. Maternal adaptation and postpartum responses to a surrogate pregnancy. *Journal of Psychosomatic Obstetrics and Gynaecology* 10(Suppl.):86

In this study of 20 surrogates receiving support services, 15 "reported at least moderate symptoms of perinatal loss"; one required hospitalization. The author concludes that these normal adaptation responses to pregnancy "may place [surrogates] at risk for perinatal grief reactions. . . ."

Reame, Nancy E. 1991. The surrogate mother as a high-risk obstetric patient. *Women's Health Issues* 1(3).

Reame looks at implications of the ACOG 1990 recommendations on ethics and surrogacy, especially that a gestational mother have the rights of a biologic mother. A surrogate mother's needs make her high risk (psychologically, legally)—perhaps this requires a multidisciplinary team.

Reame, Nancy E., and Philip J. Parker. 1990. Surrogate pregnancy: Clinical features of forty-four cases. *American Journal of Obstetrics and Gynecology* 162(5):1220–1225.

For 44 surrogate mothers, these researchers report demographic statistics, perinatal risk factors, the 14 percent pregnancy loss, and newborn characteristics. Despite contract prohibition, 41 percent smoked.

Regis, Ed. 1988. A science court. *Omni* January:41–42, 44, 92, 94, 97–100.

Eight leading male scientists are given six "cases" to arbitrate. For the case on surrogacy contracts, six give the surrogate time to change her mind; the others uphold the contract.

Reimer, Reta. 1990. Issues in surrogate motherhood: An overview. In McCuen, Section II. Summary of a report for the Library of Congress Congressional Research Service, March 1988.

Law has not kept pace with advances—couples involved must rely on legal principles that have arisen in other areas of the law.

Richard, Patricia Bayer. 1990. Rights, relationships, class, and gender: Issues in the politics of surrogate contracts. *Politics and the Life Sciences* 8(2):211–215.

The author urges, "Any policy governing surrogacy contracts should combine the ethic of care with the ethic of rights." She imagines various consequences should surrogacy become routine, for example, incorporating sex selection into contracts, having employers pay for employees' contracts.

Richardson, Herbert. 1987. God is the creator of human life: *A Calvinist defense of surrogate parenthood.* In Richardson, Section II.

The author asserts that the true purpose of science is to work with God to restore goodness to nature. He devotes more space to in vitro fertilization than surrogacy; approves both.

Robbins, Sonia Jaffe. 1990. When is a mother not a mother? The Baby M case. *Women and Language* 13:41–46.

The author analyzes the words used to characterize the man and the two women in the Baby M case from 28 news articles in the New York City press over a seven-month period.

Robertson, John A. 1990. Procreative liberty and the state's burden of proof in regulating noncoital reproduction. In Gostin, Section II.

Restriction of noncoital reproduction should be limited to cases of serious harm; interfering with paying for surrogacy is largely symbolic and moralistic; the New Jersey Supreme Court's decision (re Baby M) is incoherent and deficient.

Rothenberg, Karen H. 1990. Gestational surrogacy and the health care provider: Put part of the IVF genie back into the bottle. *Law, Medicine, & Health Care* 18:345–352.

Rothenberg provides good analyses of the Calvert/Johnson case, international events, screening, informed consent; concludes that professionals should resist temptation to expand IVF with gestational surrogacy. Good legal reference list.

Rothenburg, Karen H. 1990. Surrogacy and the health care professional: Baby M and beyond. In Gostin, Section II.

The author points out that health care professionals played no active role in the Baby M appeal; discusses some complex legal and ethical questions faced by those professionals in counseling, informed consent, insemination, prenatal care, and birth.

Rothman, Barbara Katz. 1987. Surrogacy: A question of values. *Conscience* 7(3)(May/June):1–4. Also in Bartels et al., Section II.

Rothman explains that she may be antisurrogacy like some religious leaders, but she calls on different values (such as the centrality of relationships) and objects when women are "used."

Rothman, Barbara Katz. 1988. Cheap labor: Sex, class, race—and "surrogacy." *Society* 25(3):21–23. Response to Neuhaus, this section.

Patriarchy (issues of sex) and race are intertwined with class issues in surrogacy; "surrogacy is the reductio ad absurdum of Western patriarchal capitalism."

Rothman, Barbara Katz. 1988. Reproductive technology and the commodification of life. In Baruch et al., Section II.

The "key unifying concept" in the new reproduction technology is "the increasing commodification of life..," made "dramatically clear . . . in 'surrogacy' arrangements in which . . . women sell both their 'labor' and their 'product.'"

Rowland, Robyn. 1990. At issue: Response to the draft report of the National Bioethics Consultative Committee (NBCC), *Surrogacy. Issues in Reproductive and Genetic Engineering: Journal of International Feminist Analysis* 3(2):147–157.

Rowland takes issue with several aspects of the draft report, including political use of language, failure to properly compare fatherhood to motherhood, the privileging of personal autonomy, and dismissal of the welfare of children. See also Chapter 26, this volume.

Ryan, Michael D. 1987. Sorting out motivations: *Personal integrity as the first criterion of moral action.* In Richardson, Section II.

A surrogate's motivations could be ethically noble or instrumental (an I-it relation with the uterus and pregnancy); the renting couple should not have a "throwaway" attitude toward her but should pay for postpartum therapy for her.

Sandberg, Eugene C. 1989. Only an attitude away: The potential of reproductive surrogacy. *American Journal of Obstetrics and Gynecology* 160(6):1441–1446.

In this 1988 presidential address, Sandberg strongly advocates all types of surrogacy (and provides a table of types with indication for each). To him, gestational surrogacy offers an "optimal embryological foundation for the fetus," and could "minimize the perpetuation of genetic defects," and "precipitately reduce both maternal and fetal morbidity."

Schuker, Eleanor. 1988. Psychological effects of new reproductive technologies. In Baruch et al., Section II.

Schuker expounds four psychological principles helpful in understanding the effects of the new technologies; includes some data from her own psychoanalytic interviews with a few surrogates.

Schwartz, Lita Linzer. 1987. Surrogate motherhood I: Responses to infertility. *American Journal of Family Therapy* 15(2):158–162.

"Legal 'potholes'" and "psychological 'rocks'" in the surrogacy path to parenthood are examined. Family therapists should prepare to provide services to the parties involved.

Schwartz, Lita Linzer. 1988. Surrogate motherhood II: Reflections after "Baby M." *American Journal of Family Therapy* 16(2):158–166.

For therapists, Schwartz gives suggestions for helping infertile couples from E.B. Cook's work on the crisis of infertility. She summarizes religious, sociopolitical, legal, ethical, and mental health issues. Excellent source for *Philadelphia Inquirer* coverage of Baby M case.

Schwartz, Lita Linzer. 1989. Surrogate motherhood III. The end of a saga? *American Journal of Family Therapy* 17(1):67–72.

The author criticizes that the Sterns were not given beforehand the full psychological screening report on Mary Beth Whitehead, that the proposed visitation schedule will be hard on Baby M. She summarizes views of 11 law professors in the *New Jersey Law Journal* Vol. 121 (1988).

Schwartz, Lita Linzer. 1990. Surrogate motherhood and family psychology/therapy. *American Journal of Family Therapy* 18(4):385–392.

Schwartz describes some psychological issues (motives, mental health of all parties) and legal issues and urges family psychologists and therapists to become informed in case they should be asked to evaluate participants prior to a contractual agreement.

Scutt, Jocelynne A. 1991. Whose surrogate? Surrogacy, ethics, and the law. *Issues in Reproductive and Genetic Engineering: Journal of International Feminist Analysis* 4(2):169–177.

Antisurrogacy arguments are developed through consideration of language, common law, results of the 1991 Australian national conference on surrogacy, and altruism in surrogacy.

Shanley, Mary Lyndon. 1990. A case against pregnancy contracts: Embodied selves, liberal theory and the law. *Politics and the Life Sciences* 8(2):216–220.

This argument that "contracts for pregnancy should be void and unenforceable" is a rebuttal to Hill (1990, this section). Shanley rejects "strict contractarianism" but does "not wish to return to the patriarchal models of family life."

Shannon, Thomas A. 1987. What the market will bear. *Commonweal* 24 April:234–235.

Shannon discusses commodification of people, alienation of the self.

Sheean, Leon A., James M. Goldfarb, Robert Kiwi, and Wulf H. Utian. 1989. In vitro fertilization (IVF)-surrogacy: Application of IVF to women without functional uteri. *Journal of in Vitro Fertilization and Embryo Transfer* 6(3):134–137.

Report from Cleveland on five successful pregnancies, using natural cycles, in gestational surrogates recruited by an attorney.

Shevory, Thomas C. 1990. Rethinking public and private life via the surrogacy contract. *Politics and the Life Sciences* 8(2):173–184.

The author uses insights from Critical Legal Studies scholarship to analyze weaknesses of surrogacy contracts; discusses in detail Elizabeth Kane's saga. To him, surrogacy might be a "useful practice for deconstructing the walls that divide the world into . . . very fragile and beseiged family structures."

Shinn, Roger L. 1987. High-tech birth. *Christianity and Crisis* 4 May:155–156.

This editorial criticizes the dogmatism in the Vatican's statement on human reproduction, recommends better ways of working out ethical judgments, worries about the scars borne by Baby M and the roles of money, class, and contract law in the Baby M transaction.

Singer, Linda. 1989. Bodies—Pleasures—Powers. *differences* 1(1):45–81.

This involved analysis of sexual politics and the "language of sexual epidemic" also discusses Camus, Foucault, and class-biased ads for or against motherhood. To Singer, the Baby M case "functions as the opposing pole to those issues emerging . . . from sexual disease."

Sistare, Christine T. 1988. Reproductive freedom and women's freedom: Surrogacy and autonomy. *Philosophical Forum* 19(4):227–240.

Prosurrogacy arguments, particularly concerning women's freedom and reproductive independence. To the author, social acceptance of surrogacy may prove beneficial.

Smith, David H. 1988. Wombs for rent, selves for sale? *Journal of Contemporary Health Law and Policy* 4:23–36.

Smith discusses in some detail six analogies associated with surrogacy: artificial insemination, adoption, prostitution, sales of organs, risky uses of one's body, and slavery.

Smith, George P., II. 1990. The case of Baby M: Love's labor lost. In Gostin, Section II.

Smith argues that the New Jersey Supreme Court erred in giving Whitehead visiting rights and in not allowing Mrs. Stern to adopt; middle-class standards ensure the best interests of the child.

Sokoloff, Burton Z. 1987. Alternative methods of reproduction: Effects on the child. *Clinical Pediatrics* 2:11–17.

The author discusses donor insemination and adoption, less space on surrogacy; is concerned about the effect of family secrets on children; urges using adoption experience as a guideline for the child's best interests.

Sorrel, Lorraine. 1987. Baby M again. *off our backs* July:26.

Sorrel, single with a child by artificial insemination, criticizes Whitehead for subjecting her husband and children to a highly publicized trial. Allowing Whitehead to break her contract means a "woman cannot be responsible for making reproductive decisions or motherhood is so sanctified . . . that women will rarely be allowed . . . other significant roles."

Steadman, Jennifer H., and Gillian Tennant McCloskey. 1987. The prospects of surrogate mothering: Clinical concerns. *Canadian Journal of Psychiatry* 32:545–550.

Surrogacy has hazards for "unsuspecting infants, the undefended children, and the vulnerable adults"; centers should inform participants of risks and get their agreement to take part in careful longitudinal studies.

Stein, M.L. 1990. Media crush in California. *Editor & Publisher* 20 October:12–13, 46.

Stein analyzes the media "blitz" in Southern California over the Johnson/Calvert gestational surrogacy case.

Steinbock, Bonnie. 1990. Surrogate motherhood as prenatal adoption. In Gostin, Section II.

The author examines "lessons" offered by the Baby M case, then the claims that surrogacy is exploitive, inconsistent with human dignity, and harmful to children; concludes that surrogate contracts should be restricted, not banned.

Steinfels, Peter. 1987. Surrogate-gate. *Commonweal* 30 January:35–36.

This editorial claims that the Baby M nightmare comes from a "breakdown in moral understanding," urges that noncommercial surrogacy be "opposed by moral pressure," and advocates that commercial surrogacy be banned.

Steptoe, Patrick. 1987. Surrogacy. *British Medical Journal* 294:1688–1689.

Steptoe urges not condemning surrogacy without scientific evidence; claims gestational surrogacy eases doubts about the status of the child.

Surrogacy standards set by Mt. Sinai. 1987. *CenterViews* 2(2):1, 4–5.

Interview with Wulf Utian (Mt. Sinai Medical Center, Cleveland, Ohio), the first doctor to engineer a live birth (June 1987) via gestational surrogacy.

Swan, Norman. 1990. Australian ethics committee approves surrogacy. *British Medical Journal* 301:254.

This editorial describes the committee's recommendations that surrogacy be strictly controlled under uniform legislation. See also Chapter 26, this volume.

Swerdlow, Marian. 1987. Class politics and Baby M. *Against the Current* 2 (Sept./Oct.):53.

Swerdlow discusses alienation of work and exploitation of working-class women in surrogacy; urges depriving contracts of legal validity to protect such women and their families.

Tangri, Sandra Schwartz, and Janet R. Kahn. 1989. Who is my mother? *Broadsheet* 166 (March):23–27.

Editor Pat Rosier sets forth the authors' antisurrogacy stance and calls upon "feminist principles" to prevail, especially control over one's own body.

Taub, Nadine. 1990. Surrogacy: A preferred treatment for infertility? In Gostin, Section II.

Taub urges that we redirect attention from surrogacy questions to the causes of infertility and its pain; analyzes the extent of infertility in the United States and discusses its causes in some detail.

Tauer, Carol. 1990. Essential ethical considerations for public policy on assisted reproduction. In Bartels et al., Section II.

Six criteria for establishing public policy on moral issues are listed, then three fundamental ethical principles. After applying these to surrogacy, Tauer concludes that fees should be prohibited, but not the practice of surrogacy.

Thom, Mary. 1988. Dilemmas of the new birth technologies. *Ms.* 16(11)(May):70–72, 74–76. Pages 74–76 are on surrogacy.

An even-handed analysis, with quotes, of various feminist views expressed after the Baby M case; summary of state legislation.

Tomlinson, Tom. 1989. Surrogacy revisited. *Hastings Center Report* 19(3):44–45.

This letter asserts that Annas (1988, this section) and the New Jersey justices have dismissed surrogacy "with pious denunciations that don't withstand scrutiny."

Tong, Rosemarie. 1990. The overdue death of a feminist chameleon: Taking a stance on surrogacy arrangements. *Journal of Social Philosophy* 21 (2/3):40–56

Turin, Maureen. 1991. Viewing/reading *Born to be sold: Martha Rosler reads the strange case of Baby S/M* or motherhood in the age of technological reproduction. *Discourse* 13(2):21–38.

This confusing criticism of Paper Tiger Video's 1988 tape *Born to be sold* claims that this spunky, melodramatic spectacle, with Rosler disguised as seven characters, does show how surrogacy serves patriarchal power but is often offensive, for example in its brutal treatment of middle-class women.

Utian, Wulf H., Leon Sheean, James M. Goldfarb, and Robert Kiwi. 1985. Successful pregnancy after in vitro fertilization and embryo transfer from an infertile woman into a surrogate. *New England Journal of Medicine* 313:1351–1352.

Report of the first pregnancy in a surrogate from an in vitro fertilized egg obtained from a woman without a uterus.

Walters, William A.W. 1989. Ethical aspects of surrogacy. *Australian and New Zealand Journal of Obstetrics and Gynaecology* 29:322–325.

By applying five moral principles to the actors in contract pregnancy, Walters derives an ethical "balance sheet."

Werhane, Patricia H. 1989. AGAINST the legitimacy of surrogate contracts. In Richardson, Section II.

It is a fallacy to claim that the Whitehead/Stern contract is moral or legally binding; it confuses parental rights with contract rights and threatens the rights of Baby M.

Wettstein, Robert M. 1990. Surrogate parenting contracts. *American Journal of Obstetrics and Gynecology* 163(2):679–680.

This rebuttal to La Puma et al. (1989, this section) urges that surrogacy not be condemned out of hand—it has potential benefits. Physicians should provide all medical care to all parties. Of course, they should not own or administer a surrogate parenting agency.

What Baby M is telling us. Editorial. 1987. *America* 7 February:90–91.

Children of surrogacy run a risk of growing up in an ambiguous household; recruiting women to bear children they do not want is also evil, and we should abandon "wombs for hire" now.

Whiteford, Linda M. 1989. Commercial surrogacy: Social issues behind the controversy. In Whiteford and Poland, Section II.

The author discusses social, ethical, legal issues; analyzes contradictory social values "called into focus;" claims commercial surrogacy cannot be ignored and merits thoughtful discussion.

Whitehead, Mary Beth. 1989. Women who experienced surrogacy speak out (USA). In Klein, Section II.

In this brief description of her experiences, Whitehead enumerates mistakes she made and hopes that "other women will learn from my mistakes."

Whose baby is it anyway? 1981. *Newsweek* 97(6 April):83.

On Noyes/Thrane controversy. Of historical interest.

Winkler, Ute. 1988. New U.S. know-how in Frankfurt—A "surrogate mother" agency. *Reproductive and Genetic Engineering: Journal of International Feminist Analysis* 1(2):205–207.

The author describes the attempt of American surrogacy broker Noel Keane to establish an agency, United Family International, in Frankfurt, the ensuing public protest, and the speedy closure of the agency.

Wolfram, Sybil. 1989. Surrogacy in the United Kingdom. In Whiteford and Poland, Section II.

Wolfram explains that surrogacy is "unpalatable" in Britain because of the passing of money; describes the Warnock Report's reception, parliamentary debate, Baby Cotton in 1984–85.

Woliver, Laura R. 1989. The deflective power of reproductive technologies: The impact on women. *Women & Politics* 9(3):17–47.

Woliver describes skeptical feminist views of science and the political power of reproductive technologies that "deflect pressures for social reforms by promising technological fixes." After discussing the Baby M case in detail, she emphasizes considering group impact vs. individual choice. A lengthy, useful bibliography.

Woliver, Laura R. 1990. Reproductive technologies and surrogacy: Policy concerns for women. *Politics and the Life Sciences 9(2):*185–194.

Regulation of surrogacy should be by female-informed rather than male-standardized legislatures. Good bibliography.

Wood, E. Carl, and Peter Singer. 1988. Whither surrogacy? *Medical Journal of Australia* 149:426–430.

The authors give a detailed plan for selecting surrogates in their proposal for acceptable surrogacy—a generous, loving act "one woman can carry out for another." Surrogacy also may have positive benefits by optimizing conditions for a successful pregnancy and should not be condemned on the basis of "the notorious U.S. [commercial] cases."

Wrigley, Julia. 1987. Whose baby is it anyway? *Against the Current* 2 (Sept./Oct.):53–55.

Pointing out the class bias in the Baby M case and most custody decisions, Wrigley argues that parents be allowed to raise their children whatever class differences exist; she advocates shared custody in surrogacy.

Yovich, John L. 1987. Surrogacy. *Lancet* i:1374.

Yovich is disappointed that the British Medical Association no longer supports surrogacy; on "behalf of our patients," he urges gestational surrogacy with a sister or other relative.

Zelizer, Viviana A. 1988. From baby farms to Baby M. *Society* 25(3):23–28. Response to Neuhaus, this section.

The author places the "baby market" into historical context; discusses how monetary value of children depends on connotations. Well done.

Zipper, Juliette, and Selma Sevenhuijsen. 1987. Surrogacy: Feminist notions of motherhood reconsidered. In *Reproductive technologies: Gender, motherhood and medicine*, ed. Michelle Stanworth. Minneapolis: University of Minnesota Press.

Excellent historical analysis of Dutch feminist action regarding motherhood. The authors attack the FINRRAGE position on surrogacy, without clearly taking a stance; they believe that more informal surrogacy exists than we are aware of and advocate this.

V. Bibliographies

Compiled by attorneys, legal assistants, or law students, these bibliographies (and research and resource guides) emphasize the legal literature; most also include major newspapers and news magazines. These are excellent sources for articles before 1988; for recent legal literature, see *Current Law Index* under the headings Surrogate Motherhood or Surrogate Mothers.

Adams, Marilyn. 1988. An examination of bill introductions during the 1987 legislative sessions relating to surrogacy contracts. *State Legislative Report* 13(2):1–13.

Description of 26 bills to regulate surrogacy (none of which passed); 17 bills to declare surrogacy contracts null and void (one in Louisiana passed); and 22 bills to establish task forces or commissions (of which 7 passed). Useful source.

Bach, Kathleen K. 1987. *Research guide: Surrogate motherhood.* Legal Research Guides Series, Vol. 6. Buffalo: Hein. 46 pp.

How to use legal encyclopedias, data bases, guides to state statutes; proposed legislation and some court decisions in 20 states; citations of 81 legal articles and notes, 106 popular press articles before October 1986.

Buchanan, Jim. 1987. "Baby M" and surrogate motherhood: A resource guide. Public Administration Series: P 2194. Vance Biblios. 17 pp.

Through 1986: citations to 177 articles in law journals and popular magazines, to 10 legal cases, and to 26 state laws on fees in connection with adoption.

Field, Martha A. 1988. Pp. 201–210 in her book, *Surrogate motherhood.* See Section I.

Gostin, Larry. 1990. Pp. 338–355 in his edited book, *Surrogate motherhood: Politics and privacy.* See Section II.

Jacobs, Daniel J. 1987. Surrogate motherhood: A selective bibliography. *Record of the Association of the Bar of the City of New York* 42:839–851.

Through early 1987: 180 citations to law journals and some news magazines and books.

Peritore, Laura. 1988. A select bibliography on surrogacy. *Family Law Quarterly* 22(2):213–224.

List of 12 books, 89 law journal articles, 26 law review notes, 23 newspaper articles, and 11 court cases.

Riemer, Rita Ann. 1988. *Analysis of legal and constitutional issues involved in surrogate motherhood.* Washington, D.C.: Congressional Research Service.

Robbins, Sara. 1984. *Surrogate parenting: An annotated review of the literature.* CompuBibs Series No. 3. New York: Vantage Information Consultants. 40 pp.

Through October 1983: careful summaries of 31 legal and 29 medical or popular articles; citations to 57 newspaper pieces; 6 examples of judicial activity; legislative activity in 11 states. Recommended.

Sutterlin, Edith. 1988. *Surrogate mothers: Bibliography-in-brief.* Washington, D.C.: Congressional Research Service.

Name Index

Subject Index